Serono Symposia USA
Norwell, Massachusetts

Springer Science+Business Media, LLC

PROCEEDINGS IN THE SERONO SYMPOSIA USA SERIES

THERAPEUTIC OUTCOME OF ENDOCRINE DISORDERS: Efficacy, Innovation and Quality of Life
Edited by Brian Stabler and Barry B. Bercu

EMBRYO IMPLANTATION: Molecular, Cellular and Clinical Aspects
Edited by Daniel D. Carson

SEX-STEROID INTERACTIONS WITH GROWTH HORMONE
Edited by Johannes D. Veldhuis and Andrea Giustina

MALE STERILITY AND MOTILITY DISORDERS: Etiological Factors and Treatment. A Serono Symposia S.A. Publication
Edited by Samir Hamamah, Roger Mieusset, François Olivennes, and René Frydman

NUTRITIONAL ASPECTS OF OSTEOPOROSIS. A Serono Symposia S.A. Publication
Edited by Peter Burckhardt, Bess Dawson-Hughes, and Robert P. Heaney

GERM CELL DEVELOPMENT, DIVISION, DISRUPTION AND DEATH
Edited by Barry R. Zirkin

CELL DEATH IN REPRODUCTIVE PHYSIOLOGY
Edited by Jonathan L. Tilly, Jerome F. Strauss III, and Martin Tenniswood

INHIBIN, ACTIVIN AND FOLLISTATIN: Regulatory Functions in System and Cell Biology. A Serono Symposia S.A. Publication
Edited by Toshihiro Aono, Hiromu Sugino, and Wylie W. Vale

PERIMENOPAUSE
Edited by Rogerio A. Lobo

GROWTH FACTORS AND WOUND HEALING: Basic Science and Potential Clinical Applications
Edited by Thomas R. Ziegler, Glenn F. Pierce, and David N. Herndon

POLYCYSTIC OVARY SYNDROME
Edited by R. Jeffrey Chang

IDEA TO PRODUCT: The Process
Edited by Nancy J. Alexander and Anne Colston Wentz

BOVINE SPONGIFORM ENCEPHALOPATHY: The BSE Dilemma
Edited by Clarence J. Gibbs, Jr.

GROWTH HORMONE SECRETAGOGUES
Edited by Barry B. Bercu and Richard F. Walker

CELLULAR AND MOLECULAR REGULATION OF TESTICULAR CELLS
Edited by Claude Desjardins

GENETIC MODELS OF IMMUNE AND INFLAMMATORY DISEASES
Edited by Abul K. Abbas and Richard A. Flavell

Continued after Index

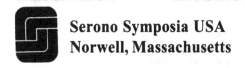

Serono Symposia USA
Norwell, Massachusetts

Brian Stabler Barry B. Bercu
Editors

Therapeutic Outcome of Endocrine Disorders

Efficacy, Innovation and Quality of Life

With 24 Figures

Springer

Brian Stabler, Ph.D.
Department of Psychiatry
School of Medicine
University of North Carolina at Chapel Hill
Chapel Hill, NC 27599
USA

Barry B. Bercu, M.D.
Department of Pediatrics
College of Medicine
University of South Florida
All Children's Hospital
St. Petersburg, FL 33701
USA

Proceedings of the International Symposium on Therapeutic Outcome of Endocrine Disorders: Efficacy, Innovation and Quality of Life, sponsored by Serono Symposia USA, Inc., held November 13 to 16, 1997, in Palm Beach Gardens, Florida.

For information on previous volumes, contact Serono Symposia USA, Inc.

Library of Congress Cataloging-in-Publication Data
Therapeutic outcome of endocrine disorders: efficacy, innovation and quality of life /
Brian Stabler, Barry B. Bercu, editors.
p. cm.
Includes bibliographical references and index.
ISBN 978-0-387-98962-4 ISBN 978-1-4612-1230-0 (eBook)
DOI 10.1007/978-1-4612-1230-0
1. Endocrine glands—Diseases—Treatment. 2. Outcome assessment (Medical care)
3. Quality of life. I. Stabler, Brian. II. Bercu, Barry B. III. International Symposium on
Therapeutic Outcome of Endocrine Disorders: Efficacy, Innovation and Quality of Life
(1997: Palm Beach Gardens, Fla.)
[DNLM: 1. Endocrine Diseases—therapy—Congresses. 2. Quality of Life—Congresses.
3. Treatment Outcome—Congresses. WK 140 T398 2000]
RC649 T47 2000
616.4'06—dc21 99-055306

Printed on acid-free paper.

Production coordinated by Chernow Editorial Services, Inc., and managed by Francine McNeill; manufacturing supervised by Jerome Basma.
Typeset by KP Company, Brooklyn, NY.

9 8 7 6 5 4 3 2 1

ISBN 978-0-387-98962-4

SYMPOSIUM ON THERAPEUTIC OUTCOME OF ENDOCRINE DISORDERS: EFFICACY, INNOVATION AND QUALITY OF LIFE

Scientific Committee

Brian Stabler, Ph.D., Chair
Barry B. Bercu, M.D., Chair
Leona Cuttler, M.D.
Dennis Drotar, Ph.D.
Louis E. Underwood, M.D.

Organizing Secretary

Leslie Nies
Serono Symposia USA, Inc.
100 Longwater Circle
Norwell, Massachusetts

Preface

Changes in the allocation of healthcare resources have raised issues related to the efficacy and outcomes of medical therapy and how such factors may be measured. The questions associated with the quality of life and functional capability of patients with chronic health conditions have been of special interest. Endocrine disorders have the potential for disrupting the general health and well-being of affected individuals and their families; thus they warrant serious attention. This symposium was convened in November 1997 at Palm Beach Gardens, Florida, to bring together medical, behavioral, and social scientists. The meeting fostered the presentation and discussion of the most current clinical research on the effects of various therapies on a wide range of endocrine disorders from diabetes to adrenal insufficiency and growth hormone deficiency. The participants, all noted national and international experts in their fields, focused their attention on both the biomedical value and effectiveness of treatment, as well as on the impact such treatments have on psychological states such as mood and cognition. Many presentations specifically emphasized the quality of life (QOL) indicators that now regularly appear in many research protocols and reports.

The pioneering work of two clinical researchers was a major highlight of the meeting and an Award of Recognition was presented to Robert Blizzard, M.D., and John Money, Ph.D., for their innovative and insightful work in pediatric endocrinology and psychosexual development. The presentations were grouped under five clinical diagnostic groups: congenital adrenal hyperplasia, Turner syndrome, diabetes mellitus, congenital hypothyroidism, and growth hormone deficiency. Attention was given to biomedical indicators and symptoms, associated social and psychological symptoms, and measurements of treatment efficacy and QOL. A special allocation of time was made for invited papers on topics of particular interest or which represented research still in early development. There was spirited discussion and interchange, leading to the conclusion that much work is yet to be done in documenting the lifetime efficacy of endocrine therapies to include comprehensive assessment of functionality and life quality.

The symposium was rated as highly successful by participants, for which appreciation is given to Leslie Nies and the dedicated professional staff at Serono Symposia USA who underwrote and organized the meetings. We sincerely hope these proceedings are helpful to clinicians and clinical investigators who seek to improve the outcome of endocrine therapy.

BRIAN STABLER
BARRY B. BERCU

Contents

Part IV. Treatment of Diabetes: Efficacy, Innovation and Quality of Life

Part V. Treatment of Congenital Adrenal Hyperplasia: Efficacy, Innovation and Quality of Life

Part VI. Treatment of Congenital Hypothyroidism: Efficacy, Innovation and Quality of Life

Contributors

KERSTIN ALBERTSSON-WIKLAND, International Pediatric Growth Research Center, Department of Pediatrics, Göteborg University, Göteborg, Sweden.

DANA E. ALLIGER, Pediatric Psychiatry, Children's Hospital of Buffalo, Buffalo, New York, USA.

SUSAN W. BAKER, Department of Pediatrics, New York Hospital–Cornell Medical Center, New York, New York, USA.

MARTHA U. BARNARD, Department of Behavioral Pediatrics, University of Kansas Medical Center, Kansas City, Missouri, USA.

JENNIFER J. BELL, Department of Pediatrics, Columbia University College of Physicians and Surgeons, and Babies and Children's Hospital, New York, New York, USA.

SHERI A. BERENBAUM, Department of Behavioral and Social Sciences, School of Medicine, and Department of Psychology, Southern Illinois University, Carbondale, Illinois, USA.

CÉSAR BERGADÁ, Division of Endocrinology, Children's Hospital Ricardo Gutierrez, Buenos Aires, Argentina.

DOROTHY BISHOP, MRC Applied Psychology Unit, Cambridge, UK.

STELLA MARIS CAMPO, Endocrinology Research Center, Children's Hospital Ricardo Gutierrez, Buenos Aires, Argentina.

PAUL V. CARROLL, Department of Medicine, St. Thomas' Hospital, London, UK.

HÉCTOR EDGARDO CHEMES, Endocrinology Research Center, Children's Hospital Ricardo Gutierrez, Buenos Aires, Argentina.

Emanuel R. Christ, Department of Medicine, St. Thomas' Hospital, London, UK.

Richard R. Clopper, Department of Psychiatry, School of Medicine and Biomedical Sciences, State University of New York at Buffalo, Buffalo, New York, USA.

Leona Cuttler, Department of Pediatrics, Rainbow Babies and Children's Hospital, and Case Western Reserve University, Cleveland, Ohio, USA.

Ralf W. Dittmann, Department of Psychiatry, Columbia University College of Physicians and Surgeons, New York, New York, USA.

Curtis Dolezal, New York State Psychiatric Institute, and Department of Psychiatry, Columbia University College of Physicians and Surgeons, New York, New York, USA.

Dennis Drotar, Department of Pediatrics, Rainbow Babies and Children's Hospital, and Case Western Reserve University School of Medicine, Cleveland, Ohio, USA.

Kate Elgar, Behavioral Sciences Unit, Institute of Child Health, London, UK.

Ann E. Erling, International Pediatric Growth Research Center, Department of Pediatrics, Göteborg University, Göteborg, Sweden.

Delbert A. Fisher, Quest Diagnostics–Nichols Institute, San Juan Capistrano, California, USA.

Caroline Fung, Pediatric Psychiatry, Children's Hospital of Buffalo, Buffalo, New York, USA.

Sonia Gidwani, Department of Pediatrics, New York Hospital–Cornell Medical Center, New York, New York, USA.

Jerome A. Grunt, Department of Pediatrics, The Children's Mercy Hospital, and The University of Missouri–Kansas City School of Medicine, Kansas City, Missouri, USA.

Juan Jorge Heinrich, Division of Endocrinology, Children's Hospital Ricardo Gutierrez, Buenos Aires, Argentina.

Campbell P. Howard, Department of Pediatrics, The Children's Mercy Hospital, and The University of Missouri–Kansas City School of Medicine, Kansas City, Missouri, USA.

ALAN M. JACOBSON, Department of Psychiatry, Harvard Medical School, and Joslin Diabetes Center, Boston, Massachusetts, USA.

SUZANNE BENNETT JOHNSON, Center for Pediatric Psychology and Family Studies, University of Florida Health Sciences Center, Gainesville, Florida, USA.

ANA CLAUDIA KESELMAN, Division of Endocrinology, Children's Hospital Ricardo Gutierrez, Buenos Aires, Argentina.

LINDA LEROUX, Pediatric Psychiatry, Children's Hospital of Buffalo, Buffalo, New York, USA.

MARGARET H. MACGILLIVRAY, State University of New York at Buffalo Medical School, and Department of Pediatrics, Children's Hospital of Buffalo, Buffalo, New York, USA.

JOHN I. MALONE, Division of Endocrinology, Diabetes and Metabolism, University of South Florida College of Medicine, Tampa, Florida, USA.

ALICIA SUSANA MARTÍNEZ, Division of Endocrinology, Children's Hospital Ricardo Gutierrez, Buenos Aires, Argentina.

TOM MAZUR, State University of New York at Buffalo Medical School, and Department of Pediatrics, Children's Hospital of Buffalo, Buffalo, New York, USA.

HEINO F.L. MEYER-BAHLBURG, New York State Psychiatric Institute, and Department of Psychiatry, Columbia University College of Physicians and Surgeons, New York, New York, USA.

CLAUDE J. MIGEON, Pediatric Endocrine Clinic, The Johns Hopkins Hospital, Baltimore, Maryland, USA.

ANDERS MÖLLER, Department of Obstetrics and Gynecology, Göteborg University, Göteborg, Sweden.

JOHN MONEY, Psychohormonal Research Unit, The Johns Hopkins University and Hospital, Baltimore, Maryland, USA.

WAYNE V. MOORE, Department of Pediatrics, The Children's Mercy Hospital, Kansas City, Missouri, and Department of Endocrinology, University of Kansas Medical Center, Kansas City, Kansas, USA.

AKIRA MORISHIMA, Department of Pediatrics, Columbia University College of Physicians and Surgeons, and Babies and Children's Hospital, New York, New York, USA.

Elena Morris, Behavioral Sciences Unit, Institute of Child Health, London, UK.

Maria I. New, Department of Pediatrics, New York Hospital–Cornell Medical Center, New York, New York, USA.

Liliana Pantano, Division of Endocrinology, Children's Hospital Ricardo Gutierrez, Buenos Aires, Argentina.

Jessica C. Roberts, Clinical Psychology Program, University of Kansas, Lawrence, Kansas, USA.

Michael C. Roberts, Clinical Child Psychology Program, University of Kansas, Lawrence, Kansas, USA.

Jane R. Robinson, Department of Psychology, Case Western University School of Medicine, Cleveland, Ohio, USA.

María Gabriela Ropelato, Division of Endocrinology, Children's Hospital Ricardo Gutierrez, Buenos Aires, Argentina.

Ron G. Rosenfeld, Department of Pediatrics, Oregon Health Sciences University, Portland, Oregon, USA.

Joanne F. Rovet, Department of Pediatrics, The University of Toronto, Toronto, Ontario, Canada.

David E. Sandberg, Departments of Psychiatry and Pediatrics, School of Medicine and Biomedical Sciences, State University of New York at Buffalo, Buffalo, New York, USA.

I. David Schwartz, Department of Pediatrics, The Children's Mercy Hospital, and The University of Missouri–Kansas City School of Medicine, Kansas City, Missouri, USA.

David Skuse, Behavioral Sciences Unit, Institute of Child Health, London, UK.

Peter H. Sönksen, Department of Medicine, St. Thomas' Hospital, London, UK.

Brian Stabler, Departments of Psychiatry and Pediatrics, University of North Carolina School of Medicine, Chapel Hill, North Carolina, USA.

Louis E. Underwood, Department of Pediatrics, University of North Carolina School of Medicine, Chapel Hill, North Carolina, USA.

Eric M. Vernberg, Clinical Child Psychology Program, University of Kansas, Lawrence, Kansas, USA.

Ulla Wide Boman, Departments of Psychology and Pediatrics, Göteborg University, Göteborg, Sweden.

Ingela K. Wiklund, Department of Public Health and Primary Health Care, The University of Bergen, Bergen, Norway; Quality of Life Research, Astra Hässle AB, Mölndal, Sweden; and International Pediatric Growth Research Center, Department of Pediatrics, Göteborg University, Göteborg, Sweden.

Tim Wysocki, Division of Behavioral Pediatrics and Psychology, Nemours Children's Clinic, Jacksonville, Florida, USA.

1

Outcome Research in Pediatric Psychoendocrinology and Sexology

JOHN MONEY

Outcome research is both biographical and statistical. The longitudinal data of biographical studies are multivariate and sequential. They provide the opportunity to tease out the conflation of factors that may be responsible for a given outcome. These factors may then be tested cross-sectionally, one or a few variables at a time, on a group of individuals statistically homogeneous for diagnosis, and for as many other variables as can be held constant. Biographical data should be collected and tabulated systematically, according to a planned schedule of inquiry, and not haphazardly. These data should include wide-ranging information, including some (e.g., handedness, color blindness, or natal sequence) that may not have self-evident significance. The computer program for processing statistical data should be planned ahead of time so as to ensure that no variable will be fortuitously overlooked and that there will be no overload of surplus data (e.g., on a questionnaire). Today, the logistics, continuity, and funding of longitudinal outcome research are more likely to be haphazard than predictably guaranteed.

Since 1951, three of the categories of outcome research for which I have been responsible have pertained to IQ and specific cognitional functioning, incidence of major psychopathology, and sexological issues. The syndromes studied have included congenital hypothyroidism, Turner syndrome, congenital adrenal hyperplasia (CAH) female hermaphroditism, androgen insensitivity syndrome, micropenis, and male hermaphroditism. Sexological issues are particularly difficult to manage because of the cultural taboos against speaking of sexual problems and the attached social stigma associated with it. The management of cases is made more difficult through faulty prescientific ideology and folk sexology that resists and limits sex education. To be fully literate in the sexological outcome of the syndromes treated by medical professionals, a formalized discipline needs to be created. Although needed, there is no specialty of pediatric sexology.

It goes without saying that long-term follow-up and outcome studies in pediatric endocrinology require long-term logistical planning and stability of personnel, both of which require a guarantee of long-term funding amounting cumulatively to very large sums of money. Meticulous attention must be given to statistical design to ensure diagnostic homogeneity and to avoid skewing so that patients with chronic or recurrent symptoms are overrepresented, and patients who become symptom free are underrepresented. Satisfying all of these criteria, especially in today's climate of research funding, is more likely to be haphazard than systematically guaranteed.

In my own case, for example, I have lived hand to mouth, from one grant renewal to the next, since I began working in pediatric psychoendocrinology under Lawson Wilkins in 1951. I became a grantee of the National Institute of Child Health and Human Development when it was chartered in 1962 (1). Even though my renewal applications have been approved continuously since then, with only one short hiatus, I have had no way of predicting that they would be, nor that the amount would progressively shrink. In recent years, in fact, I have been too underfunded and too short-staffed to do the full range of outcome studies that deserve to be done. In addition, I have encountered restrictions on the publication of sensitive sexological case history data.

Since 1951, I have published follow-up psychohormonal data on several pediatric syndromes, in some instances before and after treatment. These publications are subdivisible into three categories. Category I pertains to IQ and specific cognitional functions. In the case of hypothyroidism, for example, the data showed that in extreme cases the deficiency at birth was so severe as not to benefit from very early onset of replacement therapy. At the other extreme, there were, unexpectedly, a very few cases in which the IQ, after remaining low for several years, despite treatment, would unpredictably increase into the normal range, or in one case from below normal (IQ, 84) at age 5 to IQ 127 at age 27 (2–4).

Another Category I example is that of alleged mental retardation in Turner syndrome. Follow-up in my unit showed that the IQ deficit is not across the board, but rather that it affects nonverbal or praxic IQ only, and represents a specific cognitional defect (i.e., space-form blindness and impaired directional sense) (5–7).

Category II pertains to the incidence of major psychopathology. A history of the traumatizing sequelae of Turner syndrome was found not to be associated with major psychosis (8,9). A parallel lack of incidence of major psychosis was also found in CAH female hermaphroditism with a history of either female or male rearing, either before or after the discovery of cortisol treatment in 1950 (10,11). By contrast, an association might exist between psychosis and a subtype of those with a history of male hermaphroditism that has as yet no identifiable etiology.

Category III pertains to sexological issues (e.g., precocious and delayed puberty) and in various syndromes of birth defect of the sex organs. Here, I shall address the latter, and quote from the abstracts of four follow-up studies. The first is a study, published in 1984, entitled: "Adult Erotosexual Status and Fetal Hormonal Masculinization and Demasculinization: 46,XX Congenital Virilizing Adrenal Hyperplasia and 46,XY Androgen-Insensitivity Syndrome Compared" (11).

Among 30 young women with a history of the treated adrenogenital syndrome (CAH), 11 (37%) rated themselves as bisexual or homosexual. Among a control group consisting of 15 women with the 46,XY androgen-insensitivity syndrome (AIS) plus 12 with the Rokitansky syndrome (MRKS), the corresponding figure was 2 (7%), both bisexual. Chi-square was significant beyond the 0.01 level. In Kinsey's 1953 sample 15% of women experienced homoerotic arousal imagery by age 20, and 10% had had homoerotic partner contact. The most likely hypothesis to explain the CAH findings is that of a prenatal and/or neonatal masculinizing effect on sexual dimorphism of the brain in interaction with other developmental variables.

The second of this group of follow-up studies was published in 1985, under the title: "Micropenis: Gender, Erotosexual Coping Strategy, and Behavioral Health in Nine Pediatric Cases Followed to Adulthood" (12). All had a history since birth of living as male.

In nine cases of micropenis followed from pediatric age until adulthood (ages 22–31) the adult penis size was 2.5 SD below the mean or smaller, with one exception. Pubertal virilization was inadequate in six cases, in five of which there was also a history of neglecting follow-up and androgen-replacement therapy. In six cases there was a low incidence of erotosexual activity. In three there was a long-term pair-bonded attachment. There was one case of homosexual hustling, one of homosexual pair-bondedness, and one of homosexual attraction frustrated by the concealment of a skin-grafted phalloplasty. In the latter two cases, there was a history of agonizing over the option of possible sex reassignment and contemplating death by suicide. In one other case there was a history of paraphilic sadomasochism, in fantasy only, with a woman victim. The juvenile experience of micropenis in the family, the clinic, and the community may dislocate what should be the normal juvenile erotosexual rehearsal play and fantasy of uncomplicated heterosexual differentiation.

The third follow-up study, published in 1986, is entitled: "Gender Identity and Gender Transposition: Longitudinal Outcome Study of 32 Male Hermaphrodites Assigned as Girls" (13).

The longitudinal case histories of 32 female-assigned male hermaphrodites aged 18 or older were indexed and abstracted for evidence of variables related to gender transposition (i.e., bisexualism, lesbianism, or sex reassignment to live as male). The prevalence of transposition was biased because of the referral of cases selected for reassignment. Childhood stigmatization, either subtle or blatant, because of the birth defect of the sex organs correlated with gender transposition ($p < .001$) and was related to the age of feminizing surgery ($p < .05$), which often coincided with the age of gonadectomy. Variables not significantly correlated with gender transposition were: neonatal ambivalence regarding the sex of announcement; feminizing or masculinizing puberty; presence or absence of mullerian organs; and gross family pathology. Physicians encountered no moral problem with sex reassignment as the chromosomal and gonadal sex were male.

In 1987, the counterpart of this study was published under the title, "Gender Identity and Gender Transposition: Longitudinal Outcome Study of 24 Male Hermaphrodites Assigned as Boys" (14).

The longitudinal case histories of 24 male-assigned male hermaphrodites aged 18 or older were indexed and abstracted for the presence or absence of variables related to gender transposition, namely, bisexualism, homosexuality, or sex reassignment to live as a female. The sample was biased in favor of cases (*N* = 20) not showing signs of gender transposition. In these cases, there was no gender transposition even if the following variables were in evidence; neonatal ambivalence in announcing the sex; cosmetic inadequacy of masculine genital appearance; sitting posture for urination; and feminizing (*N* = 9) instead of virilizing (*N* = 11) puberty. Despite the small size of the minority subsample (*N* = 4), it showed a trend toward an association between gender transposition and sitting to urinate, and being stigmatized in childhood. This trend is consistent with the association between stigmatization and gender transposition found in a counterpart study of male hermaphrodites announced and reared as girls. Freedom from gender transposition did not prevent suicidal depression, drug or alcohol addiction, marital failure, or death from testicular cancer.

Follow-up data from all three of the foregoing categories and their syndromes cannot lawfully be withheld from parents or older patients. They are, however, likely to touch a raw nerve insofar as, in the terminology of popular folk medicine, they are likely to signify mental deficiency, insanity, and sexual perversion, respectively, and to be stigmatizing. The sexological category has the additional stigma of being so strongly taboo that there is no institutional recognition of pediatric sexology as a scientifically respectable specialty.

With pediatric sexology not yet made respectable, all that parents have to go by is pediatric folk sexology that is derived from a faulty prescientific ideology of the sexuality of childhood, puberty, and adolescence. According to this ideology, childhood is on the one hand a period of sexual innocence and, on the other hand, a period of being susceptible to contagion by the evils of original sin. Folk sexology has no place for the concept of developmental sexuality and eroticism beginning prenatally and continuing to unfold through the juvenile years, puberty, and adolescence.

In its more conservative version, folk sexology eschews sex education so as to preserve ostensible innocence, whereas the slightly more liberal version limits sex education to the physiology of eggs, sperms, menstrual periods, and warnings of sexually transmitted diseases (STDs), AIDS, and the so-called epidemic of teenaged pregnancy (which incidentally has the horrifying consequence of equating babies with an epidemic of germs). Doctors are acceptable for this physiological curriculum, whereas priests and pastors are the ones entrusted with the moral education of abstinence, the positive spirituality of love, and the negative carnality of lust.

The majority of children pick up the intergenerational taboo against explicit exchange of sexual information. Too much frankness may be self-incriminating to both adults and children. Even domestic bathroom nudity may get adults into trouble with false accusations of child sexual abuse. In the clinic, some children interpret the genital examination, with students and junior physicians in attendance, as nosocomial abuse and the equivalent of rape and voyeurism against which they have been warned. Explicit inquiry and the language of coition is for them the equivalent of pornography for which they may have known only threats and reprisals. They may have been indoctrinated with nothing more explicit than "good touch" and "bad touch."

Silenced by their experience with the sexual taboo, many children become afflicted with elective mutism. Children clam up at the very mention of sexual rehearsal play, for example, or even of actual sexual abuse. Parents, influenced by social contamination doctrine, are phobic about medical explicitness.

We have a long way to go as parents and as professionals in pediatric psychoendocrine outcome research. In order to be fully literate in the sexological outcome of the syndromes that we treat, we need to create a whole new specialty of pediatric sexology.

References

1. Money J. Longitudinal outcome research and strategies: career support in pediatric sexology and psychoendocrinology. J Psych Human Sex 1988;1:105–14.
2. Money J. Psychologic studies in hypothyroidism, and recommendations for case management. Arch Neurol Psychiatr 1956;76:296–309.
3. Money J, Lewis V. Longitudinal study of IQ in treated congenital hypothyroidism. In: Cameron MP, O'Connor M, eds. The Ciba Foundation Study Group No. 18, Brain-Thyroid Relationships. London: J. & A. Churchill, 1964.
4. Money J, Clarke FC, Beck J. Congenital hypothyroidism and IQ increase: a quarter century followup. J Pediatr 1978;93:432–34.
5. Shaffer JW. A specific cognitive deficit observed in gonadal aplasia (Turner's syndrome). J Clin Psych 1962;18:403–6.
6. Money J. Cytogenetics and psychosexual incongruities, with a note on space-form blindness. Am J Psychiatr 1963;119:820–27.
7. Alexander D, Walker HT, Money J. Studies in direction sense. I. Turner's syndrome. Arch Gen Psychiatr 1964;10:337–39.
8. Money J, Mittenthal S. Lack of personality pathology in Turner's syndrome: relation to cytogenetics, hormones, and physique. Behav Gen 1970;1:43–45.
9. Money J. Human behavior cytogenetics: review of psychopathology in three syndromes, 47,XXY; 47,XYY; and 45,X. J Sex Res 1975;11:181–200.
10. Ehrhardt AA, Evers K, Money J. Influence of androgen and some aspects of sexuality dimorphic behavior in women with late-treated adrenogenital syndrome. Johns Hopkins Med J 1968;123:115–22.
11. Money J, Schwartz M, Lewis VG. Adult erotosexual status and fetal hormonal masculinization and demasculinization: 46,XX congenital virilizing adrenal hyperplasia and 46,XY androgen-insensitivity syndrome compared. Psychoneuroendocrinol 1984;9:405–14.
12. Money J, Lehne GK, Pierre-Jerome F. Micropenis: gender, erotosexual coping strategy, and behavioral health in nine pediatric cases followed to adulthood. Comp Psychiatr 1985;26:29–42.

13. Money J, Devore H, Norman BF. Gender identity and gender transposition: Longitudinal study of 32 male hermaphrodites assigned as girls. J Sex Marital Ther 1986;12: 165–81.
14. Money J, Norman BF. Gender identity and gender transposition: longitudinal outcome study of 24 male hermaphrodites assigned as boys. J Sex Marital Ther 1987;13:75–92.

Part I

Treatment of Growth Hormone Deficiency: Efficacy, Innovation and Quality of Life

2

Growth Hormone Replacement in Adults: The First 10 Years

PAUL V. CARROLL, EMANUEL R. CHRIST, AND PETER H. SÖNKSEN

Introduction

Most physicians until recently considered growth hormone (GH) to have no biological relevance following the cessation of linear growth. The availability of large supplies of recombinant GH throughout the 1990s has prompted intense investigation of the effects of GH in health and disease. Particular emphasis has been paid to the study of adults with GH-deficiency, and our understanding of the consequences of GH-deficiency and the effects of GH replacement in these patients has increased greatly since the publication of the first trials of GH replacement in GH-deficient adults in 1989 (1,2).

These investigations have led to the recognition of a specific "clinical syndrome," with characteristic symptoms, signs, and investigative findings, in those with long-standing GH-deficiency. The features of this syndrome are summarized in Table 2.1. The effects of GH replacement on these symptoms and signs have been studied in both randomized placebo-controlled trials and in smaller open studies. These studies have overwhelmingly produced consistent results, demonstrating that adults with GH-deficiency are both psychologically and physically less healthy than their aged matched peers, and that GH replacement results in substantial and sustained benefits. The majority of these studies were performed over 12 months; however, long-term data detailing the effects of GH replacement over a more sustained period are now beginning to emerge. In this chapter, we will highlight the important features arising from GH-deficiency and detail the effects of GH replacement in the adult with GH-deficiency.

Body Composition

A wide range of techniques have been used to assess body composition, and most investigators have referred to a two-compartment model comprised of

TABLE 2.1. The clinical features of GH-deficiency in adults and the effect of GH replacement therapy.

Symptoms of GH-deficiency	Effect of GH replacement
Abnormal body composition	
Reduced lean body mass	Increases lean body mass
Increased abdominal adiposity	Decreases abdominal adiposity
Reduced strength and exercise capacity	Increases strength and exercise capacity
Impaired psychological well-being	Improves psychological well-being
Depressed mood	
Reduced vitality and energy	
Emotional lability	
Impaired self-control	
Anxiety	
Increased social isolation	

Signs of adult GH-deficiency	Effect of GH replacement
Overweight, with predominantly central (abdominal) adiposity	Decreases abdominal adiposity, no weight loss
Decreased Bone Mineral Density (BMD)	Increases BMD
Thin, dry skin; cool peripheries; poor venous access	Increases in skin thickness
Reduced muscle strength	Increases muscle strength
Reduction in exercise performance	Improves exercise performance
Depressed affect, labile emotions	Improves affect
Elevated plasma cholesterol, low HDL	Lowers cholesterol and increases HDL
Reduced erythropoeisis	Increases erythropoesis, plasma volume, and blood volume

lean body mass (LBM) and fat mass (FM). Despite the methodological differences in these studies, the findings are very consistent. Reduced skeletal muscle mass, the most prominent component of LBM, is an important feature of adult GH-deficiency. Several studies have demonstrated mean reduction in LBM of 7–8%, which corresponds to approximately 4 kg of lean tissue (1,4,6–8). In these studies fat mass was higher by a mean of 7% in GH-deficient patients compared with predicted values based on age, sex, and height. This figure has since been confirmed by other investigators, using a variety of techniques (7,91–2). Anthropometric and imaging studies demonstrate that this excess accumulates in a central (abdominal) distribution, mostly in the visceral component (1,3,9,10). In addition, evidence suggests that total body water (TBW), particularly the extracellular water (ECW) component, is reduced in adult GH-deficiency (8,11).

Many studies have investigated the effect of GH replacement on body composition. These have reported an increase in LBM of 2–5.5 kg with GH treatment (2,3–10,13,14) (Fig. 2.1). Parallel increase occurs in skeletal muscle

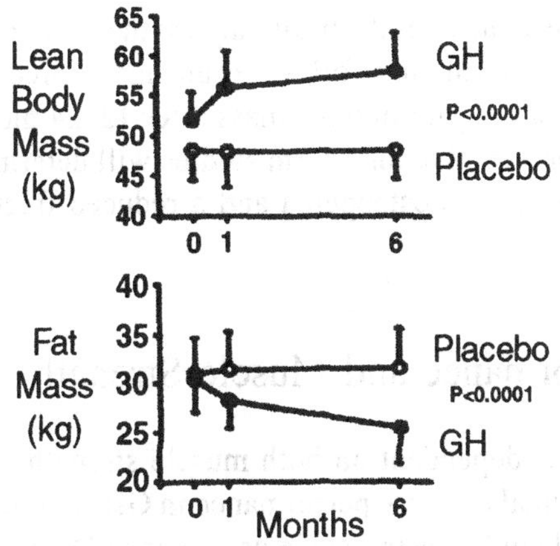

FIGURE 2.1. Changes in body composition (LBM and FM) during 6 months GH/placebo replacement in 24 adults with long-standing GH-deficiency. Modified from Salomon et al. (1).

(13). GH therapy has simultaneously resulted in a mean reduction in fat mass of approximately 4–6 kg in GH-deficient adults (2,3–10,13,14) (Fig. 2.1). The largest reduction occurs in the visceral fat of abdomen (3,10). GH is recognized to have an antinatiuretic effect, probably through direct effects of GH and/or IGF-I on renal tubular sodium absorption, in addition to stimulatory effects on the renin–angiotensin system (15). GH replacement results in an increase in TBW (4,12,16), particularly in ECW within 3–5 days (11,15).

Bone Mineral Density and Bone Metabolism

Studies of bone mineral density (BMD), despite the use of several techniques, have universally demonstrated reduced bone mass at a variety of skeletal sites in adults with GH-deficiency when compared with healthy control subjects (17–20). Data suggests that these patients are at increased risk for osteoporotic fractures (21).

Short-term studies (3–6 months) of GH replacement have failed to demonstrate an increase in bone mass (7). In several studies reduced BMD has been recorded following 6 months GH therapy (22), but after more than 12 months treatment increases of 4–10% above baseline have been demonstrated (23).

Serum bone formation (osteocalcin, alkaline phophatase, Gla) and urinary bone resorption markers (deoxypyridinoline, pyridinoline, cross-linked telopeptide of type I collagen) increased in both short-term and long-term studies, which indicates an activation of bone remodeling (7,20,22,23).

In summary, adult GH-deficiency is associated with reduced bone mass as assessed by bone mineral density measurements. The available data provide evidence that GH is an osteo-anabolic hormone when given to GH-deficient adults. The findings in most of the trials suggest that GH has a biphasic effect: Stimulation of bone formation following an initial predominance of bone resorption leads to a net gain in bone mass after 12–24 months of treatment. The results from prospective long-term studies will determine whether these changes will result in less osteopenia and a reduced fracture rate in adults with GH-deficiency.

Exercise Performance and Muscle Strength

Exercise capacity is dependent on both muscle strength and cardiovascular performance. Maximal exercise performance in GH-deficient adults has been assessed in several studies using cycle ergometry (24,25). Before treatment, values for maximum oxygen uptake were significantly reduced, being on average 72–82% of those predicted for age, sex, and height (24). Following 6 months GH treatment, maximum oxygen uptake increased significantly, virtually reaching predicted values (24). Evidence suggests that the increased performance is largely attributable to increased muscle mass (25). GH-mediated increases in erythropoesis, plasma, and blood volumes may also contribute to increased exercise capacity (12). Thus, adults with GH-deficiency have a reduced exercise performance capacity, which can be reversed with 6 months GH replacement. The decreased LBM of GH-deficiency results in a mild-to-moderate reduction in muscle strength. Isometric quadriceps force has been shown to be reduced in GH-deficient adults compared with matched normal controls (25). Six months of GH replacement increased limb–girdle force, but neither isometric quadriceps force nor quadriceps torque increased significantly in any of the studies (25–27), despite clear increases in thigh-muscle cross-sectional area. A significant increase in quadriceps force has been demonstrated only after more prolonged GH treatment (at least 12 months) with a further increase and normalization seen after 3 years (13).

Cardiovascular System

Epidemiological data suggest that adults with hypopituitarism have reduced life expectancy compared with healthy controls, with a greater than twofold increase in mortality from cardiovascular disease (28). As these patients were receiving appropriate replacement of all pituitary hormones with the exception of GH, these data support the hypothesis that long-standing GH-deficiency in adulthood predisposes to the development of premature atherosclerosis.

The mechanisms responsible for the increased cardiovascular mortality remain largely unknown, but increased intimamedial thickening, intimal plaque formation (29), and reduced arterial compliance (30) in the carotid artery have been demonstrated in hypopituitary adults on conventional replacement therapy.

Studies using both echocardiography and radionuclide scanning have demonstrated that adults with GH-deficiency have reduced left ventricular mass and impaired cardiac systolic function in adults with GH-deficiency compared with healthy controls (9,31). Treatment with GH for 6 months normalized these indexes, and cardiac function had returned to baseline 6 months after cessation of therapy. More recent studies demonstrated increased left ventricular mass (18%), stroke volume (28%), and cardiac output (43%) following 6 months GH replacement (31,32). It is important to note that these findings on cardiac performance appear to continue up to 3 years after commencement of GH (13,33).

Metabolism

Energy Expenditure

Whole-body resting energy expenditure (REE) is lower in adults with GH-deficiency than predicted values corrected for age, height, and weight (34). GH replacement results in rapid and large increases in REE (1,35,36). Restoration of LBM accounts for much of the increase observed in REE, but when changes in REE are expressed per LBM these rises are still significant, which indicates that direct increases in cellular metabolism are responsible for some of the increased REE (1). GH treatment of the GH-deficient adult results in an increase in circulating triiodothyronine levels (34), which indicates that GH is a physiological regulator of thyroid function in general, and peripheral conversion of thyroxine in particular. This alteration may contribute to the calorigenic effect of GH, as may the increases in fat oxidation (35) and protein synthesis (36) associated with GH replacement.

Protein and Carbohydrate Metabolism

Studies of protein metabolism in adults with GH-deficiency have demonstrated reduced protein flux and synthesis compared with normal matched controls (4,36). GH replacement increases protein synthesis for the first few months (4,36), with a return to baseline rates after 6 months (4), most likely as a result of achieving a new baseline rate of metabolism.

GH-deficient adults have hyperinsulinemia, which indicates insulin resistance in keeping with the clinical features of increased central obesity (37–39). GH replacement has been demonstrated to increase insulin resistance further over a 6-week period of therapy (39). Although hyperinsulinemia persists, however, carbohydrate metabolism returns to baseline following 3 months GH treatment (37,39).

Lipid and Lipoprotein Metabolism

Elevated concentrations of total cholesterol (TC), low-density lipoprotein-cholesterol (LDL-C), and apolipoprotein B (ApoB) have been observed patients with GH-deficiency (16,40,41). High-density lipoprotein-cholesterol (HDL-C) levels tend to be low and triglyceride (TG) levels high when compared with healthy controls (42). Thus, GH-deficiency is associated with a lipid profile known to be related to premature atherosclerosis and cardiovascular disease.

GH replacement results in decreases in TC concentration (16,41,43–45), LDL-C, and ApoB levels (43). In these studies GH therapy was associated with an increase in HDL-C (16,46), without alteration in concentration of plasma triglycerides (41,43,44). These "favorable" effects of GH replacement on the plasma lipid and lipoprotein profile are sustained up to 3 years after commencement of GH (16,45).

The exception to the trend of normalization of cardiovascular risk factors following GH treatment is lipoprotein(a), a proposed independent risk factor for the development of atherosclerosis and myocardial infarction (47). Studies have inconsistently demonstrated a rise in lipoprotein (a) levels following GH replacement (43–46). The importance of this observation is not yet clear.

Psychological Well-Being and Quality of Life

The psychological well-being and quality of life (QOL) of GH-deficient patients and the effects of GH replacement have been addressed in several studies, which have used validated questionnaires. Although several types of questionnaires have been used, the results have been remarkably consistent.

Decreased psychological well-being has been reported in hypopituitary adults despite replacement of all hormone deficiencies with the exception of growth hormone (48). Adults with long-standing GH-deficiency reported lower openness, less assertiveness, less energy, greater emotional lability, more difficulties with sexual relationships, and a greater sense of social isolation, than matched controls (48,49).

McGauley was the first to demonstrate in a double blind placebo controlled study that GH replacement was associated with an improvement in mood and energy levels in GH-deficient adults (50). These findings have been confirmed in subsequent studies (51,52) (Fig. 2.2).

The direct mechanism behind alterations in perceived QOL remains unknown. GH treatment of GH-deficient adults has been shown to alter levels of vasoactive intestinal polypeptide and the dopamine metabolite, homovanillic acid, as well as to elevate β-endorphin levels in cerebrospinal fluid, but whether these changes are responsible for improvement in mood and well-being is not yet known (53). GH, IGF-I, and the IGF-binding proteins may have direct effects on the nervous system.

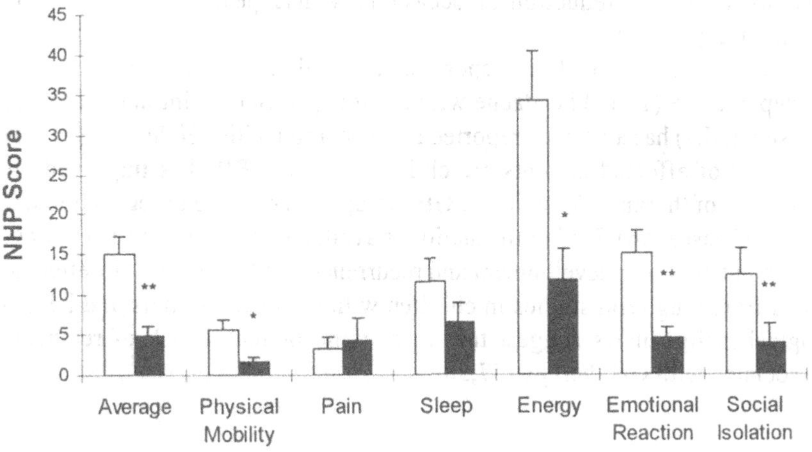

FIGURE 2.2. Changes in the psychological well-being of 38 adults during 6 months GH replacement assessed using the Nottingham Health Profile. A decrease in NHP score indicates an improvement in psychological well-being. $*p < 0.05$, $**p < 0.01$. Taken from Carroll et al. (52) with permission. © Society of the European Journal of Endocrinology.

Reported "Adverse" Effects of GH Replacement

Biosynthetic GH has an identical structural sequence to naturally occurring GH, thus adverse effects arise solely as a consequence of the use of excessive doses of GH. Early studies in adults with GH-deficiency employed similar doses to those used in pediatric populations and it is now recognized that these doses are too high and are associated with adverse effects that are in most cases avoided by a more cautious dosing protocol with monitoring of serum IGF-I levels. It is recommended that therapy should start with a low dose, 0.15–0.30 mg/day (0.45–0.90 IU/day). The dosage should be increased gradually on the basis of clinical and biochemical responses and no more frequently than at monthly intervals. The maintenance dose may vary considerably from person to person, and seldom exceeds 1.0 mg/day (3 IU/day).

The most common reported side effects following GH replacement in GH-deficient adults are those arising from sodium and water retention, and evidence suggests that those patients most at risk from adverse effects of GH replacement are the elderly and obese (54). Because patients with GH-deficiency are salt-depleted, these "effects" are to be expected (8,11). Weight gain, dependent edema, a sensation of tightness in the hands, or symptoms of carpal tunnel compression occur within days or weeks. A study of GH replacement in 233 hypopituitary adults, with GH doses ranging from 0.08 to 0.3 IU/kg/week, reported fluid retention (37.4%), arthralgia (19.1%), and muscle pains (15.7%) in the first 6 months of treatment (55). These symptoms resolve rapidly with dose reduction or occasionally disappear over several weeks without any action.

There have been isolated reports of cerebral side effects, in the form of encephalocele (1) and headache with tinnitus (3). Benign intracranial hypertension (BIH) has also been reported in association with GH therapy (56). The majority of affected patients are children, and the BIH has improved with cessation of therapy. Cessation of GH therapy has resulted in regression in all reported cases (56). Little information is available regarding the effect of GH treatment on tumor development and recurrence in adults with GH-deficiency. Data from long term studies in children with both solid tumors and hematological malignancies suggest that there is no increased risk of recurrence associated with GH therapy (57,58).

Conclusions

The importance of GH in adult life is no longer in question. GH-deficiency is recognized to result in alterations in body composition, physical performance, psychological well-being, and substrate metabolism. Many of these alterations can be improved or corrected with GH replacement. It is likely that GH replacement will, in the near future, become as routine as steroid, thyroid hormone, and sex hormone replacement in the management of the hypopituitary adult.

Several issues relating to GH replacement in adults have yet to be clarified. These include the identification of patients who may benefit from GH therapy. Current studies have focused on those with severe GH-deficiency, and little data is available in cases of partial GH-deficiency. The selection of patients is further complicated by the marked age-associated decline in GH secretion (59). Many elderly patients would meet diagnostic criteria for GH-deficiency. Whether or not such patients would benefit from GH therapy is unknown. It is also important that the units of GH replacement are universally accepted, both in the pediatric and adult spheres. The most widely used unit in adult medicine currently is international units per day, whereas many pediatric endocrinologists continue to use microns per kilogram per day. The issues of GH replacement dose and monitoring of response to therapy have been comprehensively addressed in the Port Stevens Manifesto (1997) of the Growth Hormone Research Society, published in the *Journal of Clinical Endocrinology and Metabolism* (60). The use of either microns per day or international units per day is currently recommended.

In the majority of studies, the effect of GH replacement has been rigorously assessed over 6- or 12-month periods. Although data are emerging, studies detailing the long-term effects of GH replacement are necessary to demonstrate whether the benefits are sustained. In particular, it remains to be seen whether GH treatment will reduce the incidence of cardiovascular and bone disease over a period of years. Rigorous monitoring of patients on long-term GH will provide further information regarding the issue of safety, but it will also determine whether GH replacement is associated with an increase in life expectancy for the GH-deficient adult.

References

1. Salomon F, Cuneo RD, Hesp R, Sönksen PH. The effects of treatment with recombinant human growth hormone on body composition and metabolism in adults with growth hormone deficiency. N Eng J Med 1989;321:1797–803.
2. Jorgensen JOL, Pedersen SA, Thuesen L, et al. Beneficial effects of growth hormone treatment in GH-deficient adults. Lancet 1989;i:1221–25.
3. Bengtsson B-A, Eden S, Lonn L, Kvist H, Stokland A, Lindstedt G, et al. Treatment of adults with growth hormone deficiency with recombinant human GH. J Clin Endocrinol Metab 1993;76:309–17.
4. Binnerts A, Swart GR, Wilson JHP, Hoogerbrugge N, Pois HAP, Birkenhager JC, et al. The effect of growth hormone administration in growth hormone deficient adults on bone, protein, carbohydrate and lipid homeostasis, as well as body composition. Clin Endocrinology 1992;37:79–87.
5. Chong PKK, Jung RT, Scrimgeour CM, Rennie MJ, Paterson CR. Energy expenditure and body composition in growth hormone deficient adults on exogenous growth hormone. Clin Endocrinology 1994;40:103–10.
6. Hoffman DM, O'Sullivan AJ, Freund J, Ho KK. Adults with growth hormone deficiency have abnormal body composition but normal energy metabolism. J Clin Endocrinol Metab 1995;80:72–77.
7. Beshyah SA, Freemantle C, Thomas E, Rutherford O, Page B, Murphy M, et al. Abnormal body composition and reduced bone mass in growth hormone deficient hypopituitary adults. Clin Endocrinology 1995;42:179–89.
8. Rosen T, Bosaeus I, Tolli J, Lindstedt G, Bengtsson BA. Increased body fat mass and decreased extracellular fluid volume in adults with growth hormone deficiency. Clin Endocrinol 1993;38:63–71.
9. Amato G, Carella C, Fazio S, La Montagna G, Cittadini A, Sabatini D, et al. Body composition, bone metabolism and heart structure and function in growth hormone-deficient adults before and after GH replacement therapy at low doses. J Clin Endocrinol Metab 1993;77:1671–76.
10. Snel YE, Doerga ME, Brummer RM, Zelissen PM, Koppeschaar HP. Magnetic resonance imaging-assessed adipose tissue and serum lipid and insulin concentrations in growth hormone-deficient adults. Effect of growth hormone replacement. Arter Thromb Vasc Biol 1995;15:1543–48.
11. Moller J, Frandsen E, Fisker S, Jorgensen JOL, Christiansen JS. Decreased plasma and extracellular volume in growth hormone-deficient adults and the acute and prolonged effects of GH administration: a controlled experimental study. Clin Endocrinol 1996;44:533–39.
12. Christ E, Cummings MH, Westwood NB, Sawyer BM, Pearson TC, Sönksen PH, et al. The importance of growth hormone in the regulation of erythropoiesis, red cell mass and plasma volume in adults with growth hormone deficiency. J Clin Endocrinol Metab 1997;82:2985–90.
13. Jorgensen JOL, Thuesen L, Muller J, et al. Three years of growth hormone treatment in growth hormone-deficient adults: near normalization of body composition and physical performance. Eur J Endocrinol 1994;130:224–28.

14. Beshyah SA, Freemantle C, Shahi M, Anyaoku V, Merson S, Lynch S, Skinner E, Sharp P, Foale R, Johnston DG. Replacement therapy with biosynthetic human growth hormone in growth hormone-deficient hypopituitary adults. Clin Endocrinol 1995;42:73–81.
15. Hoffman DM, Crampton L, Sernia C, Nguyen TV, Ho KKY. Short term growth hormone (GH) treatment of GH-deficient adults increases body sodium and extracellular water, but not blood pressure. J Clin Endocrinol Metab 1996;81:1123–28.
16. Attanasio AF, Lamberts SWJ, Matranga AMC, Birkett MA, Bates PC, Valk NK, et al. Adult growth hormone-deficient patients demonstrate heterogenity between childhood onset and adult onset before and during human GH treatment. J Clin Endocrinol Metab 1997;82:82–88.
17. O'Halloran DJ, Tsatsoulis A, Whitehouse RW, Holmes SJ, Adams JE, Shalet SM. Increased bone density after recombinant human growth hormone therapy in adults with isolated GH deficiency. J Clin Endocrinol Metab 1993;76:1344–48.
18. Kaufman JM, Taelman P, Vermeulen A, Vandeweghe M. Bone mineral status in growth hormone-deficient males with isolated and multiple pituitary insufficiencies of childhood onset. J Clin Endocrinol Metab 1992;74:118–23.
19. Holmes SJ, Economou G, Whitehouse RW, Adams JE, Shalet SM. Reduced bone mineral density in patients with adult onset growth hormone deficiency. J Clin Endocrinol Metab 1994;78:669–74.
20. Degerblad M, Bengtsson BA, Bramnert M, Johnell O, Manhem P, Rosen T, et al. Reduced bone mineral density in adults with growth hormone deficiency: increased bone turnover during 12 months of GH substitution. Eur J Endocrinol 1995; 133:180–88.
21. Wüster CHR, Slenczka E, Ziegler R. Increased prevalence of osteoporosis and arteriosclerosis in patients with conventionally substituted pituitary insufficiency: Is there a need for additional growth hormone substitution? Klin Wochenschrift 1991;69:769–73.
22. Beshyah SA, Kyd P, Thomas E, Fairney A, Johnston DG. The effects of prolonged growth hormone replacement on bone metabolism and bone mineral density in hypopituitary adults. Clin Endocrinol 1995;42:249–54.
23. Vandeweghe M, Taelman P, Kaufman JM. Short and long-term effects of growth hormone treatment on bone turnover and bone mineral content in adult growth hormone-deficient males. Clin Endocrinol 1993;39:409–15.
24. Cuneo RC, Salomon F, Wiles CM, et al. Growth hormone treatment in growth hormone-deficient adults. II. effects on exercise performance. J Appl Physiol 1991;70:695–700.
25. Cuneo RC, Salomon F, Wiles CM, et al. Skeletal muscle performance in adults with growth hormone deficiency. Horm Res 1990;33 (suppl 4):55–60.
26. Cuneo RC, Salomon F, Wiles CM, et al. Growth hormone treatment in growth hormone-deficient adults. I. Effects on muscle mass and strength. J Appl Physiol 1991;70:688–94.
27. Degerblad M, Almkvist O, Grunditz R, et al. Physical and psychological capabilities during substitution therapy with recombinant growth hormone in adults with growth hormone deficiency. Acta Endocrinologica 1990;23:185–93.
28. Rosen T, Bengtsson B-Å. Premature mortality due to cardiovascular disease in hypopituitarism. Lancet 1990;336:285–88.
29. Markussis V, Beshyah SA, Fisher C, Sharp P, Nicolaides AN, Johnston DG. Detection of premature atherosclerosis by high-resolution ultrasonography in symptom-free hypopituitary adults. Lancet 1992;340:1188–92.

30. Lehmann ED, Hopkins KD, Weissberger AJ, Gosling RG, Sönksen PH. Aortic distensibility in growth hormone deficient adults. Lancet 1993;341:309.
31. Cuocolo A, Nicolai E, Colao A, Longobardi S, Cardei S, Fazio S, et al. Improved left ventricular function after growth hormone replacement in patients with hypopituitarism: assessment with radionuclide angiography. Eur J Nucl Med 1996;23:390–94.
32. Caidahl K, Edén S, Bengtsson B-Å. Cardiovascular and renal effects of growth hormone. Clin Endocrinol 1994;40:393–400.
33. Thuesen L, Jorgensen JOL, Muller JR, et al. Short and long-term cardiovascular effect of growth hormone therapy in growth hormone deficient adults. Clin Endocrinol 1994; 41:615–20.
34. Jorgensen JOL, Pedersen SA, Laurberg P, et al. Effects of growth hormone therapy on thyroid function of growth hormone-deficient adults with and without concomitant thyroxine-substituted central hypothyroidism. J Clin Endocrinol Metab 1989;69:1127–32.
35. Hussain MA, Schmitz O, Mengel A, Glatz Y, Christiansen JS, Zapf J, et al. Comparison of the effects of growth hormone and insulin-like growth factor I on substrate oxidation and on insulin sensitivity in growth hormone-deficient humans. J Clin Invest 1994;94:1126–33.
36. Russell-Jones DL, Weissberger AJ, Bowes SB, et al. The effects of growth hormone on protein metabolism in adult growth hormone deficient patients. Clin Endocrinol 1993;38:427–31.
37. O'Neal DN, Kalfas A, Dunning PL, et al. The effect of 3 months of recombinant human growth hormone (GH) therapy on insulin and glucose-mediated glucose disposal and insulin secretion in GH-deficient adults: a minimal model analysis. J Clin Endocrinol Metab 1994;79:975–83.
38. Hew FL, Koschmann M, Christopher M, Rantzau C, Vaag A, Ward G, et al. Insulin resistance in growth hormone-deficient adults: defects in glucose utilization and glycogen synthase activity. J Clin Endocrinol Metab 1996;81:555–64.
39. Fowelin J, Attvall S, Lager I, Bengtsson BA. Effects of treatment with recombinant human growth hormone on insulin sensitivity and glucose metabolism in adults with growth hormone deficiency. Metab Clin Exp 1993;42:1443–47.
40. De Boer H, Blok GJ, Voerman HJ, Phillips M, Schouten JA. Serum lipid levels in growth hormone-deficient men. Metab Clin Exp 1994; 43:199–203.
41. Cuneo RC, Salomon F, Watts GF, Hesp R, Sönksen PH. Growth hormone treatment improves serum lipids and lipoproteins in adults with growth hormone deficiency. Metab Clin Exp 1993;42:1519–23.
42. Rosen T, Eden S, Larson G, Wilhelmsen L, Bengtsson B-Å. Cardiovascular risk factors in adult patients with growth hormone deficiency. Acta Endocrinologica 1993;129:195–200.
43. Russell-Jones DL, Watts GF, Weissberger A, Naumova R, Myers J, Thompson GR, et al. The effect of growth hormone replacement on serum lipids, lipoproteins, apolipoproteins and cholesterol precursors in adult growth hormone deficient patients. Clin Endocrinol 1994;41:345–50.
44. Johansson G, Oscarsson J, Rosen T, Wiklund O, Olsson G, Wilhelmsen L, et al. Effects of 1 year of growth hormone therapy on serum lipoprotein levels in growth hormone-deficient adults. Influence of gender and Apo(a) and Apo(E) phenotypes. Arter Thromb Vasc Biol 1995;15:2142–50.
45. Garry P, Collins P, Devlin JG. An open 36 month study of lipid changes with growth hormone in adults: lipid changes following replacement of growth hormone in adult acquired growth hormone deficiency. Eur J Endocrinol 1996;134:61–66.

46. Eden S, Wiklund O, Oscarsson J, Rosen T, Bengtsson B-A. Growth hormone treatment of growth hormone-deficient adults results in a marked increase in Lp(a) and HDL cholesterol concentrations. Arter Thromb 1993;13:296–301.
47. Angelin B, Rudling M. Growth hormone and hepatic lipoprotein metabolism. Curr Opin Lipidol 1994.5:160–65.
48. Stabler B, Turner JR, Girdler SS, Light KC, Underwood LE. Reactivity to stress and psychological adjustment in adults with pituitary insufficiency. Clin Endocrinol 1992;6:467–73.
49. Rosen T, Wiren L, Wilhelmsen L, Wiklund I, Bengtsson BA. Decreased psychological well-being in adult patients with growth hormone deficiency. Clin Endocrinol 1994;40:111–16.
50. McGauley GA. Quality of life assessment before and after growth hormone treatment in adults with growth hormone deficiency. Acta Paediatr Scand 1989;356 (suppl):55–59.
51. Burman P, Broman JE, Hetta J, Wiklund I, Erfurth EM, Hagg E, et al. Quality of life in adults with growth hormone (GH) deficiency: response to treatment with recombinant human GH in a placebo-controlled 21-month trial. J Clin Endocrinol Metab 1995;80:3585–90.
52. Carroll PV, Littlewood R, Weissberger AJ, Bogalho P, McGauley G, Sönksen PH, Russell-Jones DL. The effects of two doses of replacement growth hormone on the biochemical, body composition and psychological profiles of growth hormone-deficient adults. Eur J Endocrinol 1997;137:146–53.
53. Johansson JO, Larson G, Andersson M, Elmgren A, Hynsjo L, Lindahl A, et al. Treatment of growth hormone-deficient adults with recombinant human growth hormone increases the concentration of growth hormone in the cerebrospinal fluid and affects neurotransmitters. Neuroendocrinology 1995;61:57–66.
54. Holmes SJ, Shalet SM. Which adults develop side-effects of growth hormone replacement? Clin Endocrinol 1995;43:143–49.
55. Mårdh G, Lundin K, Borg G, Jonsson B, Lindeberg A. Growth hormone replacement therapy in adult hypopituitary patients with growth hormone deficiency: combined data from 12 European placebo-controlled trials. Endocrinol Metab 1994;1 (suppl A):43–49.
56. Malozowski S, Tanner LA, Wysowski D, Fleming GA. Growth hormone, insulin-like growth factor-I, and benign intracranial hypertension. N Engl J Med 1993;329:665–66.
57. Taback SP, Dean HJ. Mortality in Canadian children with growth hormone (GH) deficiency receiving GH therapy 1967–1992. The Canadian Growth Hormone Advisory Commitee. J Clin Endocrinol Metab 1996;81:1693–96.
58. Moshang T Jr., Rundle AC, Graves DA, Nickas J, Johanson A, Meadows A. Brain tumor recurrence in children treated with growth hormone: the National Cooperative Growth Study experience. J Pediatr 1996;128:S4–7.
59. Rudman D, Kutner MH, Rogers CM, et al. Impaired growth hormone secretion in the adult population: relation to age and adiposity. J Clin Invest 1981;67:1361–69.
60. Consensus guidelines for the diagnosis and treatment of adults with growth hormone deficiency: summary statement of the Growth Hormone Research Society Workshop on adult growth hormone deficiency. J Clin Endocrinol Metab 1998;83:379–81.

3

Quality of Life in Children and Adults with Growth Hormone Deficiency

INGELA K. WIKLUND, ANN E. ERLING, AND KERSTIN ALBERTSSON-WIKLAND

Introduction

There has been a growing recognition among clinicians of the importance of learning more about how patients view the effects of their condition and its treatment. The concept of health-related quality of life represents a method that is commonly used to assess the views of the patients in terms of the physical, social, and emotional aspects of living with their condition (1). *Quality of life* is an important component of research into outcomes, which is directed toward verifying the extent to which patients are compromised by their current state, and whether they benefit from the health care given. There is growing scientific awareness that clinical indicators are inadequate for explaining health-related quality of life (2). This particularly applies to conditions where there may be few biological markers of disease activity. In fact, in this situation it has been suggested that the ultimate goal of treatment is to maintain or to improve the patients' quality of life. Outcomes in growth hormone (GH) deficiency include objective measures of height, weight, body composition or bone diameter. In children, intellectual functioning is estimated in addition to the physiological outcomes. These measures, however, do not necessarily reflect the impact of the condition. Neither do changes in these parameters represent valid indicators of health-related quality of life. It is therefore essential to measure quality of life alongside conventional clinical parameters.

Assessment of Quality of Life

By definition, *quality of life* reflects a subjective perception, and direct questioning is therefore a simple and appropriate way of collecting information on how patients feel and function. It has previously been argued that subjective outcomes, such as quality of life, are often measured with less quantitative rigor. The assessment of quality of life, however is typically performed today by using standard questionnaires which ensure that the psychometric properties are well documented (3,4). There are two basic types of questionnaire: generic and disease- or treatment-specific (5). The generic scales show many similarities, covering a range of outcomes that makes them applicable to most health problems. They can be used to compare the scores among GH-deficient patients with corresponding scores from a normal population, or score values obtained from patients with other somatic conditions. Specific questionnaires, on the other hand, have been designed to capture the problems of relevance to a particular condition such as GH deficiency. The provision of adequate methods for describing the impact of GH deficiency, and for monitoring and evaluating treatment effects in those who receive therapy, is a key issue (6,7).

Quality of Life in Children with GH Insufficiency

Impact of Short Stature and/or GH Deficiency

Although it is often assumed that a short stature causes considerable disability and distress to the person affected, there is little scientific evidence to support this notion, at least with regard to short normal children (8). In fact, young children of short stature have quite favorable scores for aspects of well-being, and do not deviate from ratings made by young children of normal stature (9,10). In terms of their own height, children of short stature, that is below –2 standard deviations (SDs), tended to give a fairly accurate description of their actual height, indicating that they were aware of being very short (11). The children were less realistic, however, in terms of their future height and their height expectations far exceeded what could be expected to be achieved by treatment.

A different picture of the impact of being short was derived from studies employing projective techniques. By using such methods, the children unconsciously revealed how they were affected by their short stature. Problems with alienation from peers, fear of physical and psychological danger, and poor self-esteem were described (10). Information obtained in interviews similarly showed that 60% of the children reported problems arising from their short stature and young appearance. A lack of social contacts, discrimination against them, and a lack of strength were mentioned, whereas others referred to having fewer friends, problems with relationships, and spending their leisure time alone.

In terms of academic achievement, the work by Stabler and his colleagues has consistently indicated that both children with GH deficiency (–2.7 SDs) and children with idiopathic short stature are disadvantaged (12). In a large multicenter study addressing the educational and behavioral functioning of short children referred for GH treatment, both those with isolated GH insufficiency and those with idiopathic short stature showed a significant discrepancy between intelligence quotients and achievement scores in reading, spelling, and arithmetic. In other words, despite average intelligence, an advantaged social background, and an absence of significant family dysfunction, a large number of children were considered to suffer from academic underachievement, which are findings that have serious implications for the children's future life and career. The same study also showed significantly elevated scores for problems with psychosocial adjustment compared with normal values, which indicate high levels of anxiety and depression, aggression, and hyperactivity. Children with a clinically more pronounced degree of GH insufficiency complain about lack of energy and being low in vitality (i.e., the same type of problems reported by adults).

Treatment Effects

There are comparatively few studies that evaluate the effects of GH therapy on different aspects of functioning in children. There is evidence that alertness and cognitive function are important, and may be beneficially affected by treatment (13), at least in children with below-average scores for intellectual performance (14). Treatment also resulted in a more favorable perception in the children of themselves and of their stature (15). Another study showed that for children referred for GH treatment, there was an increase in problems with school achievement and behavioral problems, such as anxiety, depression, and somatic complaints, and a lack of social skills (16). A follow-up 3 years after initiation of GH therapy showed an improvement in overall combined psychosocial problems in both children with GH insufficiency and children with idiopathic short stature (16). Despite a good growth response, however, many children showed a less-than-average quality of life in young adulthood, which suggests that short stature per se may not be the cause of this outcome.

Confounding Variables

The impact of a short stature is related to both gender and age. In terms of gender, the majority of the young children referred to the hospital because of short stature are boys (9,12). This suggests that problems with height are interpreted as being more disabling and distressing for boys than for girls, and short boys do in fact complain more frequently of verbal and physical abuse, which may explain reports of low self-esteem (17). There is also a relationship between a number of psychosocial indicators, height, and age (18). Age was significantly associated with perceived social acceptance, physical appearance, and global self-worth, which suggests that the older the child, the more pronounced problems, distress, and dysfunction tend to become.

Another study in a large unselected group of 18-year-old students showed a marked discrepancy between adolescent boys of normal and short stature, which indicates that the short boys were compromised in terms of poor self-esteem, alertness, and mood (19). This supports the notion that preadolescence and early adolescence represent particularly difficult periods for short children, as problems relating to juvenization and looking inappropriately young have become more obvious at this stage.

Quality of Life in Adults with GH Deficiency

Even though there is inconclusive evidence of an adverse impact arising from short stature and/or GH insufficiency in children, data obtained from GH-deficient adults are more clear cut. Among a group of adults who were GH-insufficient as children, a high incidence of social phobia and psychiatric distress was linked with the lack of GH secretion (16). These individuals in many cases also had a poor quality of life. Similar findings were noted in a further study, whereas the psychiatric status was assessed in 21 GH-deficient adults who had been treated with GH for short stature during childhood (20). Compared with healthy controls, a high rate of previously undiagnosed social phobia, 38%, was found. The scores corresponded closely with scores derived from a matched group of psychiatric patients with social phobia. As these psychiatric symptoms have deleterious effects on quality of life, social function, and productivity, physicians should be alert to the potential psychiatric problems in patients with GH deficiency.

Other expressions of psychosocial maladjustment compared with healthy controls were observed among GH-deficient adults, who complained of low self-esteem, more fatigue and depression, and less fulfillment in life (21). A comparison of adults of short stature with or without GH deficiency showed that the GH-deficient individuals reported significantly higher degrees of social anxiety and distress, fear of negative events, and fear in general, as well as higher scores on a depression scale (22). Evidence of an impaired quality of life, based on the results of clinical trials, has also been shown in GH-deficient adults compared with matched controls (23). The psychiatric distress scores were lower than they were in patients with anxiety disorders; in fact, they were as low as in subjects suffering from insomnia, a highly disabling problem. The same study also showed that the GH-deficient adults suffered in terms of emotional distress and a lack of energy compared with matched controls. Yet another study confirmed that GH-deficient adults, in addition to emotional distress and a lack of energy suffered in terms of social isolation and sexual problems (24). This study also indicated that sexual functioning, a neglected but nevertheless essential issue, was impaired.

Treatment Effects

In patients with adult onset of GH deficiency, pretreatment values indicated an impairment in quality of life in terms of fatigue and poor well-being. After a 6-month period of substitution, however, those supplied with GH reported more pronounced benefits in energy and mood than those given placebo treatment (24). Results from different studies also suggest an improvement in cognitive function (25), sleep (26), and physical capacity (27). A crossover trial comparing the effects of GH substitution and placebo over 6 months in adult GH-deficient patients showed a more pronounced improvement for dimensions depicting energy and emotions during active therapy compared with placebo (24). In terms of well-being, GH treatment provided a greater improvement than placebo, even though the scores did not reach values shown in normal populations. On a psychiatric rating scale, the overall score showed a significant benefit with GH therapy. The subscales depicting anxiety, fearfulness, and cognition were the indicators most sensitive to treatment changes.

In a small study of only eight adults with childhood onset of GH deficiency, the scores before treatment indicated that the patients tended to underestimate their body size by 30% (28). The study also showed that the patients had a low level of self-esteem, were socially withdrawn, and displayed a pessimistic attitude with a tendency toward depression. After 6 months of GH treatment, the patients presented an overall improvement in intellectual ability. There was also a clear improvement in emotional control. It is important to note that 6 months after stopping therapy the psychological problems reverted to pretreatment levels, which suggests that the observed effects were GH dependent. An analysis was carried out on the scores derived during treatment from 12 European placebo-controlled studies in GH-deficient adults (29). A corresponding favorable effect for GH substitution was observed in terms of emotional distress and social isolation. Additional benefits included a decrease in fat body mass, whereas lean body mass increased.

Discussion

There is little doubt that GH-deficient adults suffer from an impaired quality of life, and that substantial benefits may be derived from treatment with GH. A corresponding impairment is not so discernable in young GH-insufficient children. There is evidence, however, that they are at a disadvantage intellectually. There is also evidence that they suffer from social and behavioral problems, which become more manifest and pronounced during adolescence, particularly in boys.

Nonetheless, there is a discrepancy between observations obtained from GH-deficient adults, on the one hand, and those from GH-insufficient children, on the other. There are several possible explanations. It has been suggested that the tools used to assess health-related quality of life and the psychosocial consequences of short stature in children may not be sensitive enough. If the impact of short stature is comparatively small, as may be the case at least in young children, a ceiling effect may ensue. The discriminative ability of the rating scales with regard to subjects with relatively modest deviations from normal, such as in young children of short stature, may therefore be jeopardized.

Standardized questionnaires focus on distress and dysfunction; therefore, they lack a specific focus on issues that may be related to short stature or GH deficiency. Important areas such as energy deficits or difficulties in concentrating, to which there is a potential link with intellectual underachievement, are not always addressed. The same applies to embarrassment, frustration, or specific experiences perceived to be a direct result of short stature because these domains are not normally included on the standardized questionnaires.

Results derived from using projective techniques suggest that denial may confound the detection of the true impairment of being short. Denial of problems in combination with inappropriate coping strategies might explain why no discrepancies are found between children of short and normal stature, at least in the younger age groups (30). An advantage associated with the use of projective methods is that they provide a means by which the child can more easily share and disclose frustrating, embarrassing, or anxiety-provoking experiences.

It is important to find standardized routes for obtaining direct answers from the children because the agreement between how parents and the children themselves rate height and aspects of well-being is only modest (11). Moreover, children tend to volunteer less information on problems than do their parents (9). In particular, they avoid mentioning painful experiences and behavioral problems relating to somatic complaints and social withdrawal.

Attention to study design issues is important. The sample sizes are generally small, and they typically include a heterogeneous population with regard to diagnoses as well as age range. Other methodological difficulties found in studies both of adults and of children relate to inappropriate or nonexistent control groups. The follow-up period seldom extends beyond 2 or 3 years. Longitudinal studies provide a better description of the course of children's adjustment to short stature because problems induced by a short stature do not generally appear until later in life. Longitudinal studies that follow the child to final height during therapy, therefore are probably the best way of deriving detailed information about potential treatment effects, or potential benefits in terms of the prevention of problems during adolescence as well as in adult life (31,32).

There seems to be a strong belief among endocrinologists that GH therapy is of value in GH-deficient children and adults by having a positive influence on well-being (33). There is substantial agreement (84%) among pediatric endocrinologists that short stature has a dysfunctional emotional impact on children and adults, and one third of the clinicians indicated that GH therapy is also likely or very likely to have a positive impact on emotional well-being in non–GH-deficient children, even in the absence of any major influence on adult height.

In conclusion, short stature is a problem for many individuals, irrespective of whether a GH insufficiency is present or not. As short stature may reflect underlying morbidity, it requires further medical attention and examination. Young patients and their families, as well as adult patients, need close and careful monitoring throughout the treatment process in order to check the effects and to promote compliance. Clinical parameters are important, but they constitute an insufficient basis for efficacy evaluation. Good subjective measurement tools, applied longitudinally, are therefore indispensable. Improvement should not be regarded as the only key to successful treatment because prevention may represent a far more desirable goal.

References

1. Spitzer WO. State of science 1986; quality of life and functional status as target variables for research. J Chron Dis 1987;40:465–71.
2. Whitehead WE, Burnett CK, Cook EW, Taub E. Impact of irritable bowel syndrome on quality of life. Dig Dis Sci 1996;41:2248–53.
3. Shumaker S, Anderson R, Czajhowski S. Psychological tests and scales. In: Spilker B, ed. Quality of life assessments in clinical trials. New York: Raven Press, 1990:95–113.
4. Testa MA, Simonson DC. Assessment of quality of life outcomes. N Engl J Med 1996;334:835–40.
5. Patrick DL, Deyo RA. Generic and disease-specific measures in assessing health status and quality of life. Med Care 1989;27:217–32.
6. Fitzpatrick R, Fletcher A, Gose S, Jones D, Spiegelhalter D, Cox D. Quality of life measures in health case. I: Applications and issues in assessment. Br Med J 1992;305:1074–77.
7. Kirshner B, Guyatt G. A methodological framework for assessing health indices. J Chron Dis 1985;38:27–36.
8. Voss LD, Mulligan J. The short normal child in school: self-esteem, behavior, and attainment before puberty. In: Stabler B, Underwood LE, eds. Growth, stature, and adaptation. Chapel Hill: The University of North Carolina. 1994:47–64
9. Sandberg DE, Brook AE, Campos SP. Short stature: a psychosocial burden requiring growth hormone therapy? Pediatrics 1994;94:832–40.
10. Rotnem D, Genel M, Hintz RL, Cohen DJ. Personality development in children with growth hormone deficiency. J Am Acad Child Psychiatr 1977;16:412–26.
11. Erling A, Wiklund I, Albertsson-Wikland K. Prepubertal children with short stature have a different perception of their well-being and stature than their parents. Qual Life Res 1994;3:425–29.
12. Stabler B, Clopper RR, Siegel PT, Stoppani C, Compton PG, Underwood LE. Academic achievement and psychological adjustment in short children. Dev Behav Pediatr 1994;15:1–6.
13. Westphal O. Experiences of Somatonorm in Sweden. Acta Paediatr Scand 1986;325 (suppl):41–44.

14. Siegel PT, Clopper RR, Stoppani C, Stabler B. The psychological adjustment of short children and normal controls. In: Stabler B, Underwood LE, eds. Growth, stature, and adaptation. Chapel Hill: The University of North Carolina. 1994: 123–34.
15. Boulton TJ, Dunn SM, Quigley CA, Taylor JJ, Thompson L. Perceptions of self and short stature: effects of two years of growth hormone treatment. Acta Paediatr Scand 1991;377(suppl):20–27.
16. Stabler B, Clopper RR, Siegel PT, Nicholas LM, Silva SG, Tancer ME, et al. Links between growth hormone deficiency, adaptation and social phobia. Horm Res 1996;45:30–33.
17. Law CM. The disability of short stature. Arch Dis Child 1987;62:855–59.
18. Zimet GD, Cutler M, Litvene M, Dahms W, Owens R, Cuttler L. Psychological adjustment of children evaluated for short stature. A preliminary report. J Dev Behav Pediatr 1995;16:264–70.
19. Svensson B, Wiklund I, Albertsson-Wikland K. Well-being in a population of 18 year old high school students in Göteborg, Sweden, 1993. Abstract. Growth, stature and adaptation. Chapel Hill: The University of North Carolina. October 1993.
20. Stabler B, Tancer ME, Ranc J, Underwood LE. Evidence for social phobia and other psychiatric disorders in adults who were growth hormone deficient during childhood. Anxiety 1996;2:86–89.
21. Nicholas LM, Tancer ME, Silva SG, Underwood LE, Stabler B. Short stature, growth hormone deficiency, and social anxiety. Psychosom Med 1997;59:372–75.
22. Burman P, Broman JE, Hetta J, Wiklund I, Erfurth EM, Hagge E, et al. Quality of life in adults with growth hormone (GH) deficiency: response to treatment with recombinant human GH in a placebo controlled 21-month trial. J Clin Endocrinol Metab 1995;80:3585–90.
23. Rosén T, Wirén L, Wilhelmsen L, Wiklund I, Bengtsson BÅ. Decreased psychological well-being in adult patients with growth hormone deficiency. Clin Endocrinol 1994;40:111–16.
24. McGauley GA. Quality of life assessments before and after growth hormone treatment in adults with growth hormone deficiency. Acta Paediatr Scand 1989;356(suppl):70–72.
25. Almqvist O, Thorén M, Sääf M, Eriksson O. Effects of growth hormone substitution on mental performance in adults with growth hormone deficiency: a pilot study. Psychoneuroendocrinology 1986;11:347–52.
26. McKenna SP, Doward LC. Quality-of-life assessment of adults with growth hormone efficiency. Implications for drug therapy. Pharmacoeconomics 1994; 6:434–41.
27. Degerblad M, Almkvist O, Grunditz R, Hall K, Kaijser L, Knutsson E, et al. Physical and psychological capabilities during substitution therapy with recombinant growth hormone in adults with growth hormone deficiency. Acta Endocrinol 1990;123:185–93.
28. Sartorio A, Molinari E, Riva G, Conti A, Morabito F, Faglia G. Growth hormone treatment in adults with childhood onset growth hormone deficiency: effects on psychological capabilities. Horm Res 1995;44:6–11.
29. Mårdh G, Lundin K, Borg G, Jonsson B, Lindeberg A on behalf of the investiga-

tors. Growth hormone replacement therapy in adult hypopituitary patients with growth hormone deficiency: Combined data from 12 European placebo-controlled clinical trials. Endocrinol Metab1994;1(suppl):A:43–49.
30. Rotnem D, Cohen DJ, Hintz R, Genel M. Psychological sequelae of relative treatment failure for chidlren receiving human growth hormone replacement. Am Acad Child Psychiatr 1979;18:505–20.
31. Holmes CS, Karlsson JA, Thompson RG. Longitudinal evaluation of behavior patterns in children with short stature. In: Stabler B, Underwood LE, eds. Slow grows the child: psychosocial aspects of growth delay. Hillsdale, NJ: Lawrence Erlbaum Associates, 1986:1–12.
32. Molinari E, Coretti E, Morabito F, Sartorio A, Peri G. Personality development follow-up in subjects with GH deficiency. Acta Med Auxolog 1990;22:171–80.
33. Cuttler L, Silvers JB, Singh J, Marrero U, Finkelstein B, Tannin G, et al. Short stature and growth hormone therapy. JAMA 1996;276:531–37.

4

Treatment of Childhood Growth Hormone Deficiency: Efficacy and Innovation

LEONA CUTTLER

This chapter reviews the efficacy of treatment for childhood growth hormone (GH) deficiency in the context of the natural history of the condition. Data on the effects of GH therapy on the multidimensional morbidity of GH deficiency will be discussed, and emerging innovations in treatment of childhood GH deficiency will be reviewed.

The Natural History of Childhood Growth Hormone (GH) Deficiency: Implications for Assessment of Treatment Efficacy

Evaluating current outcomes of treatment for childhood GH deficiency may best be undertaken in relation to the natural history of the condition. As early as 1903, the medical literature reported adults with "ateleiotic dwarfism" who had many of the classical features of congenital GH deficiency, including extreme short stature, childlike physiognomy and body proportions, a high-pitched voice, delayed osseous development, and markings on the face suggestive of aging (1).

In such early publications, affected adults had heights of 3–4 feet. More recently, Wit et al. reported adult heights of untreated GH-deficient adults as, on average, 4.7 standard deviations (SDs) below the mean for those with spontaneous puberty and 3.1 SDs below the mean for those with induced puberty (2).

In addition to extreme short stature, the natural history of childhood GH deficiency (Table 4.1) includes decreased bone mineral density (3–5), the potential for hypoglycemia, increased body fat (6,7), decreased muscle mass, pubertal abnormalities (including delayed puberty in those with isolated GH deficiency, failure of pubertal development in those with panhypopituitar-

TABLE 4.1. Natural history of childhood GH deficiency.

Extreme short stature	Pubertal abnormalities
Hypoglycemia	Decreased bone mineral content
Abnormal body composition	Psychosocial dysfunction
Premature aging	

ism, and precocious puberty in those with associated organic hypothalamic–pituitary lesions), and psychosocial dysfunction (8–11).

The natural lifespan of individuals with childhood GH deficiency is not well understood. Taback and colleagues, reviewing the Canadian experience including the early years of GH therapy, reported no increase in mortality except that due to hypoglycemia or adrenal insufficiency (12). Rosen et al. (13) reported increased mortality due to cardiovascular disease in GH deficient adults (including those who acquired GH deficiency after childhood), but comparable data specifically for childhood GH deficiency are not available.

Full assessment of therapeutic outcomes in childhood GH deficiency are therefore complex. The multidimensional morbidity of childhood GH deficiency requires that complete evaluation of treatment efficacy be multifaceted, including assessment of short-term and long-term growth, body composition, bone mineralization, metabolic parameters, and psychosocial function. Even targeted assessments of the effect of treatment on adult height are potentially confounded by differing definitions of final height, variations in subjects and treatment regimens, unclear compliance and drop-out rates, and co-morbid conditions. Moreover, the assessment of therapeutic efficacy to some degree depends on the outcome measure chosen. In the case of adult height, options include height expressed as SDs from the mean, in centimeters, as a proportion of patients who achieve adult heights in the "normal" range, in relation to originally predicted adult height, or in relation to target adult height.

Efficacy of GH Therapy in the Treatment of Childhood GH Deficiency

Since the late 1950s, GH has been the classical treatment for childhood GH deficiency. Initial reports about its impact on growth velocity in children with GH deficiency were very enthusiastic, and recent reports using biosynthetic GH in current doses and treatment regimens substantiate the dramatic effect of GH on growth velocity in children. During the first year of GH therapy, children with GH deficiency increase their growth rates, on average, from 4.5 cm/year or less to approximately 9 cm/year (14,15). The younger the child, the greater the growth velocity during initial GH therapy. Other predictors of initial growth response to GH therapy include the maximal GH response to provocative stimuli and the GH treatment regimen (14). Regarding the treatment regimen, daily GH therapy results in dramatically greater growth than would the same weekly dose divided into three injections per week: After 4 years of GH therapy, children on daily treatment regimens may be expected to have gained almost 10 cm more than those treated with regimens involving thrice weekly injections (16).

In terms of adult height after GH therapy, series involving patients treated (at least in part) during the hGH era have reported increased adult height over that predicted by natural history analyses, although the mean adult height achieved still remained relatively low at 2–4 SDs below the mean (e.g., 17–22; Fig. 4.1). Although they are very important in understanding GH therapy from a historical context, many of these studies are limited as indexes of adult height potential following GH treatment because they involved intermittent GH therapy, GH doses below current standards, a mixture of prepubertal and pubertal children at onset of therapy, a high proportion of individuals who ceased GH therapy before meeting existing guidelines, relatively short durations of GH treatment, and/or low participation rates for follow-up studies.

More recent studies, involving children treated with current doses and treatment regimens, have yielded a much more optimistic view of the effectiveness of GH therapy in improving the adult height of children with GH deficiency. For example, Blethen et al. reported that adult height in a cohort of prepubertal GH deficient children treated with rGH (0.3 mg/kg/week) as, on average, 0.7 SDs below the mean (23). The mean adult heights achieved by men and women in that study were 171.6 cm (SD 8.2 cm) and 158.5 cm (SD 7.1 cm), respectively. It is interesting to note that the development of puberty spontaneously during the course of therapy did not affect adult height achieved, which is in contrast with earlier studies. Although the adult heights exceeded those originally predicted using the Bayley-Pinneau method, they did not reach target midparental height scores. Predictors of adult height

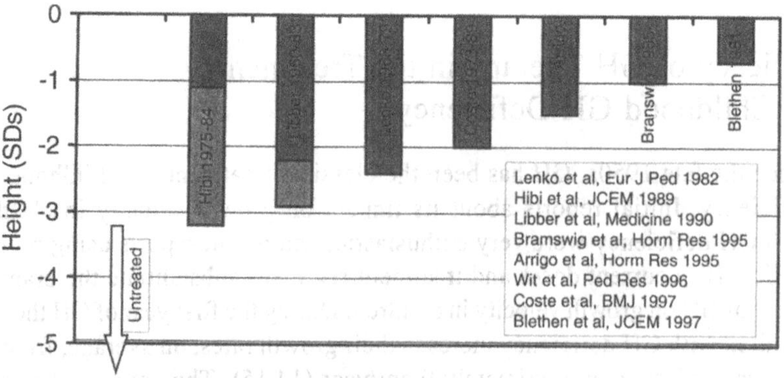

FIGURE 4.1. Effect of GH therapy for childhood GH deficiency on adult height (in SDs from the mean), as reported in seven separate studies.

included duration of GH treatment and young age at onset of treatment. Because the mean age of children at the onset of GH therapy was 10–11 years in that study, it is likely that the results still do not represent the optimal impact of GH therapy on adult height in children with GH deficiency.

Decreased bone mineral density in children with GH deficiency can be improved or normalized with GH therapy (4,5); however, young adults with GH deficiency of childhood onset, who have stopped GH therapy, demonstrate reduced bone mineral density (5), which suggests that GH may be needed for normal mineralization beyond cessation of linear growth. This is particularly important because peak bone mass (the highest level of bone mass achieved as a result of normal growth), a major factor in determining bone mass later in life), develops in late adolescence at approximately 18–20 years of age (24).

Regarding body composition, it is clear that GH therapy decreases body fat and increases muscle mass in children with GH deficiency (6,7,25). After completion of GH therapy in childhood, however, young adults exhibit increased body fat and decreased muscle mass compared with controls (26). These findings suggest that earlier treatment regimens, which often involve relatively low doses of GH and/or discontinuous therapy, were suboptimal in improving body composition or, perhaps more likely, that GH continues to be needed for metabolic functions beyond the age at which linear growth has ceased. It may also be that previously reported poor energy levels and poor quality of life in affected individuals reduce their level of physical activity, compounding abnormalities of body composition. Long-term follow-up of body composition in children treated with GH using current regimens will be needed to resolve these issues. It is interesting to note that data suggest that the effectiveness of GH therapy in modifying body composition in adults may depend, in part, on whether the GH deficiency is of childhood onset or adult onset (26).

The effectiveness of GH therapy in improving psychosocial status and quality of life is an important issue particularly in view of earlier studies that suggest lack of independence and poor outcomes (11). Stabler et al. have suggested that GH treatment may reduce overall behavior problems in children with GH deficiency (27); however, data are lacking on adult psychosocial outcomes in GH-deficient children who have received current treatment regimens.

Assessments of the efficacy of GH therapy must consider measures of risk as well as benefit. Potential side effects of GH therapy have been reviewed (28,29), but their likelihood in children with GH deficiency is not clear. Adverse effects of GH therapy include idiopathic intracranial hypertension, edema or lymph edema, carpal tunnel syndrome, diabetes mellitus, slipped capital femoral epiphysis, the growth of nevi, benign gynecomastia, acute pancreatitis, and the development of antibodies to GH. The risk of neoplasms in children treated with GH appears to be mainly a problem for those with underlying conditions that predispose to malignancy, although continuing monitoring is needed for final data due the relatively small numbers of children involved.

Innovations in Therapy for Childhood GH Deficiency

Several interesting alternatives or adjuncts to GH therapy have emerged, although much less is known about their efficacy or therapeutic potential than is known for GH treatment. In view of the burden of daily GH injections over several years, alternative GH preparations are under development (30,31). For example, Johnson et al. found that an injectable, sustained release form of GH, developed by stabilizing and encapsulating GH protein in biodegradable microcapsules, resulted in sustained elevation of serum GH, insulinlike growth factor I (IGF-I), and insulinlike growth factor binding protein 3 (IGF-BP3) for more than 1 month in nonhuman primates (30). Such approaches are in an early stage, and efficacy in humans is not known.

GH therapy has been combined with gonadotropin-releasing hormone agonists in treating children with GH deficiency and precocious puberty, and this combination appears to improve height predictions (32,33). To our knowledge there are no data on the effect of such combinations in children with isolated GH deficiency and normal onset of puberty; however, inordinate iatrogenic delay of puberty may pose intrinsic risks to psychosocial adaptation.

IGF-I has been effective in increasing growth of children with defects in the GH receptor (34,35). IGF-I also promotes growth in children with GH deficiency who have developed neutralizing antibodies to GH (35); therefore, it provides a therapeutic alternative for such children.

GH-releasing hormone (GHRH), administered daily, also significantly increases growth rates in children with GH deficiency (36), without major adverse effects.

GH-releasing peptides and related analogs, when administered orally or parenterally, have been found to stimulate GH release in normal individuals and in a proportion of children with GH deficiency (37). Children who have anatomic defects of the pituitary may be less responsive to these agents. Although GHRH may contribute to the GH secretory response to GH releasing peptides (38), the GH releasing peptides appear to act, at least in part, through distinct intracellular pathways and may promote pulsatile GH secretion. Initial studies suggest that they may be effective in promoting growth in children with GH deficiency (39), although long-term studies are currently underway and are necessary for full evaluation of efficacy.

Conclusions

Childhood GH deficiency has multidimensional morbidity. Full evaluation of the effectiveness of treatment for GH deficiency, therefore, requires short-term and long-term assessment of many variables. GH is clearly beneficial for improving growth in childhood GH deficiency. More comprehensive analyses are needed; however, as treatment aims expand beyond an increase in height. Potential innovations in therapy for GH-deficient children are emerging: Their value (and use) will likely be based on comparative analyses among treatment options.

Acknowledgments. This work was supported in part by the NIH.

References

1. Gilford H. Ateliosis: a form of dwarfism. Practitioner 1903;70:797–819.
2. Wit JM, Kamp GA, Rikken B. Spontaneous growth and response to growth hormone treatment in children with growth hormone deficiency and idiopathic short stature. Pediatr Res 1996;39:295–302.
3. Shore RM, Chesney RW, Mazess RB, Rose PG, Bargman GJ. Bone mineral status in growth hormone deficiency. J Pediatr 1980;96:393–96.
4. Zamboni G, Antoniazzi F, Radetti G, Musumeci C, Tato L. Effect of two different regimens of recombinant human growth hormone therapyon the bone mineral density of patients with growth hormone deficiency. J Pediatr 1991;119:483–85.
5. Saggese G, Baroncelli GI, Bertelloni S, Barsanti S. The effect of long-term growth hormone (GH) treatment on bone mineral density in children with GH deficiency. Role of GH in the attainment of peak bone mass. J Clin Endocrinol Metab 1996;81: 3077–83.
6. Novak LP, Hayles AB, Cloutier MD. Effect of hGH on body composition of hypopituitary dwarfs. Mayo Clin Proc 1972;47:241–46.
7. Parra A, Argote RM, Garcia G, Cervantes C, Alatorre S, Perez-Pasten E. Body composition in hypopituitary dwarfs before and during human growth hormone therapy. Metabolism 1979;28:851–57.
8. Stabler B, Siegel PT, Clopper RR. Growth hormone deficiency in children has psychological and educational co-morbidity. Clin Pediatrics 1991;3:156–60.
9. Drotar D, Owens R, Gotthold J. Personality adjustment of children and adolescents with hypopituitarism. Child Psych Hum Dev 1980;11:59–65.
10. Stabler B, Clopper RR, Seigel PT, Stoppani C, Compton PG, Underwood LE. Academic achievement and psychological adjustment in short children. J Dev Behav Pediatr 1994;15:1–6.
11. Dean HJ, McTaggart TL, Fish DG, Friesen HG. The educational, vocational, and marital status of growth hormone-deficient adults treated with growth hormone during childhood. Am J Dis Child 1985;139:1105–10.
12. Taback S, Dean HJ, and members of the Canadian growth hormone advisory committee. Mortality in Canadian children with growth hormone (GH) deficiency receiving GH therapy 1967–1992. J Clin Endocrinol Metab 1996;81:1693–96.
13. Rosen T, Bengtsson BA. Premature mortality due to cardiovascular disease in hypopituitarism. Lancet 1990;336:285–88.
14. Blethen SL, Compton P, Lippe BM, Rosenfeld RG, August GP, Johanson A. Factors predicting the response to growth hormone (GH) therapy in prepubertal children with GH deficiency. J Clin Endocrinol Metab 1993;76:574–79.

15. Ranke MB, Guilbaud O. Growth response in prepubertal children with idiopathic growth hormone deficiency during the first two years of treatment with human growth hormone. Analysis of the Kabi Pharmacia International Growth Study. Acta Paediatr Scand 1991;379(suppl):109–15.
16. MacGillivray MH, Baptista J, Johanson A, on behalf of the Genentech Study Group. Outcome of a four-year randomized study of daily versus three times weekly somatotropin treatment in prepubertal naïve growth hormone-deficient children. J Clin Endocrinol Metab 1996;81:1806–09.
17. Hibi I, Tanaka T, Tanae A, Kagawa J, Hashimoto N, Yoshizawa A, et al. The influence of gonadal function and the effect of gonadal suppression treatment on final height in growth hormone (GH)-treated GH-deficient children. J Clin Endocrinol Metab 1989;69:221–26.
18. Lenko HL, Leisti S, Perheentupa J. The efficacy of growth hormone in different types of growth failure. Eur J Pediatr 1982;138:241–49.
19. Arrigo T, DeLuca F, Bernasconi S, Bozzola M, Cavallo L, Crisafulli G, et al. Catch-up growth and height prognosis in early treated children with congenital hypopituitarism. Horm Res 1995;44(suppl):26–31.
20. Bramswig JH, Schlosser H, Kiese K. Final height in children with growth hormone deficiency. Horm Res 1995;43:126–28.
21. Libber SM, Plotnick LP, Johnason AJ, Blizzard RM, Kwiterovich PO, Migeon CJ. Long-term follow-up of hypopituitary patients treated with human growth hormone. Medicine 1990;69:46–55.
22. Coste J, Letrait M, Carel JC, Tresca JP, Chatelain P, Rochiccioli P, et al. Long-term results of growth hormone treatment in France in children of short stature: population, register based study. Br Med J 1997;315:708–13.
23. Blethen SL, Baptista J, Kuntze J, Foley T, LaFranchi S, Johanson A. On behalf of the Genentech Growth Study Group. Adult height in growth hormone (GH)-deficient children treated with biosynthetic GH. J Clin Endocrinol Metab 1997;82:418–20.
24. Saggese G, Baroncelli GI. Bone and mineral density and biochemical parameters of bone turnover in children with growth hormone deficiency. Horm Res 1996;45(suppl):67–68.
25. Bonnet F, Vanderschueren-Lodeweyckx, Eeckels R, Malvaux P. Subcutaneous adipose tissue and lipids in blood in growth hormone deficiency before and after treatment with human growth hormone. Pediatr Res. 1974;8:800–5.
26. Attanasio AF, Lamberts SWJ, Matranga AMC, Birkett MA, Bates PC, Valk NK, et al. Adult growth hormone (GH)-deficient patients demonstrate heterogeneity between childhood onset and adult onset before and during human GH treatment. J Clin Endocrinol Metab 1997;82:82–88.
27. Stabler B, Clopper RR, Nicholas LM, Silva SG, Tancer ME, Underwood LE. Links between growth hormone deficiency, adaptation and social phobia. Horm Res 1996;45:30–33.
28. Blethen SL, Allen DB, Graves D, August G, Moshang T, Rosenfeld R. Safety of recombinant deoxyribonucleic acid-derived growth hormone: the National Cooperative Growth Study Experience. J Clin Endocrinol Metab 1996;81:1704–10.
29. Malazowski S, Hung W, Scott DC. Acute pancreatitis associated with growth hormone therapy for short stature. N Engl J Med 1995;332:401–2.
30. Johnson OFL, Cleland JL, Lee HJ, Charnis M, Duenas E, et al. A month-long effect from a single injection of microencapsulated human growth hormone. Nat Med 1996;2:795–99.

31. Leone-Bay A, Ho K-K, Agarwal R, Baughman RA, Chaudhary K, Demorin F, et al. 4-[4-[(2-Hydroxybenzoyl)amino]phenyl]butyric acid as a novel oral delivery agent for recombinant human growth hormone. J Med Chem 1996;39:2571–78.
32. Cara JF, Kreiter ML, Rosenfield RL. Height prognosis of children with true precocious puberty and growth hormone deficiency: Effect of combination therapy with gonadotropin releasing hormone agonist and growth hormone. J Pediatr 1992;120:709–15.
33. Adan L, Souberielle JC, Zucker JM, Pierre-Kahn A, Kalifa C, Brauner R. Adult height in 24 patients treated for growth hormone deficiency and early puberty. J Clin Endocrinol Metab 1997; 82:229–33.
34. Guevara-Aguirre J, Vasconez O, Martinez V, Martinez AL, Rosenbloom AL, Diamond FB, et al. Randomized, double blind, placebo-controlled trial on safety and efficacy of recombinant human insulin-like growth factor-1 in children with growth hormone receptor deficiency. J Clin Endocrinol Metab 1995;80:1393–98.
35. Backeljauw PF, Underwood LE, and the GHIS collaborative group. J Clin Endocrinol Metab 1996;81:3312–17.
36. Thorner M, Rochiccioli P, Colle R, Lanes R, Grunt J, Galazka A, et al. Once daily subcutaneous growth hormone-releasing hormone therapy accelerates growth in growth hormone-deficient children during the first year of therapy. J Clin Endocrinol Metab 1996;81:1189–96.
37. Loche S, Cambiaso P, Merola B, Colao A, Faedda A, Imbibo BP. The effect of hexarelin on growth hormone (GH) secretion in patients with GH deficiency. J Clin Endocrinol Metab 1995;80:2692–96.
38. Bercu BB, Yang SW, Masuda R, Walker RF. Role of selected endogenous peptides in growth hormone-releasing hexapeptide activity: analysis of growth hormone-releasing hormone, thyroid hormone-releasing hormone, and gonadotropin-releasing hormone. Endocrinology 1992;130:2579–86.
39. Mericq F, Cassorla F, Slazar T, Avila A, Iniguez G, Bowers CY, et al. Increased growth velocity during prolonged GHRP-2 administration to growth hormone deficient children. Presented at the 1997 meeting of the Endocrine Society (OR30-3) (Abstract).

5

Quality of Life Among Adults with Childhood Onset Growth Hormone Deficiency: A Comparison with Siblings

David E. Sandberg, Margaret H. MacGillivray, Richard R. Clopper, Dana E. Alliger, Caroline Fung, and Linda LeRoux

Introduction

The endocrine management of growth failure and short stature has changed dramatically since the introduction of biosynthetic growth hormone (GH). To date, however, there are no published studies concerning the behavioral outcomes of individuals who had been treated entirely within the new era of biosynthetic GH therapy. Insofar as improvements in the treatment regimen have resulted in better growth and adult height outcomes (1), there is good reason to speculate that the psychosocial adjustment of individuals treated entirely in this new era will also be superior to that of patients who were treated when supplies of GH were limited. This belief is so pervasive that it has contributed to the expanded prescribing of GH to non–GH-deficient patient groups with short stature (2,3). Until behavioral outcome studies of these newer cohorts are completed, there remains much to be learned from the experiences and quality of life (QOL) outcomes of patients, now young adults or older, who have completed treatment, regardless of treatment era.

Nine studies conducted between 1985 and 1995 have focused on the psychosocial adaptation of formerly treated patients with child-onset GH deficiency (GHD) (4–12). Studies of GH replacement in adult GHD patients were not included. The nine studies vary markedly in terms of sample sizes, the final adult height achieved, and the research design and data analyses used to assess QOL outcomes. Quality of life is a multidimensional construct that includes, but is not limited to, the social, physical, and emotional functioning of the individual (13). Most studies of former GH-treated patients have included an assessment of educational attainment, employment and marital status, and living situation. A review of these studies is presented elsewhere (14).

Several problems exist in this follow-up literature that make it difficult to interpret the findings. First, selection criteria for subject eligibility are not always explicitly stated and vary across studies. Previous studies have also commonly relied upon a postal survey methodology that provides little control over the circumstances under which (and by whom) forms are completed. An alternative would be telephone interviews that have been shown to be equivalent to in-person interviews in terms of reliability, validity, and response rates (15,16).

Given the amount of attention directed in the endocrine management of individuals with GHD toward improving growth velocity and optimizing adult height, it is surprising that only three of the nine cited QOL follow-up studies assessed the relationship between final height and psychosocial outcomes (4,6,9), and then for only selected dependent variables. Finally, the aforementioned studies provide a broad mixture of control and comparison groups against which the psychosocial adaptation of the GHD samples are evaluated. In some studies, and for some measures, no comparisons to physically healthy control subjects are provided; thus, the results are of a totally descriptive nature (e.g., 11). In other cases, "population" norms are invoked for an estimation of expected demographic parameters within the GHD sample without adjusting for differences in potentially influential background differences between the clinic-based sample and the general population (e.g., 5). Along the same lines, questionnaire norms are adopted for comparison purposes with little consideration given to the suitability of such norms (e.g., 12). Although an attractive alternative to "norms," the potential methodological benefits of utilizing a healthy sibling control group has not been maximized in previous studies because same- and opposite-sex siblings are lumped together and given without consideration to potential age differences between probands and siblings (6,9,11). Data regarding siblings are also based upon proxy reporting by GHD patients or parents (6,9,11). In the case of comparisons between subgroups of GHD patients, analyses do not adjust for potential background differences (e.g., age, gender, SES) that could influence the results.

The present study revisits the question of the adult psychosocial adjustment of formerly treated, child-onset, GHD individuals, but it does so in a relatively large and endocrinologically well-defined GHD sample. Telephone administration of psychometrically robust questionnaires is introduced as a methodological innovation in order to enhance both the reliability and validity of the data collected. In addition to comparisons with published norms for the selected questionnaires, this study is the first directly to contrast the adaptive functioning of GHD patients to unaffected, same-sex siblings. The study also addressed the relationship between adult height, patient diagnosis, and QOL. Finally, case-sibling comparisons for the two eras of GH therapy—pituitary GH (pGH) and recombinant human GH (rGH)—will be presented.

Subjects and Methods

Target Subjects

The potentially eligible sample ($N = 212$) comprised all formerly treated GHD patients from one endocrinology program at a regional pediatric hospital in a moderate-size city in the northeastern United States who were 18 years or older at the start of this follow-up study (November 30, 1993). All patients had exhibited a peak GH response to two standard provocative GH stimulation tests of less than 10 ng/ml (polyclonal antibody) prior to initiating therapy. The presence of mental retardation (IQ £ 70 on standardized testing) or a chronic physical disability/disease (e.g., blindness, insulin-dependent diabetes mellitus) served as exclusion criteria ($N = 17$). An additional 10 cases were deceased at the time of the follow-up. Forty-five cases (24.3%) were either lost to follow-up, did not respond to repeated requests by mail to participate, or refused. A total of 140 former patients (75.7%; 117 male, 23 female) participated. The mean age at follow-up was 26.1 (± 6.5) years (18.8–46.9 years). Sixty-five percent of the GHD families of origin fell within social strata I (major business and professional) and II (medium business, minor professional, technical) (17). Some 42.8% of the GHD sample completed GHD therapy prior to 1985 (i.e., pGH era). The treatment for 22.9% spanned both the pGH and rGH eras. Finally, 34.3% started and completed their GH therapy during the rGH era of treatment. Patients whose treatment spanned the two eras were recoded for purposes of particular data analyses as being treated in the pGH era if they received pGH for 68.9% or more of their time on GH. All others were recoded as receiving treatment in the rGH era. After the recoding, 67 (47.9%) and 73 (52.1%) patients were classified as having received treatment in the pGH and rGH eras, respectively. Eighty-four percent of the patients in each of these groups were male. The mean age of pGH patients was 31.0 (± 6.0) years (20.9–46.9 years). rGH patients had a mean age of 21.5 (± 2.2) years (18.8–26.8 years). Patients treated in the pGH era were significantly older ($p < .001$) than those treated in the rGH era. Final height was ascertained by one of two methods: (1) excerpts from the patient's endocrine chart at that visit when growth velocity was less than 2cm/yr and bone age exceeded 16 yrs for boys or 14 yrs for girls; or (2) height was measured during the period of the follow-up study either in the endocrine clinic or in the office of the subject's primary physician. Selected diagnostic and treatment-related anthropometric variables are summarized in Table 5.1.

TABLE 5.1. Selective diagnostic and anthropometric variables for total GHD sample and subset of patients with a same-sex sibling participating in study.

Variable	Total GHD sample			
	Total (N = 140)	pGH (N = 67)	rGH (N = 73)	GHD with sibling (N = 53)
Isolated GHD (vs. MPHD) (%)[†]	67.9%	53.7%***	80.8%	58.5%
Idiopathic GHD (vs. Organic) (%)	87.1%	85.1%	89.0%	83.0%
Age at start of GH therapy (years)				
Mean (SD)	12.3 (3.4)	11.6 (3.5)*	13.0 (3.1)	12.2 (3/5)
Range	2.6–18.1	2.6–18.1	3.3–17.2	2.6–18.1
Height at start of GH therapy (SD)				
Mean (SD)	−3.1 (1.2)	−3.6 (1.3)***	−2.7 (0.8)	−3.2 SD (1.3)
Range	−7.2 to −0.5	−7.3 to −1.2	−6.4 to −0.5	−7.2 to −0.5
Duration of GH therapy (years)				
Mean (SD)	4.5 (3.1)	5.1 (3.4)*	3.9 (2.7)	4.5 (3.3)
Range	0.9 to 4.3	1.0 to 14.3	0.9 to 13.9	0.9 to 14.3
Final height (SD)				
Mean (SD)	−1.5 (1.0)[2]	−1.7 (1.0)*[3]	−1.3 (1.0)[4]	−1.5 (1.0)[5]
Range	−4.7 to −0.8	−4.7 to −0.8	−3.5 to −0.4	−4.7 to −0.1
Change in Height Over Rx (SD)				
Mean (SD)	1.6 (1.2)[2]	1.8(1.5)*	1.3 (0.9)	1.7 (1.3)[3]
Range	−2.0 to −6.0	−1.0 to −6.0	−2.0 to −4.4	−2.0 to −5.1

[†]Abbreviations: IGHD = isolated growth hormone deficiency; MPHD = multiple pituitary hormone deficiency; pGH = pituitary era; rGH = recombinant human GH era; [2] N = 132; [3] N = 63; [4] N = 69; [5] N = 51.

* Statistically significant ($p < .05$); **($p < .01$); ***($p < .001$).

Control Subjects

Sixty-three GHD subjects had an unaffected, same-sex sibling 18 years or older; 53 siblings (84%) agreed to participate. The mean age at follow-up was 29.7 (± 7.6) years (18.4–52.9 years). The GHD patients were significantly younger: 27.9 ± 6.8, 19.0–45.5 years, paired t, $p < .01$.41 (77%) of the GHD-sibling pairs were male. 34 pGH and 19 rGH era patients had siblings take part in the study.

Study Protocol

The study was conducted in several steps. First, a letter describing the study was mailed to all eligible GHD subjects by the study coordinator. Those agreeing to participate were subsequently mailed several color-coded, questionnaire-specific, response keys to facilitate the completion of questionnaires over the telephone. An interview appointment, lasting approximately 45 minutes, was then scheduled and performed by an interviewer who was blind to the medical history of the subject. After completion of the interview, the study coordinator requested permission of GHD subjects to contact their same-sex siblings. The letter to siblings stated that the investigators were conducting a study of former patients who had received GH therapy as well as their siblings who were not treated. It was not stated in the letter to siblings that they were included in order to serve as "control" subjects for their GHD brothers/sisters. This strategy was adopted to reduce the likelihood that siblings would bias their reports in the direction of positive psychological adjustment in concordance with them being labeled "control" subjects by the investigators (18). Contact letters to all subjects (and a reminder at the outset of the interview) requested that they not disclose to the interviewer any aspects of their medical background unless requested so that data collection would less likely be biased. This instruction was only partially successful: 77.9% and 86.8% of the interviews with GHD subjects and siblings, respectively, were conducted blindly. Participating subjects received a $25 honorarium.

SF-36 Health Survey

The SF-36 is a generic QOL measure assessing eight health concepts relevant to functional status and well-being (19). The psychometric properties of the SF-36 have been extensively documented and demonstrate it to be both reliable and valid in a range of medical and physically healthy populations. Age- and gender-specific norms are available for a sample of the general U.S. population.

Social Relationship Scale (SRS)

This SRS (20) was developed to assess both the structures and processes of social relationships. Five social support constructs were assessed: perceived availability of support, validation, conflict, objective social integration, and subjective social integration. Chronbach alphas (a measure of internal consistency of items within a scale) ranged from .78 to .89. Norms for the general population are not available.

Social Adjustment Scale-Self Report (SAS-SR)

The SAS-SR (21) measures either instrumental or expressive role performance in six major areas of functioning. The internal consistency (mean Chronbach alpha = .74) and test–retest stability (mean coefficient of .80) of the SAS-SR demonstrate its reliability, and its ability to differentiate between psychiatric patient and nonpatient groups provides evidence of its discriminant validity (22). In order to make SAS-SR items applicable to the majority of subjects in the present study, and also to reduce the overlap in content between the SAS-SR and SRS (see earlier), only the items (13 in total) from the following role areas were assessed: work as a student, and social and leisure. The latter scale includes two items regarding frequency of and interest in romantic dating, which, in the present study, were broken out for data analysis. Questionnaire norms were not used because only a limited set of SAS-SR items were incorporated in the present protocol.

Brief Symptom Inventory

The Brief Symptom Inventory (BSI) (23) is a self-report symptom inventory assessing the psychological symptom patterns of psychiatric and medical patients as well as community nonpatient respondents. The scoring of the BSI generates nine primary symptom dimensions and three global indexes of distress. Chronbach alpha coefficients are very good, ranging from .71 to .85. Test-retest coefficients over a 2-week interval were comparably high (.68–.91). Strong discriminant and convergent validity for the BSI has also been demonstrated.

Results*

Educational Attainment, Employment and Marital Status, and Current Living Arrangements

GHD Versus Same-Sex Siblings

Restricting the data analysis to those GHD and sibling pairs not currently attending school ($N = 30$), GHD subjects did not differ in their level of educational attainment from sibling control subjects (paired *t*-test; $p > .05$). The mean level of education attained for both groups was approximately equivalent to partial completion of a college degree (or specialized training). There was also no difference in the proportion of cases (91.9%) and control subjects (95.5%) who were gainfully employed at the time of the study (χ^2 with Yates' correction). A comparable proportion of GHD subjects (67.9%) and siblings (77.4%) were living independently from their parents and relatives ($p > .383$). In contrast, a higher proportion of siblings (50.9%) than GHD subjects (26.4%) were married at the time of the study ($p < .05$). Because the same-sex siblings were significantly older than the GHD cases at the time of the study, supplementary multiple (or logistic) regression analyses were conducted in which subject's age was controlled. Because these secondary analyses did not uncover results at variance with those of the χ^2 or paired *t*-tests, they will not be discussed further.

*A complete set of data-analytic tables are available from the authors upon request.

Isolated GHD (IGHD) Versus Multiple Pituitary Hormone Deficiency (MPHD)

Hierarchical (or logistic) regression analyses, statistically controlling for differences between the subgroups in subject's age and duration of GH therapy, did not reveal significant differences in mean educational attainment (IGHD: 4.9 ± 1.0, $N = 58$ vs. MPHD: 5.0 ± 0.9, $N = 34$), percent employed (IGHD = 91.4% and MPHD = 79.4%), married (IGHD = 15.8% and MPHD = 28.9%), or living independently (IGHD = 56.8% and MPHD = 51.1%).

Health-Related Quality of Life

Transformed SF-36 scores, where the lowest and highest possible scores on each scale are converted to zero and 100, respectively, were used in all data analyses. Scores between these values represent the percentage of total possible score achieved (19).

GHD Versus Same-Sex Siblings

The GHD sample differed significantly from the sibling control group on only one of eight QOL scales: GHD cases scored more negatively than control subjects (72.8 ± 21.4 vs. 80.7 ± 20.3) on the General Health scale (paired *t*-test; $p < .05$). General Health assesses perceptions of current health, resistance to illness, and health outlook.

GHD Versus Questionnaire Norms

The total sample of GHD cases (those with and without a same-sex sibling in the study) was compared by *t*-test to population norms for the SF-36 Health Survey. In order to calculate relative effect sizes for the differences between the GHD and normative samples, we used the measure *d* (24), which estimates how far apart the means for samples are in terms of standard deviation (SD) units. For instance, a *d* of .50 would mean that the means were .5 SD apart. Norms for the SF-36 are reported separately for each gender and by age group. Because the number of female GHD subjects falling into any one age range was too small for statistical analysis, comparisons to norms on this instrument are restricted to males. Compared with the normative sample of males, ages 18–44 years (weighted means were calculated for the age groupings 18–24, 25–34, and 35–44 years, $N = 509$), the male GHD sample ($N = 115$) scored higher (indicating *better* functioning) on the *Bodily Pain* (86.9 ± 19.8 vs. 80.9 ± 20.1; $d = .30$) and *Emotional Role* (93.6 ± 18.3 vs. 84.5 ± 29.5; $d = .31$) scales (both $p < .01$). *Bodily Pain* assesses the intensity of bodily pain experienced in the past 4 weeks and the extent to which pain interferes with normal work. *Emotional Role* assesses problems with work or other daily activities as a result of emotional problems.

IGHD Versus MPHD

Hierarchical multiple regression analyses controlling for subject's age and social class revealed that the MPHD subgroup received significantly lower scores (i.e., indicating poorer functioning) on five of eight scales (*Physical Functioning*, 89.2 ± 14.9 vs. 97.2 ± 6.7, R^2 change = .078, $p < .001$; *General Health*, 70.0 ± 18.6 vs. 80.9 ± 18.4, R^2 change = .053, $p < .01$; *Emotional Role*, 85.0 ± 27.2 vs. 94.7 ± 17.8, R^2 change = .051, $p < .01$; *Social Functioning*, 84.3 ± 19.8 vs. 91.9 ± 16.5, R^2 change = .038, $p < .05$; and *Mental Health*, 72.9 ± 18.5 vs. 78.4 ± 14.9, R^2 change = .028, $p < .05$). *Physical Functioning* assesses limitations in performing physical activities due to health problems; the influence of either physical health or emotional problems upon the quantity and quality of social activities is rated on the *Social Functioning* scale; and *Mental Health* incorporates items concerned with depression, anxiety, and psychological well-being.

Social Adjustment

GHD Versus Same-Sex Siblings

Statistically significant differences were not detected between the GHD-sibling pairs on any of the five SRS scales. The same was true for the *Social and Leisure* scale of the SAS-SR, including the items assessing romantic dating. A comparison of GHD patients and siblings on the *Work as Student* scale of the SAS-SR was precluded because there were no pairs in which both the case and control were attending school at the time of study.

IGHD Versus MPHD

With the exception of the *Subjective Integration* scale of the SRS, significant differences between the IGHD and MPHD subgroups (controlling for subject's age and social class) were not detected. IGHD patients expressed feeling more a part of a group of friends than did those with MPHD (28.6 ± 4.6 vs. 26.0 ± 4.4, R^2 change = .045, $p < .01$). Differences in the same direction were observed on the *Social and Leisure* scale (1.8 ± 0.5 vs. 2.1 ± 0.6, R^2 change = .059, $p < .01$) and the two combined dating items (IGHD: 1.9 ± 0.9, $N = 74$ vs. MPHD: 2.9 ± 1.4, $N = 30$, R^2 change =.142, $p < .001$) of the SAS-SR.

Emotional Distress

GHD Versus Same-Sex Siblings

GHD subjects were not statistically distinguishable on any of the nine primary symptom dimensions or three global indexes of distress.

GHD Versus Questionnaire Norms

Comparisons to gender-specific norms were performed for both males and females (BSI norms are not broken down by age group). In marked contrast to the GHD-sibling comparisons, both the male and female GHD patients (those with and without siblings combined) reported significantly more distress than gender-specific nonclinical norms. The male GHD patients scored higher than did norms on eight of nine primary symptom dimensions and on two global indexes of distress. The effect sizes of the significant differences ranged from .28 (phobic anxiety) to .78 SD units (paranoid ideation) (mean $d = .62$). According to the recommended definition of (psychiatric) caseness (23), 23.9% of the male GHD sample would be classified as "cases" based upon the *Global Severity Index* score and 40.2% according to the method utilizing primary dimension scores. The GHD females received significantly higher symptom scores on five of nine symptom dimensions and the same two of three global indexes of distress as the males. The effect sizes of the significant differences ranged from .56 (obsessive-compulsive) to 1.14 SD units (interpersonal sensitivity) (mean $d = .85$). These relatively large effect sizes are reflected in the numbers of subjects classified as "cases": 30.4% and 52.2%, according to the *Global Severity Index* and elevated primary dimensions schemes, respectively.

IGHD Versus MPHD

Controlling for subject's age and social class, MPHD patients scored higher than those with IGHD on only one primary symptom dimension scale, *Somatization* (0.4 ± 0.4 vs. 0.2 ± 0.3, R^2 change = .034, $p < .05$). The *Somatization* dimension reflects distress from perceptions of bodily dysfunction.

Relationship Between Anthropometric/Treatment Variables and Outcome Variables

Patient's adult height and growth response to GH therapy (as measured by change in relative height [SD units] from the start of treatment until adult height was achieved) were regressed on all psychosocial variables in separate hierarchical multiple (or logistic) regression analyses. The potential confounding influences of subject's age, family of origin's socioeconomic status, subject's diagnosis (IGHD vs. MPHD), and whether or not the subject had a same-sex sibling ≥18 years†, were statistically controlled by entering these variables into the regression model first, followed either by the variable *final height* or *growth response to GH therapy*. Subjects' change in relative height was not a statistically significant predictor for any of the psychosocial outcome variables. The same was true for the relationship between adult height and educational attainment, marital status, whether or not the GHD patient was living indepen-

†GHD patients with same-sex siblings ≥ 18 years exhibited poorer psychosocial adaptation on several outcome variables.

dently or was gainfully employed, and scale scores on the SF-36 and BSI. A taller adult height was predictive, however, of higher (better) scores on the *subjective integration* scale of the SRS (R^2 change = .028, $p < .05$). This scale assesses perceptions of feeling part of a group of friends. Taller patients similarly scored higher on the *social and leisure* scale of the SAS-SR (R^2 change = .032, $p < .05$), but there was no effect seen on the two dating items.

pGH Versus rGH Eras of GH Therapy

Comparisons between subjects from the two eras were restricted to those involving cases versus same-sex siblings. A direct comparison of the GHD subgroups was considered inappropriate because of the substantial differences between the two in age, diagnostic, and GH treatment outcomes (Table 5.1) that could potentially confound interpretation of the analyses. The patient subgroups were not significantly different from their respective siblings in terms of educational attainment (pGH: 5.2 ± 0.8 vs. 5.4 ± 1.0 and rGH: 4.6 ± 0.8 vs. 4.8 ± 1.2), the proportions that were married (after statistically controlling for age differences by logistic regression) (pGH: 32.4% vs. 55.9% and rGH: 15.8% vs. 42.1%), living independently (pGH: 82.4% vs. 85.3% and rGH: 42.1% vs. 63.2%), or who were gainfully employed (pGH: 96.3%, $N = 27$ vs. 100.0%, $N = 30$) and rGH: 80.0%, $N = 10$ vs. 85.7%, $N = 14$). In addition, neither paired t-tests nor multiple regression analyses controlling for subject's age revealed statistically significant differences on any of the eight health-related QOL (SF-36) or social adjustment scales (SRS and SAS-SR). Finally, on the multiscale measure of emotional distress (BSI), only one significant difference emerged in comparisons between former patients and their siblings: Patients from the pGH era received significantly higher distress scores on the *phobic anxiety* scale (55.0 ± 9.3 vs. 50.5 ± 6.8, paired t-test; $p < .05$).

Discussion

Replicating earlier reports (5–9,11), the educational attainment of GHD patients in this study appears to be unaffected by clinical status. This observation is particularly noteworthy in view of findings from other studies that indicate that subgroups of GHD patients exhibit lower IQ scores (8,25) and/or cognitive deficits (26–27). These latter effects might be related to the observation that GHD patients are at risk for experiencing academic underachievement and grade retention (for review, see 28). The apparent discrepancy between the different sets of findings might be understood as indicating that GHD is a better predictor of academic achievement during the early years of schooling than it is of the *ultimate* level of educational attainment. A comparison between GHD cases and sibling controls also did not reveal differences in the proportions of each group who were gainfully employed at the time of the study, or who were living independently from parents or other relatives. In the case of marriage, however, a significantly lower proportion of GHD cases than siblings were married. Scores on social support and adjustment measures, however, did not differentiate GHD cases from sibling control subjects. Further research is needed to explain why, in this and several other studies, marriage rates for GHD patients are lower than expected despite apparent similarities between GHD and non-GHD cases on several other indexes of psychosocial adjustment.

When GHD cases were compared with general population norms for the SF-36 Health Survey, a health-related QOL measure, an unexpected finding emerged: Former patients scored higher (indicating better functioning) on two of eight scales, without any significant differences in the opposite direction. In contrast, a comparison of GHD cases with norms for the BSI, a measure of psychological distress, revealed much higher symptom rates within the patient group. A more consistent and interpretable picture developed from comparisons between GHD cases and same-sex siblings. In the case of both the SF-36 and BSI, there were very limited differences between the groups. The one statistically significant difference that did emerge was predictable and relatively easy to understand: The GHD cases reported more problems than did the siblings on the *general health* scale of the SF-36. These findings suggest that the choice of control or comparison groups in studies of GHD patients can have profound effects on the results and thus the conclusions drawn from the study. We favor those comparisons utilizing same-sex siblings because of the greater ability to control for genetic and social-environmental factors within individual families, which could influence the psychosocial adaptation as assessed by the questionnaires used in this study.

IGHD and MPHD patients could not be differentiated based upon educational attainment, percentage employed, or marital or living status. Similar findings have been reported in some studies (5–7,9), but not in another (4). Similarities between these GHD patient subgroups were not uniform when they were compared on the SF-36, social support and adjustment, and BSI scales. In all domains, the IGHD patients described themselves as higher functioning than did patients with MPHD. The effect sizes of the group differences on five of eight SF-36 scales, although statistically significant, were relatively small (between 2.8% for *mental health* and 7.8% of the variance for *physical functioning*). The IGHD group also reported more positive self-perceptions regarding their integration within a network of peers and involvement in spare-time activities (SRS and SAS-SR questionnaires). These findings contrast with those of Björk and colleagues (12), who did not detect differences between these subgroups on similar measures, although their sample size was substantially smaller ($N = 23$) than seen in this study. In the area of emotional distress, as assessed by the BSI, the MPHD subgroup reported more distress than did those with IGHD on only one scale, *somatiza-*

tion. This difference should be interpreted cautiously. The *somatization* scale is designed to assess distress arising from perceptions of bodily dysfunction in generally healthy individuals. The higher scores among the MPHD than IGHD patients may reflect true differences in somatic symptoms attributable to the patient's clinical status rather than a tendency to somatize psychological difficulties. One potential explanation for the differences between the IGHD and MPHD subgroups involves compliance with recommended hormone replacement. One of the telephone interview items concerned self-ratings of compliance. Statistically significant correlations between these self-ratings and scores on the outcome variables were not detected. In view of the common observation that adherence to medical regimens is typically far from perfect (29), future studies ideally will include laboratory assessments to verify patients' self reports.

One of the goals of GH therapy for GHD is to allow the child to achieve his/her full genetic growth potential. Furthermore, it is often assumed that increases in growth velocity and adult height will translate into enhanced QOL (3). It is thus surprising that only a minority of studies of formerly treated GHD patients have directly assessed the relationship between adult height or magnitude of catch-up growth over the course of therapy and QOL outcomes in adulthood (4,6,9). Findings from these analyses do not support the presence of a statistically significant relationship between adult height and psychosocial adjustment. The present study generally confirms this finding in a relatively large and complete sample of GHD patients. Although final height (but not change in relative height over the course of therapy) was related to a limited set of variables, the effect sizes were rather small (between 2 and 3% of the variance in outcome scores). This was the case despite the very wide range in adult heights (from –4.7SD to +0.8SD) and changes in relative height with treatment (–2.0SD to +6.0SD). It would thus appear that maximizing adult height outcomes does not automatically translate into improved QOL outcomes. This statement should not be interpreted as suggesting that GH treatment was ineffective in enhancing patients' QOL as adults. In order to make such a statement, one would need to compare treated and *untreated* GHD patients after a similar follow-up, an option that is both unrealistic as well as unethical. On the other hand, the observation that GH-induced increases in relative height are not associated with improved psychosocial adjustment may be relevant to the ongoing debate regarding the benefits of providing GH to patient groups who do not exhibit clear evidence of a GHD state (1,2). The present findings are discouraging of the expectation that improvements in psychosocial adjustment will track increases in the individual's relative height.

Finally, GHD patients from both the pGH and rGH eras of GH therapy were both largely indistinguishable from their respective sibling control groups. The sole exception was on the *phobic anxiety* scale of the BSI, where patients from the pGH era received higher (i.e., more symptomatic scores). This finding is similar to a report that social anxiety is frequently observed among GHD patients and that this effect is not attributable to short stature (30).

In conclusion, it appears that adult GHD patients are functioning better than one would have expected based upon findings from other studies using different control or comparison groups. This observation is relevant to the controversy regarding the risks and benefits of maintaining GHD patients on GH therapy beyond the point of skeletal maturation. A cautionary note regarding the QOL of adults with GHD is in order: The GHD of all patients in this study was of *childhood onset*. One report indicates that individuals with GHD of *adult onset* are more severely impacted by their clinical status, both psychologically and metabolically. They may in turn benefit from replacement of GH in adulthood to a greater degree than individuals with childhood onset GHD (31).

Acknowledgments. We wish to thank the patients and siblings who participated in the study. This research was supported in part by grant from the Genentech Foundation for Growth and Development, Inc. Portions of this work were presented at the Fifth Joint Meeting of the European Society for Pædiatric Endocrinology and the Lawson Wilkins Pediatric Endocrine Society, June 22–26, 1997, Stockholm, Sweden.

References

1. Allen DB, Johanson AJ, Blizzard RM. Growth hormone treatment. In: Lifshitz F, editor. Pediatric endocrinology, 3rd ed. New York: Marcel Dekker, 1996:61–81.
2. Allen DB, Fost NC. Growth hormone for short stature: panacea or Pandora's box? J Pediatr 1990;117:16–21.
3. Cuttler L, Silvers JB, Singh J, et al. Short stature and growth hormone therapy: a national study of physician recommendation patterns. JAMA 1996;276:531–37.
4. Takano K, Tanaka T, Saito T, and the Committee for the Study Group of Adult GH Deficiency. Psychosocial adjustment in a large cohort of adults with growth hormone deficiency treated with growth hormone in childhood: summary of a questionnaire survey. Acta Pædiatr 1994;399(suppl):16–19.
5. Clopper RR, MacGillivray MH, Mazur T, Voorhess ML, Mills BJ. Post-treatment follow-up of growth hormone deficient patients: psychosocial status. In: Stabler B, Underwood LE, eds. Slow grows the child: psychosocial aspects of growth delay. Hillsdale, NJ: Lawrence Erlbaum Associates, 1986:83–96.
6. Sartorio A, Peri G, Molinari E, Grugni G, Morabito F, Faglia G. The psychosocial outcome of adults with growth hormone deficiency. Acta Med Auxol 1986; 18:123–28.
7. Rikken B, van Busschbach J, le Cessie S, et al. Impaired social status of growth hormone deficient adults as compared to controls with short or normal stature. Clin Endocrinol 1995;43:205–11.
8. Galatzer A, Aran O, Beit-Halachmi N, et al. The impact of long-term therapy by a multidisciplinary team on the education, occupation and marital status of growth

hormone deficient patients after termination of therapy. Clin Endocrinol 1987; 27:191–96.
9. Dean HJ, McTaggart TL, Fish DG, Friesen HG. The educational, vocational, and marital status of growth hormone-deficient adults treated with growth hormone during childhood. Am J Dis Child 1985;139:1105–10.
10. Frisch H, Häusler G, Lindenbauer S, Singer S. Psychological aspects in children and adolescents with hypopituitarism. Acta Pædiatr Scand 1990;79:644–51.
11. Mitchell CM, Joyce S, Johanson AJ, et al. A retrospective evaluation of psychosocial impact of long-term growth hormone therapy. Clin Pediat 1986;25:17–23.
12. Björk S, Jönsson B, Westphal O, Levi J-E. Quality of life of adults with growth hormone deficiency: a controlled study. Acta Pædiatr Scand 1989;356(suppl): 55–59.
13. Gill TM, Feinstein AR. A critical appraisal of the quality-of-life. JAMA 1994; 272:619–26.
14. Sandberg DE, MacGillivray MH, Clopper RR, Fung C, LeRoux L, Alliger DE. Quality of life among formerly treated childhood-onset growth hormone-deficient adults: a comparison with unaffected siblings. J Clin Endocrinol Metab 1998; 83:1134–42.
15. Bauman LJ. Collecting data by telephone interviewing. J Develop Behav Pediat 1993;14:256–57.
16. Wells KB, Burnam MA, Leake B, Robins LN. Agreement between face-to-face and telephone-administered versions of the depression section of the NIMH Diagnostic Interview Schedule. J Psychiat Res 1988;22:207–20.
17. Hollingshead AB. Four factor index of social status. Unpublished manuscript, New Haven, CT: Department of Sociology, Yale University, 1975.
18. Kazdin AE. Research design in clinical psychology, 2nd ed. Boston: Allyn and Bacon, 1992.
19. Ware JE, Snow KK, Kosinski M, Gandek B. SF-36 health survey. Manual and interpretation guide. Boston: The Health Institute, New England Medical Center; 1993.
20. O'Brien K, Wortman CB, Kessler RC, Joseph JG. Social relationships of men at risk for AIDS. Soc Sci Med 1993;36:1161–67.
21. Weissman MM, Bothwell S. Assessment of social adjustment by patient self-report. Arch Gen Psychiatr 1976;33:1111–15.
22. Weissman MM, Prusoff BA, Thompson WD, Harding PS, Myers JK. Social adjustment by self-report in a community sample and in psychiatric outpatients. J Nerv Ment Dis 1978;166:317–26.
23. Derogatis LR. Brief symptom inventory. Administration, scoring, and procedures manual, 3rd ed. Minneapolis: National Computer Systems, 1993.
24. Glass GV, McGaw B, Smith ML. Meta-analysis in social research. Beverly Hills, CA: Sage, 1981.
25. Meyer-Bahlburg HFL, Feinman JA, MacGillivray MH, Aceto T, Jr. Growth hormone deficiency, brain development, and intelligence. Am J Dis Child 1978; 132:565–72.
26. Siegel PT, Hopwood NJ. The relationship of academic achievement and the intellectual functioning and affective conditions of hypopituitary children. In: Stabler B, Underwood LE, eds. Slow grows the child: psychosocial aspects of growth delay. Hillsdale, NJ: Lawrence Erlbaum Associates, 1986:57–71.

27. Deijen JB, de Boer H, Blok GJ, van der Veen EA. Cognitive impairments and mood disturbances in growth hormone deficient men. Psychoneuroendocrinology 1996;21:313–22.
28. Sandberg DE. Short stature: intellectual and behavioral aspects. In: Lifshitz F, ed. Pediatric endocrinology, 3rd ed. New York: Marcel Dekker, 1996:149–62.
29. Meichenbaum D, Turk DC. Facilitating treatment adherence. A practitioner's guide. New York: Plenum Press, 1987.
30. Nicholas LM, Tancer ME, Silva SG, Underwood LE, Stabler B. Short stature, growth hormone deficiency, and social anxiety. Psychosom Med 1997;59:372–75.
31. Attanasio AF, Lamberts SWJ, Matranga AMC, et al. Adult growth hormone (GH)-deficient patients demonstrate heterogeneity between childhood onset and adult onset before and during human GH treatment. J Clin Endocrinol Metab 1997;82:82–88.

6

Quality of Life in Adults with Growth Hormone Deficiency Diagnosed During Childhood

An Invited Contribution

Ana Claudia Keselman, Alicia Susana Martínez, Liliana Pantano, César Bergadá, and Juan Jorge Heinrich

Introduction

The aim of treatment of hypopituitary children is the achievement of final adult height as near to normal ranges as possible, correct signs and symptoms due to other hormone deficiencies, and increase the sense of well-being. In this way, a satisfactory physical, psychological, and social adjustment is anticipated. A good physical outcome has been reported by many authors, but poor psychosocial adaptation is not yet resolved. The aim of this study was to evaluate the degree of social integration of a group of adult hypopituitary patients diagnosed and treated during childhood by analyzing educational achievement, employment, and personal adjustment (1–3).

Patients and Methods

One hundred and sixty three adults formerly treated for idiopathic hypopituitarism at the Division of Endocrinology of the "Ricardo Gutiérrez" Children's Hospital of Buenos Aires were contacted by phone or letter. Forty-six refused participation, but 117 individuals (81 males and 36 females) finally participated in a personal interview. Patient's clinical data were obtained from their medical records. Pituitary hormone deficiencies are shown in Table 6.1. Hypopituitary patients due to organic lesions were not included.

TABLE 6.1. Clinical data of hypopituitary patients.

N		117 Males 81 Females 36
Chronological age at interview (years)		25.3 ± 6.9 (range, 18–50)
Chronological age at start of treatment (years)		12.9 ± 3.8
Bone age at start of treatment (years)		8.4 ± 3.5
Chronological age at onset of sex steriod replacement (years)	Males	17.2 ± 3.1
	Females	18.0 ± 2.1
Final height cm (SDS)	Males	156.3 ± 8.9 (–2.7 ± 1.3)
	Females	142.6 ± 8.5 (–3.2 ± 1.4)
Deficiencies		
IGHD		23%
MPHD without Gonadotrophic deficiency		14%
MPHD with Gonadotrophic deficiency		63%

Data are expressed as mean ± SD.

One hundred and seven patients had been treated with GH for different periods of time; 10 had never received GH. In the older patients, treatment was irregular due to difficulties in GH supply at that time. Patients improved on average one SD of height at the end of the treatment.

All patients were interviewed by the same person (AK) at a mean age of 25.30 ± 6.9 years (range, 18–50 years). They answered a semistructured questionnaire specially designed to evaluate social integration by parameters related to educational achievement, social life attitudes and recreational activities, and work and personal experiences, as well as comments about therapy. The Beck Depression Inventory test (BDI) (4) was completed by 91 patients. Scores above 9 indicate positive signs of depression.

Data were compared with those of the population registry of INDEC of Argentina (5). In a subgroup of 43 patients comparison with the nearest-age sibling was performed for the evaluation of maximal educational achievement, rate of employment, and marital status. For this group statistical analysis was performed using χ^2 to estimate differences between groups.

Results

Educational Achievements

Seventeen percent of the subjects completed elementary school, whereas 2% only completed some grades of it. Twenty-three percent finished high

TABLE 6.2. Maximal educational achievement of hypopituitary patients.

Level	Total group (N =117) %	Selected (N = 43) %	Siblings (N = 43) %	Statistical differences*
Incomplete elementary school	1.7	0	0	NS
Complete elementary school	17	14	9.3	NS
Incomplete high school	29.9	18.6	18.6	NS
Complete high school	23	25.6	16.3	NS
Post high school	9.5	21	25.6	NS
Incomplete university	9.5	11.6	18.6	NS
Complete university	9.5	9.3	11.6	NS

*Selected patients versus siblings.

school, 9.5% finished post–high school studies, 9.5% finished or were still university students, and 9.5% gave up their university studies without finishing them. Fifty-five subjects were trained in different skilled occupations. Sixty-four percent of the subjects repeated at least one grade, mostly in elementary school. We did not find differences between patients and siblings in maximal educational achievement (Table 6.2).

Social Life

Eighty percent of the subjects still live with their parents or other members of their families. Only 15% live with their heterosexual partners, whereas 6% live alone. More than 50% of the patients have very few friends and 13% reported being completely alone. One third of the interviewed patients have younger friends (up to 15 years of difference in age) due to the feeling that their peers confront different living situations. Sixty-five percent of the subjects had no social organized activities or involvement in team sport activities. Almost 50% had no dating experiences, and 55% had not had sexual intercourse. Late onset of sexual intercourse was common, in some of the patients after 30 years of age, and almost all of them practice it sporadically. Only 15 subjects got married (5 females and 10 males). Nine of them (2 females and 7 males) have biologic children (Fig. 6.1). Significantly more married siblings were found ($p < .05$).

Employment and Work

Thirty-nine percent of the subjects were unemployed. (The unemployment rate in Argentina in 1996–97 was around 17%). Thirteen percent were students and would not be expected to be employed. Fifty-eight percent of those employed work within their family group, 11% of them without receiving a salary. Twenty-one percent were self-employed, 60% in private service, 4.2% in public service, and 3.8% as housekeepers. The distribution in these categories is similar to that of the general population, except for those working

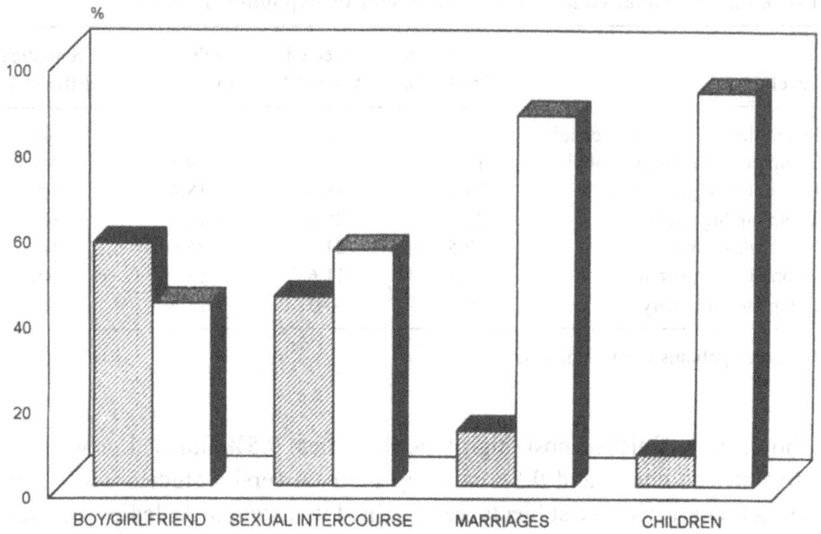

FIGURE 6.1. Social and marital status in 117 hypopituitary patients. Hatched bars, yes; solid bars, no.

without receiving a salary (5.4% in the general population). Employment levels did not differ when compared with siblings.

Personal and Adjustment Problems

Forty-five percent of the subjects felt that their peers regarded them as different: Some of them (18%) felt overprotected and 50% teased. An equal proportion had the same feelings coming from family members, complaining mainly about overprotection. Thirty-seven percent of the patients reported overprotection by their teachers, mainly during the first grade in elementary school. Most of the patients were not satisfied with their appearance: Common complaints were being overweight by females, poor virilization and muscle strength by men, and height and juvenilization by both sexes. Sterility worried older subjects of both sexes. Fifty-eight percent of the hypogonadotrophic patients considered that sex hormone replacement therapy was started late, and that this delay in sexual development had modified their relationship with their peers. At this time they started to meet younger people, with whom they felt closer. Despite being disappointed with their attained height, 85% of the patients thought that GH treatment had helped them and they would recommend it to younger patients. Depression was common. As shown in Figure 6.2, out of 91 subjects who completed the BDI, 29% with IGHD and 48% with MPHD had scores greater than 9. Depression was more common in patients with gonadotrophic deficiency of both sexes. No correlation between depression score and age or attained height was found.

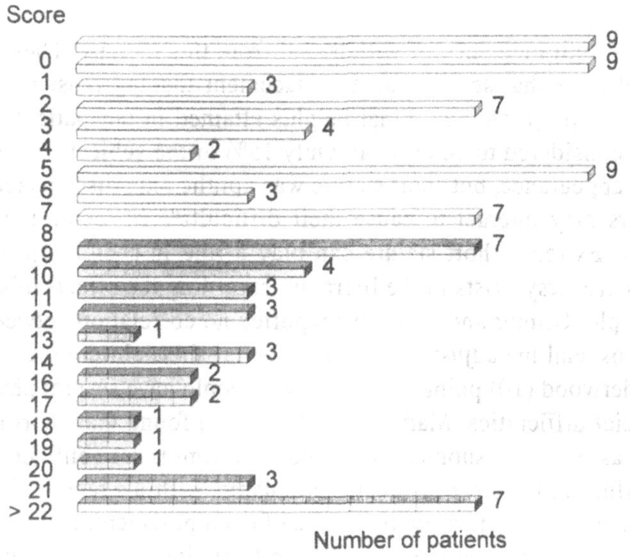

FIGURE 6.2. Beck Depression Inventory test in 91 hypopituitary patients. A score above 9 indicates depression. The number of patients for each score is indicated at the end of bars.

Discussion

As reported by others (6) we found in our adult hypopituitary patients, diagnosed and treated during childhood, difficulties in adult life according to social parameters, low self-esteem, low rates of marriages, high degrees of depression, and social isolation. Unemployment was high, and getting an independent job was difficult. There was a high incidence of dependent life style, with an enhanced tendency in continuing to live with their parents until older ages. Although a high degree of school drop-out and grade repetition was observed in patients compared with siblings, we did not find any differences in educational achievements and levels of employment. This suggests that day-to-day performance is not as disadvantaged as the psychosocial functioning seems to be.

Adolescence was a remarkably difficult period in the life of these patients; short stature and delayed puberty made them feel different from peers. As already reported by Siegel et al. (7) and Holmes et al. (8) we found a tendency to give up sports and social activities at this age. They had difficulties in attaining sexual partners and depression was common, particularly among gonadotrophic-deficient patients. Although the majority of patients complained about the late onset of sex hormone replacement, paradoxically we found a high incidence of withdrawal from this therapy. These observations emphasize that sex hormone replacement therapy must be started at the earliest appropriate age. Final heights attained in our patients were below those considered to be optimal. Only 15% of the subjects were satisfied with their appearance, but short stature was not the only dissatisfaction. Several factors may interact to cause their difficulties in social and personal adaptation. Extreme short stature can play a role in social adjustment, although controversy exists in the literature regarding the effects of short stature on people. Gilmur and Skuse (9) reported no correlation between stature and psychosocial maladjustment in prepubertal short children. On the other hand, Underwood (10) points out that short people have several physical and psychosocial difficulties. Martell and Biller (11) found that short men were perceived as insecure, submissive, withdrawn, timid, not confident, passive, unsuccessful, and more pessimistic compared with average and tall men. Sartorio et al. (12) found more incidence of unemployment, fewer marriages, and more dependency on their families in GHD individuals compared with those of a control group. These controversial data might be due to the degree of shortness of the different group of patients, as well as to the reversibility or not of the condition causing the short stature. Extremely short individuals might find more difficulties in adaptation.

Some authors have suggested that neuroendocrine hormones may play a role in emotional and behavioral problems. It has been reported that GH affects vitality, muscle tone, strength, mood, and the feeling of positive well-being (13,14) and by the involvement of other neurotransmitters GH may affect various brain functions directly or indirectly. GH might have action on neuroendocrine centers that regulate mood and affects that also have cognitive and psychoactive properties, improving memory, attention, and response to stress. In GHD patients, Stabler et al. (15) found a poor response to behavioral stress, suggesting that this inhibited social behavior, especially in patients with MPHD, due to the impact of hormonal deficiency rather than to short stature.

The impact of having a chronic disease is another fact or that might play a role. Daily injections and frequent medical controls since early childhood may predispose them to difficulties in adult life. Medically ill children are assumed to be more vulnerable by parents and society, leading them to have difficulties in autonomy, independence, security, and relation with peers (16).

Despite having different social background our patients share common handicaps with hypopituitary patients from other countries. The handicap due to their physical problems secondary to GH and other pituitary hormone deficiencies can be resolved by adequate and early replacement treatment. Family and society attitudes that surround these subjects, however, must be taken into consideration. Early parental guidance and realistic expectations about the treatments results and possible final heights should be informed (17,18).

Conclusion

Hypopituitarism is a multifactorial chronic disorder involving short stature, neuroendocrine hormone disturbances, and emotional problems. It seems that living with GHD since childhood induces difficulties in developing independence from parents, interaction with peers, sexual maturation, education, and employment.

Patients show a more dependent life style, a high degree of depression, and social isolation. These findings emphasize that hypopituitary children and their families need much early medical and psychological support to achieve a normal social integration.

References

1. Dean H, McTaggart T, Fish D, Friesen H. Long-term social follow-up of growth hormone deficient adults treated with growth hormone during childhood. In: Stabler B, Underwood L, eds. Slow grows the child: psychosocial aspects of growth delay. Hillsdale, NJ: Lawrence Erlbaum Associates, 1986:73–82.
2. Clopper R, MacGillivray M, Mazur T, Voorhess M, Mills B. Post-treatment follow-up of growth hormone deficient patients: psychosocial status. In: Stabler B, Underwood L, eds. Slow grows the child: psychosocial aspects of growth delay. Hillsdale, NJ: Lawrence Erlbaum Associates, 1986:83–96.
3. Meyer-Bahlburg HF. Short stature: psychosocial issues. In: Fima Lifshitz, ed. Pediatric endocrinology: a clinical guide, 2nd ed. New York: M. Dekker, 1990:173–96.
4. Beck AT, Ward CH, Mendelson M, Mock J, Erbaugh J. An inventory for measuring depression. Arch Gen Psych, 1961;4:561–71.
5. Instituto Nacional de Estadísticas y Censos, INDEC, República Argentina. Situación y Evolución Social, Síntesis Nro. 3, 1995.
6. Stabler B. Growth hormone insufficiency during childhood has implications for later life. Acta Paed Scand 1991;(suppl)377:9–13.
7. Siegel PT, Clopper R, Stabler B. Psychological impact of significantly short stature Acta Paediatr Scand 1991;(suppl)377:14–18.
8. Holmes H, Kalsson J, Thompson R. Longitudinal evaluation of behavior patterns in children with short stature. In: Stabler B, Underwood L, eds. Slow grows the child: psychosocial aspects of growth delay. Hillsdale, NJ: Lawrence Erlbaum Associates,1986:1–12.
9. Gilmour J, Skuse D. Short stature—the role of intelligence in psychosocial adjustment. Arch Dis Child 1996;45:25–31.
10. Underwood LE. The social cost of being short: social perceptions and biases. Acta Paediatr Scand 1991;(suppl)377:3–8.
11. Martell LF, Biller HB. Stature and stigma: the biopsychosocial development of short males. Lexington, MA: DC Heath, 1987.
12. Sartorio A, Morabito F, Conti A Gaglia G. The social outcome of adults with constitutional growth delay. J Endocrinol Invest 1990;13:593–95.
13. Rosén T, Johannsson G, Bengtsson BA. Consequences of growth hormone defi-

ciency in adults and effects of growth hormone replacement therapy. Review paper. Acta Paediatr 1994;(suppl)399:21–24.
14. Bengtsson BA, Edén S Lonn LJ, Kvist H, Stokland A, Lindtedt BA, et al. Treatment of adults with growth hormone (GH) deficiency with recombinant human GH. J Clin End Metab 1993;76:309–17.
15. Stabler B, Turner JR, Girdler SS, Ligth KC, Underwood L. Reactivity to stress and psychological adjustement in adults with pituitary insufficiency. Clin Endoc 1992;36:467–73.
16. Rotnem D. Size versus age: ambiguity in parenting short statured children. Slow grows the child: psychosocial aspects of growth delay. In: Stabler B, Underwood L, eds. Slow grows the child: psychosocial aspects of growth delay. Hillsdale, NJ: Lawrence Erlbaum Associates, 1986:178–90.
17. Grew RS, Stabler B, Williams RW, Underwood L. Facilitating patient understanding in the treatment of growth delay. Clin Pediatr 1993;22:685–90.
18. Galatzer A, Aran O, Beith Halachmi N, Nofar E, Rubitchek J, Pertzelan A, et al. The impact of long-term therapy by multidisciplinary team on the education, occupation and marital status of growth hormone deficient patients after termination of therapy. Clin Endocrinol 1987;27:191–96.

Part II

Treatment of Turner Syndrome: Efficacy, Innovation and Quality of Life

7

The Impact of Growth Hormone Therapy on Turner Syndrome

Ron G. Rosenfeld

Introduction

Turner syndrome (TS) affects approximately 1:2000 live-born females (1). Thus, it has a prevalence only one fourth that of Klinefelter syndrome, although it is a far more frequent cause of referral to pediatric endocrinologists. This can be attributed to the fact that the Turner phenotype is much more evident during childhood than is the case for Klinefelter syndrome. Congenital heart abnormalities or lymphedema may be evident prenatally (as ascertained by ultrasonography) or at birth; growth abnormalities may be apparent during childhood, and pubertal delay is observed in approximately 80% of TS girls. Any of these abnormalities should alert the physician to the possible diagnosis of TS.

Initiation of appropriate therapy during childhood can have significant impact during childhood, adolescence, and adult life. Growth hormone (GH) treatment, ideally, can facilitate (1) acceleration of growth and normalization of height during childhood, (2) attainment of an adult height within the normal range, (3) initiation of estrogen replacement at a physiologically appropriate age, and (4) psychosocial adjustment. Although adequate long-term analysis of the effects of therapy on quality-of-life issues is necessary, it is apparent that the overall outlook for TS girls has improved considerably over the last two decades.

Acceleration of Growth

A variety of hormonal therapies have been employed in an effort to accelerate growth in girls with TS, including anabolic steroids, estrogen preparations, and GH. In 1983, a multicenter, prospective, randomized trial of hGH, alone or in combination with oxandrolone, was begun in the United States.

Preliminary 1-year (2), 3-year (3), and 6-year reports (4) confirmed that both GH alone and the combination of GH plus oxandrolone accelerate short-term growth. As has been observed with GH treatment of GH deficiency, a waning response to GH was observed with prolonged treatment, but even out to 6 years of therapy, most TS girls continued to grow faster than anticipated for age-matched, untreated TS girls (4). Bone-age acceleration was modest, and the anticipated adult height of the majority of subjects was found to be significantly improved, when compared with the pretreatment projected adult heights.

Adult Height

The multicenter trial begun in 1983 has been completed (5). Adult height data have substantiated the interpretations of the earlier reports and have confirmed a positive impact of both GH and GH plus oxandrolone on adult height (Table 7.1 and Fig. 7.1). Sixteen of the 17 girls who received GH alone exceeded their baseline-projected adult heights. Of the 45 recipients of combination GH plus oxandrolone, 42 attained adult heights greater than their initial projected adult heights; the three subjects who did not surpass their original projected adult heights were only 0.7–3.1 cm below the original projections.

Figure 7.1 shows each subject's adult height, relative to her original projected adult height. For girls who received GH alone, the mean increment in adult height was 8.4 cm (range, –0.9 to +15.9 cm). In the group receiving combination GH plus oxandrolone, the mean increment in height was 10.3 cm (range, –0.7 to –17.9 cm). By comparison, the retrospective control group experienced no improvement in final height over their projected adult heights. All told, the recipients of GH alone reached a mean adult height of 150.4 cm, whereas recipients of combination therapy reached a mean adult height

TABLE 7.1. Response to GH treatment.

	GH-Rx (*N*=25)	Combination Rx (*N*=17)	American historical controls (*N*=43)
Baseline age (years)	9.1 (2.1)	9.9 (2.3)	9.2 (1.7)
Baseline height (cm)	114.6 (9.5)	117.3 (10.4)	117.1 (8.9)
Baseline TS SDS[1]	–0.2 (0.9)	–0.2 (0.9)	–0.2 (0.9)
Baseline Lyon PAH[2] (cm)	142.0 (5.9)	141.8 (5.9)	144.2 (5.6)
Target height[3] (cm)	164.5 (3.7)	162.6 (4.0)	164.3 (5.6)
Duration GH Rx (years)	7.6 (2.2)	6.1 (1.9)	—
Last age (years)	18.0 (2.2)	17.4 (1.7)	22.1 (3.1)
Last height (cm)	150.4 (5.5)	152.1 (5.9)	144.2 (6.0)

Data are presented as mean (SD). [1]Turner syndrome height SDS based upon data of Lyon et al. (12). [2]Turner syndrome projected adult height based upon the data of Lyon et al. (12). [3]Midparental target height for females.
Table adapted from Reference 5.

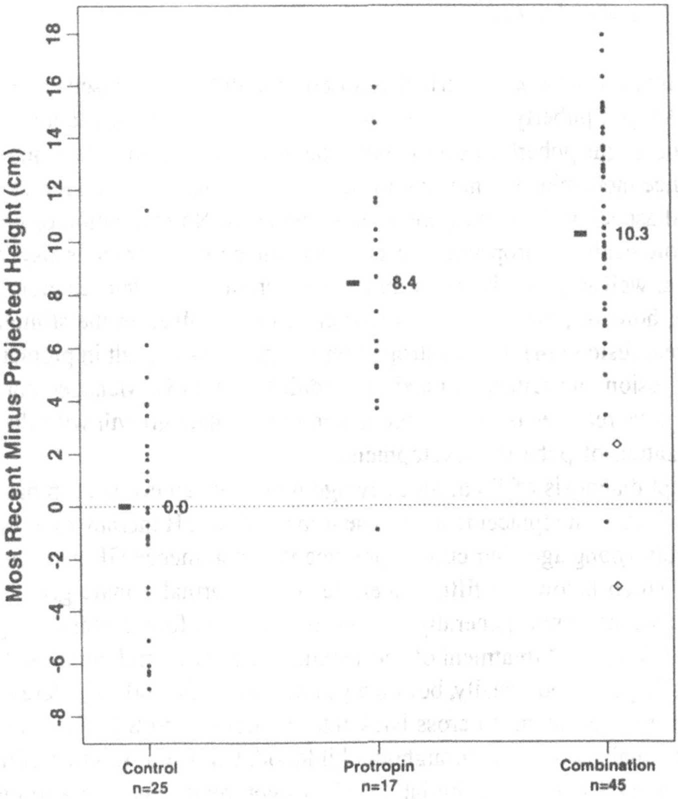

FIGURE 7.1. The most recent height of each subject (or American historical control) relative to each subject's projected adult height (indicated by the dotted line through "Zero." The mean increment in height (centimeters) relative to projected adult height is indicated. The diamond symbols in the "Combination" group indicate two early stoppers of treatment. (From Ref. 5, with permission, The Journal of Pediatrics, Rosenfeld et al., Growth hormone therapy of Turner' syndrome: beneficial effect on adult height, 1998;132:319–24.)

of 152.1 cm. These final heights compare favorably with (1) the subjects' initial projected adult heights, (2) the final heights achieved by the retrospective control group (144.2 cm), and (3) the final heights for untreated Turner girls reported from Italy (142.5 cm) (6), Germany (143.8 and 146.8 cm) (7,8), Japan (137 cm) (9), Denmark (146.6 cm) (10), the United States (11), and the study of Lyon et al. (12), in which the mean final height of 138 untreated TS girls over 20 years of age was 142.9 cm. Furthermore, the data are supported by preliminary results from a second study in which 29 TS girls receiving GH achieved a mean height at age 16.3 years of 150.4 cm, 8.4 cm greater than their mean pretreatment projected adult height (13). These findings thus indicate that short-term acceleartion of growth velocity with GH treatment can in most cases result in an improvement in adult height.

Estrogen Replacement

Approximately 80% of TS girls diagnosed in childhood/adolescence will experience delayed puberty or a complete failure to initiate feminization. Of those girls who begin pubertal development, only a few will complete puberty and experience menarche and normal, cyclic menses. Thus, estrogen replacement is a critical aspect of the management of TS patients. Normalization of puberty at a physiologically appropriate age is important both for obvious psychosocial reasons as well as, possibly, to maximize the accretion of skeletal calcium. Studies indicate, however, that estrogen is also critically involved in the stimulation of epiphyseal fusion (14). Early estrogen replacement may result in premature epiphyseal fusion and failure to maximize adult height (13). Management of girls with TS thus requires balancing the desire to stimulate growth with the goal of normalization of pubertal development.

Prompt diagnosis of TS at an early age may have an eventual impact on the timing of estrogen replacement because it may allow GH therapy to be started at a relatively young age. Our current practice is to commence GH as soon as a TS girl has fallen below the fifth percentile of the normal female growth curve, although we have not, generally, started treatment before 2 years of age (15). The initiation of GH treatment of short stature in early to mid-childhood (before the age of 8 years and, ideally, before 5 years) may sufficiently accelerate growth to permit the TS patient to cross back into the normal growth curve and maintain a "normal" percentile throughout childhood. Clinical responses of this kind may allow consideration of initiation of estrogen replacement at a more physiologically appropriate age than has been generally used for TS, where estrogens have been withheld frequently until 15–16 years of age, to allow the patient to attain maximal height gain before stimulation of epiphyseal fusion. This does not imply that estrogens are begun at age 10.6 years (the mean age for Tanner B2 stage in American girls), but, nevertheless, it can permit commencement of estrogen therapy by 12–13 years. The use of GH and estrogens in TS patients ideally should be individualized, with appropriate consideration given to the patient's growth pattern, target height, bone age, and desire for pubertal development. Early diagnosis and appropriate management should permit most TS girls to achieve relatively normal growth, as well as pubertal progression at an age within the broad normal range.

Psychosocial Adjustment

Inadequate data are currently available to allow evaluation of the impact of GH treatment on psychosocial, educational and vocational aspects of life for the girl with TS. It has certainly been the anecdotal impression of most observers that TS patients have benefited psychosocially from GH treatment and have a more optimistic outlook on life. Such observations, however, must be supported by appropriate studies because any therapy can have its own disabling ramifications, which must be weighed against its benefits. The use of medications to enhance growth and to stimulate pubertal development unfortunately can add to a TS girl's sense of inadequacy. All therapy accordingly should be administered together with psychosocial support and counseling, and with the goal of reinforcing the TS girl's self-esteem and ability to remain in the mainstream of social, school, and vocational activities.

Outlook for Adults with TS

The limited data available concerning the long-term outlook for women with TS are unsettling and concerning: Death rates from cardiovascular and renal complications, as well as from suicide, are significantly greater than they are in the normal female population. All adult women with TS require careful medical follow-up by physicians experienced in the care of this disorder, with particular attention paid to cardiac problems, hypertension, renal function, bone mineral density, thyroid function, gynecologic issues, hearing, and psychosocial function. Even though the use of GH has had a significant impact on the care of girls with TS, the underlying chromosomal abnormality and its associated phenotype remain unaltered. Table 7.2 summarizes some of the critical issues in the outlook for adult women with TS.

TABLE 7.2. Factors involved in the outlook for Turner syndrome.

Maximizing growth (factors involved)
Parental heights
Age of initiation of GH treatment
Duration of GH treatment
Age at initiation of estrogen replacement
Unknown factors
Medical problems of adult women with Turner syndrome
Thyroid dysfunction
Hearing loss
Osteoporosis
Carbohydrate intolerance
Cardiovascular abnormalities
Hypertension
Renal failure
Reproductive issues in Turner syndrome
Counseling
Adoption
in vitro fertilization of donor eggs
in vitro fertilization of frozen eggs harvested from patient
Potential issues concerning reproduction by TS women with intact ovarian function
Psychosocial issues in Turner syndrome
Personality and social adjustment
Cognitive and academic performance
Careers
Marriage and family

References

1. Robinson A. Demography and prevalence of Turner syndrome. In: Rosenfeld RG, Grumbach MM, eds. Turner syndrome. New York: Marcel Dekker, 1990:93–100.
2. Rosenfeld RG, Hintz RL, Johanson, AJ, Brasel JA, Burstein S, Chernausek SD, et al. Methionyl human growth and oxandrolone in Turner syndrome: preliminary results of a prospective randomized trial. J Pediatr 1986;109:936–43.
3. Rosenfeld RG, Hintz RL, Johanson AJ, Sherman B, Brasel JA, Burstein S, et al. Three-year results of a randomized prospective trial of methionyl human growth hormone and oxandrolone in Turner syndrome. J Pediatr 1988;113:393–400.
4. Rosenfeld RG, Frane J, Attie KM, Brasel JA, Burstein S, Cara JF, et al. Six-year results of a randomized, prospective trial of human growth hormone and oxandrolone in Turner syndrome. J Pediatr 1992;121:49–55.
5. Rosenfeld RG, Attie KM, Frane J, Brasel JA, Burstein S, Cara JF, et al. Growth hormone therapy of Turner's syndrome: Beneficial effect on adult height. J Pediatr 1998;132:319–24.
6. Bernasconi S, Giovanelli G, Volta C, Aicardi G, Balestrazzi P, Benso L, et al. Spontaneous growth in Turner syndrome: preliminary results of an Italian multicenter study. In: Ranke MB, Rosenfeld R, eds. Turner's syndrome and growth-promoting therapies. Amsterdam: Elsevier, 1991:53–57.
7. Ranke MB, Pfluger H, Rosendahl W, Stubbe P, Enders H, Bierich JR, et al. Turner syndrome: Spontaneous growth in 150 cases and review of the literature. Eur J Pediatr 1983;141:81–88.
8. Hausler G, Schemper M, Frisch H, Blumel P, Schmitt K, Plochl E, et al. Spontaneous growth in Turner syndrome: evidence for a minor pubertal growth spurt. In: Ranke MB, Rosenfeld R, eds. Turner's syndrome and growth-promoting therapies. Amsterdam: Elsevier, 1991:67–73.
9. Hibi I, Tanae A, Tanaka T, Yoshizawa A, Miki Y, Ito J. Spontaneous puberty in Turner syndrome: its incidence, influence on final height and endocrinological features. In: Ranke, MB, Rosenfeld R, eds. Turner's syndrome and growth-promoting therapies. Amsterdam: Elsevier, 1991:75–81.
10. Naeraa RW, Nielsen J. Standards for growth and final height in Turner's syndrome. Acta Paediatr Scand 1990;79:182–90.
11. Lippe B, Plotnick L, Attie K, Frane J. Growth in Turner syndrome: updating the United States experience. In: Hibi I, Takano K, eds. Basic and clinical approach to Turner syndrome. Amsterdam: Elsevier, 1993:77–82.
12. Lyon AL, Preece MA, Grant DB. Growth curve for girls with Turner syndrome. Arch Dis Child 1985;60:932–35.
13. Attie KM, Chernausek S, Frane J, Rosenfeld RG, Genentech Study Group. Growth hormone use in Turner syndrome: a preliminary report on the effect of early vs. delayed estrogen. In: Albertsson-Wikland K, Ranke M, eds. Turner syndrome in a life-span perspective: research and clinical aspects. Amsterdam: Elsevier. 1995: 175–81.
14. Smith EP, Boyd J, Frank GR, Takahashi H, Cohen RM, Specker B, et al. Estrogen resistance caused by a mutation in the estrogen-receptor gene in man. N Engl J Med 1994;331:1056–61.
15. Rosenfeld RG, Tesch L-G, Rodriguez-Rigau LJ, McCauley E, Albertsson-Wikland K, Asch R, et al. Recommendations for diagnosis, treatment, and management of individuals with Turner synrome. Endocrinologist 1994;4:351–58.

8

Phenotype–Karyotype Relationships in Turner Syndrome

DAVID SKUSE, DOROTHY BISHOP, KATE ELGAR, AND ELENA MORRIS

Turner syndrome (TS) is a chromosomal disorder in which all, or a substantial part, of one X chromosome is missing due to nondisjunction, or chromosome loss, during gametogenesis or early cleavage of the zygote. The condition is associated with a range of psychosocial difficulties, primarily involving immaturity and problems with social relationships, although intelligence is usually entirely normal for verbal skills (1–4). Girls with this disorder have been described as characteristically immature, with a poor self-concept, relative to normal comparisons of similar age. There is some evidence that self-esteem declines as they pass from earlier childhood into adolescence. Within-group differences in stature, relative to the normal range, are not predictive of social adjustment, which suggests that whatever factors do contribute to poor social adjustment, short stature as such is unlikely to be of major significance (5,6). The problems in social adjustment do persist over time. Studies of older individuals have found that impairment in the ability to make and sustain friendships, which often becomes apparent during adolescence, often continues into adult life (4).

Females with Turner syndrome also have a characteristic pattern of deficiencies in their cognitive abilities. In general they have a poorer overall performance (nonverbal) than verbal IQ (7). The magnitude of verbal-performance discrepancies found varies, from 11 to 20 points on average. The deficit is in spatial cognition, and it may be identified by tasks from the Wechsler battery of intelligence tests (8,9) such as object assembly (equivalent to a simple jigsaw puzzle) and block design (10). Females with Turner syndrome often have difficulty with drawing tasks such as Draw-a-Man (11), and they also find it hard accurately to copy a complex shape such as the Rey Figure. Their visual memory for such complex shapes may also be impaired (12). Several strands of research have suggested there is a consistent deficit in skills known as *executive functions* that are usually considered to be mediated by the frontal lobes. These include a heightened distractibility to irrelevant sources of information, as in the stimuli presented by the Stroop task which requires the reading of the names of colors that are spelled (e.g., "red," "green") in letters of a different color (13). Nevertheless, they may have normal performance on a task that requires the child to plan ahead and to order and sequence a series of moves (the Tower of Hanoi) (14,15).

Apart from those with a small ring X chromosome, which has been associated with mental retardation (16), TS is not characterized by a diminished overall level of verbal intelligence. It has even been suggested that TS girls may have a small advantage in verbal abilities relative to norms, and that they may have better reading skills than would be predicted for their age (17); however, there may be impaired verbal fluency despite good verbal intelligence and a vocabulary that is normal for the child's age (18).

It has also been proposed that the degree of cognitive deficit in those with essentially normal intelligence might vary with the specific chromosomal abnormality. Temple and Carney (18) followed up a report by Salbenblatt et al. (19) that TS individuals with mosaicism had less marked motor difficulties than those with the 45,X variant, and they queried whether the intellectual profile would also vary with the karyotype. Their results were consistent with the hypothesis that the cognitive phenotype of the condition was indeed less deviant when the karyotype was mosaic rather than strictly monosomic. That is examination of the chromosomal make-up of a large number of cells (usually white blood cells) finds two or more different karyotypes are present in different cell lines. Temple and Carney have more recently claimed that patterns of spatial cognition also vary with karyotype (20). McCauley et al. (2) made an attempt to link, conceptually, the cognitive and social difficulties encountered in Turner syndrome. They suggested that because TS girls have specific cognitive deficits indicating right hemisphere dysfunction (21) they may also have problems processing affect, particularly in discriminating between facial expressions. In turn, the facial affect processing deficits could be causally linked to the development of behavior problems and poor peer relationships. Their results indicated that TS girls, aged between 9 and 12 years with verbal IQs over 79, did indeed perform more poorly than did short stature controls on tests of spatial and attentional functioning. They were also less accurate in their discrimination of facial expressions of affect. There was no direct and simple relationship, however, between spatial ability and affective discrimination.

There is considerable variability in the cognitive and behavioral phenotype in TS. We hypothesized that this could be related to systematic differences both in the nature of the structural abnormalities of the X or Y chromosome that are found in about 50% of subjects, or to the parental origin of the single normal X chromosome in cases of X monosomy. In 70% of monosomic (45,X) TS the single X chromosome is maternal in origin (22); it is paternal in origin in the remainder. Normal females (46,XX) possess both a maternally derived X chromosome (Xm) and a paternally derived X chromosome (Xp), one of which is randomly inactivated in any given somatic cell (23). In monosomy X the single chromosome is never inactivated. In this investigation we aimed to discover whether differences in physical or behavioral phenotype between 45,Xp and 45,Xm TS subjects might indicate the existence of an imprinted genetic locus.

The term *genomic (gametic) imprinting* refers to different expression of a normal gene, depending on the sex of the parent who transmits it. When this is observed, it implies that the gene or the chromosomal region carries a "tag" or imprint that was placed during spermatogenesis or oogenesis and which can modulate gene expression in the developing embryo. The imprint may act to silence the allele from one parent, so that normal development is dependent solely on the function of the allele from the other parent. That this silencing is not a DNA mutation is shown by the fact that the same gene transmitted in a later generation by someone of the opposite sex is no longer silenced; rather, the imprint has been erased at some time between generations. An imprint may also act to prevent repression of gene expression by blocking the binding of a repressor, and thereby be associated with the active allele. Genomic imprinting raises several important questions. First, what is the nature of the gametic imprint that marks the chromosome as paternal or maternal? Second, how does this result in differential allele expression in the next generation? Third, why has imprinting evolved and been maintained in humans? When we undertook our study no imprinted gene had been described on the X chromosome in humans, but we felt a study of monosomic TS presented an ideal model by which such a mechanism could be uncovered.

Most published studies on the behavioral and psychosocial aspects of the TS have focused upon relatively small samples, almost invariably less than 25 cases. We aimed to take advantage of our links with pediatric endocrinologists throughout the United Kingdom who were members of the British Society for Paediatric Endocrinology (BSPE), in order to recruit a far larger sample. Such a large sample, which is nationally representative, would allow a variety of within-group comparisons to be made; for example, of age trends in psychosocial difficulties and also karyotype–phenotype correlations.

Methods

Subject Selection

A national register was compiled of all cases of TS known to members of the BSPE, as well as those members of a parent support organization, the Child Growth Foundation. The total number of cases on this register is presently 756. They are drawn from throughout the United Kingdom (including Northern and Southern Ireland). The sociodemographic distribution of our sample closely reflects that of the general population. In this account of our research we will confine our report to findings on 80 monosomic (45,X) females with TS, age range 6–25 years. They were selected both from our national survey of the condition and from the records of the Wessex Regional Genetics Laboratory.

Behavioral and Cognitive Measures

Initial screening of all subjects on our TS database was conducted by postal questionnaires using a well-standardized set of instruments (24–26) that were completed by parents, teachers, and the Turner subjects themselves (11 years and over). Parents were asked to complete the Child Behavior Checklist (CBCL), 1991 revision (24), which is a standardized assessment procedure for obtaining parents' ratings on a broad range of clinically relevant problem behaviors in children. We used the 4–18 year version, which was appropriate for all the children in our survey. The CBCL consists of 20 competence items and 118 problem items. Parents are requested to circle a 0 if the problem item is not true of the child, 1 if the item is somewhat or sometimes true, and 2 if it is very true or often true.

The girls themselves were asked to compute the Youth Self Report (YSR) (26) if over 11 years of age. This instrument is designed to obtain 11–18 year olds reports of their own competencies and problems in a similar format to the parent-rated CBCL/4–18. The instrument comprises 20 competence items and 112 problem and socially desirable items.

For those girls who were of school age we asked teachers to return a Teacher Report Form (TRF) (25) which is designed to obtain reports of pupil's adaptive functioning and problems, and is modeled on the CBCL/4–18. The adaptive functioning score reflects teachers' ratings of performance in academic subjects, plus general characteristics of their behavior at school. In addition, there are 118 specific problem items from which syndrome subscales can be obtained. Most of the problem items have counterparts on the CBCL and YSR, but teachers are asked to base ratings on the preceding 2 months, in contrast to the 6-month baseline used on the CBCL and YSR.

From all three instruments it is possible to generate total scores, standardized population *T*-scores, and clinical *T*-scores, in respect of a range of core syndromes comprising problem items that are common to syndromes derived from separate analyses of each sex in each age range on a particular instrument. The clinical *T*-scores have been standardized with a mean of 50, with scores above this indicating that the child's problem is probably of clinical significance, and is at least of an equivalent degree of severity to that seen in a clinical population of psychiatric clinic-referred children. Seventy parents completed the CBCL (24), 40 subjects over 11 years of age completed the YSR (26), and 45 teachers completed the TRF (25). Clinical significance of social problems was estimated from the Achenbach instruments according to clinical *T*-scores (24–26).

We also developed a 42-item questionnaire from interviews with girls with the condition, their parents, and their teachers, which summarized many of the social adjustment problems they had encountered in their everyday lives. Many of the questions concerned behaviors that could have been influenced by impaired social-cognitive skills, such as the ability to perceive emotional states in others. Scoring was similar to the standardized behavioral screening measures, on a 0–2 scale.

The complete set of screening instruments was first distributed in 1992–1993 when we had returns from 325 families (27). An identical set of instruments was circulated to the same families in 1995–1996, and we have had a response from 84.3% of the sample to date. It was possible, therefore, to compare the factorial structure of the 42-item questionnaire on social adjustment using a principal components analysis on both occasions. We found great similarity in the outcome of this analysis, with one factor accounting for between 38 and 39% of the variance in the questionnaire on both occasions. We took those 12 variables from the questionnaire whose factor scores loaded higher than 0.5 onto this factor on both occasions. Only the analysis of this subset of our larger questionnaire will be discussed here. The 12-item social cognition questionnaire (Table 8.1) was completed only by parents. It has remarkably high internal consistency: Cronbach's Alpha was 0.94. The single most discriminating question was whether the girl in question picked up on (in other words understood) others' body language.

In our survey of 175 TS subjects for whom we obtained parental ratings on two occasions, a mean of 2.7 years apart, the intraclass correlation coefficient for this set of 12 questions was 0.81 ($p < .01$), which shows remarkable

TABLE 8.1. Scale measuring social cognition.

Complete the following section by circling 0 if the statement is not at all true of your child, 1 if it is quite or sometimes true of your child, and 2 if it is very or often true of your child:

Lacking an awareness of other people's feelings	0	1	2
Does not realize when others are upset or angry	0	1	2
Is oblivious to the effect of his/her behavior on other members of the family	0	1	2
Behavior often disrupts normal family life	0	1	2
Very demanding of people's time	0	1	2
Difficult to reason with when upset	0	1	2
Does not seem to understand social skills (e.g., interrupts conversation)	0	1	2
Does not pick up on body language	0	1	2
Unaware of acceptable social behavior	0	1	2
Unknowingly of fends people with behavior	0	1	2
Does not respond to commands	0	1	2
Has difficulty following commands unless they are carefully worded	0	1	2
Internal consistency for set of 12 questions:	Standardized item alpha 0.94		

consistency in the scores obtained by our subjects. Scores on the 12-item social cognition questionnaire correlated with the self-rated social problem subscale of the YSR (26) 0.58 ($p < .002$), with the teacher rating on the TRF (25) 0.54 ($p < .001$), and with the parent-rated CBCL (24) 0.69 ($p < .001$). The range of scores was 0–23 in the Turner sample (maximum possible score was 24).

Our measures of cognition included the Wechsler Intelligence Scales for Children (WISC III-UK) (9) and the Wechsler Adult Intelligence Scales-Revised (WAIS-R) (28). We did not administer all the subscales for want of time. All subjects were given the similarities and vocabulary subscales from the verbal subtest, and block design and object assembly subscales from the performance subtest. Cognitive testing was conducted in our laboratories at the Institute of Child Health, or in subject's homes if they lived a considerable distance from London. All assessments were video-recorded so that we could check on the reliability of their administration.

In view of previous research that has demonstrated executive function deficits in TS (15) we conducted a number of more focused neuropsychological assessments. First, although verbal abilities are moderately good predictors of social cognition, we hypothesized that higher order cognitive skills would be better predictors. These are not measured directly by conventional intelligence tests. The executive functions of the prefrontal cortex (29) exert a key influence upon social interactions. They comprise skills that allow for the development of strategies of action, and the inhibition of distracting impulses when striving toward a goal. Developmental disorders of social adjustment and language are associated with impairment in executive function measures (30). We chose tests of both planning ability (Tower of Hanoi) and behavioral inhibition (the Same-Opposite World subtest from the Test of Everyday Attention for Children) (31). Only these two tests of executive functions were used, and both were chosen on the basis that the abilities they measured reflected different aspects of frontal skills. Previous work by Temple and colleagues (15) has found in Turner females a dissociation in task performance with deficits on the Stroop (13) and Verbal Fluency (32) tasks, but intact performance on the Wisconsin Card Sort Test (33) and the Tower of London (34), which suggests that there is fractionation of executive control systems in development.

The behavioral inhibition task yields a time measure that ascertains the difference in latency for a subject responding to a series of stimuli on a task of sequential responses, which are named both as they appear and then opposite to their appearance. The subject reads a random series of numbers (1 and 2) saying "one" to 1, and "two" to 2. The subjects then repeat the task on a new series, but this time they have to inhibit the prepotent response and instead say "two" to 1, and "one" to 2, correcting any errors before proceeding. Test–retest reliability on a sample of 70 normal children gave an intraclass correlation coefficient of 0.62 ($p < .001$). The Tower of Hanoi task was based on the procedure described by Borys, Spitz and Dorans (35) and is approximately similar to the Tower of London task used by Temple et al. (15). It was scored according to the most complex level of the problem the child could reliably solve. Test–retest reliability gave an intraclass correlation coefficient for the highest level achieved of 0.45 ($p < .001$), which is in line with expectations for a test that makes novel demands of this nature (36).

Karyotypes

A very important aspect of our investigation was the accurate karyotyping of our subjects. Even though this may have been done adequately at the time the diagnosis was suspected in many cytogenetic laboratories, we wished to have a uniform assessment using the same cytogenetic techniques for all girls. We therefore aimed to rekaryotype all subjects. For details see Jacobs et al. (37). The work was undertaken at the Wessex Regional Genetics Laboratory under the direction of Professor Patricia Jacobs. Ethical permission for this aspect of the investigation was obtained on the basis that sensitive PCR procedures were used for the identification of Y chromosome material that may have been missed at the time of the original karyotyping (38). The proportions of karyotypes identified in each category of monosomic subject were in line with previous reports on epidemiologically ascertained samples (37). We karyotyped 80 monosomic (45,X) females. We determined the parental origin of the normal X chromosome by comparing proband and parental DNA polymorphisms located on distal Xp, in a region that was deleted in both 45,X and 46,XXp- patients. Of the 80 45,X females, 25 were 45,Xp and 55 were 45,Xm with ages from 6 to 25 years. Clinical records did not reveal any significant group differences in terms of physical phenotype. The mean age of the 45,Xm females was 162.3 months (SD 57.6), and that of the 45,Xp females was 164.5 months (SD 57.7).

Anthropometry and Treatment

Parents were asked to record their child's current height and weight. For the girls considered here, data were obtained on subjects for height and weight for 36 out of 55 of those with a maternal X chromosome and for 18 out of 25 of those with a single paternal X chromosome. Because these data refer to values obtained at a wide range of different ages, weights and heights have been standardized for age and are expressed in standard deviation (SDS) scores. SDS scores represent the extent of a value above or below the mean of weight for age or length for age or weight for height of the current U.K. standards (39). Computation of the SDS scores was undertaken by the Castlemead Growth Program (40). In practice a SDS score of −1.88 corresponds to the third percentile. We found that the mean value of height and weight for age were very similar in each of the karyotyped samples. The mean for the 45,Xm subjects was −1.8 SDS (SD 1.5) and that for the 45,Xp subjects was −1.9 SDS (SD 1.14). The small difference was not statistically significant. Some 84.4% of 45,Xm subjects were being treated with growth hormone, and 43.6% were on estrogen replacement therapy, 85.7% of 45,Xp subjects were being treated with growth hormone, and 61.9% were on estrogen replacement therapy, with this rather greater proportion reflecting the fact that adolescents and young women were represented more strongly in this group. All subjects were healthy, with no significant neurological disease.

Results

From a first stage screening survey (27) of parents and teachers, using standardized instruments (24–26) we discovered that 40% of 45,Xm girls of school age had received a statement of special educational needs, indicating academic failure, compared with 16% of 45,Xp subjects ($p < .05$). The general population figure is just 2%. We also found that clinically significant social difficulties, as measured by clinical *T*-scores on the CBCL, YRF, and TRF affected 72.4% of the 45,Xm subjects over 11 years of age (21 out of 29) compared with 28.6% of 45,Xp females (4 out of 14) ($p < .02$).

Such phenotypic variability between the two classes of monosomy X subjects could indicate the existence of an imprinted genetic locus, at which gene(s) that influence social adjustment are expressed only from the paternally derived X chromosome. On the maternally derived X chromosome the corresponding locus would be silenced. This could account for the excess of social and learning difficulties among 45,Xm females compared with the 45,Xp variant. Pilot interviews and observations showed 45,Xm females in particular lacked flexibility and responsiveness in social interactions. An imprinted locus is not the only possible explanation for our findings. Among the 45,Xp females there may have been a greater degree of cryptic mosaicism (with a normal 46,XX cell line) than among those who were 45,Xm. Some degree of mosaicism in apparently monosomic females may be essential for the fetus to avoid spontaneous abortion (41). We looked in both blood and cheek cells and tissues of mesodermal and ectodermal origin, respectively, and found two cryptic mosaics, but both were from the 45,Xm group.

Figure 8.1 shows the scores on the social cognition questionnaire for subjects 6–18 years of age, which confirm that there are significant differences between 45,Xm and 45,Xp females in the predicted direction. 45,Xm subjects obtained significantly higher scores than 45,Xp females on the measures of social-cognitive dysfunction. Mean values are shown with 1 standard error. Higher scores indicate poorer social cognitive skills. 45,Xm TS females score higher than 45,Xp females and normal females ($p < .0001$). The overall higher scores for the TS subjects, compared with normal females, may reflect the contribution made by visuospatial abilities to social cognition (2). These abilities are equally impaired in both monosomic groups. No information regarding parental origin of the normal X chromosome was made available to parents, their consultants or members of the research team gathering these or other data.

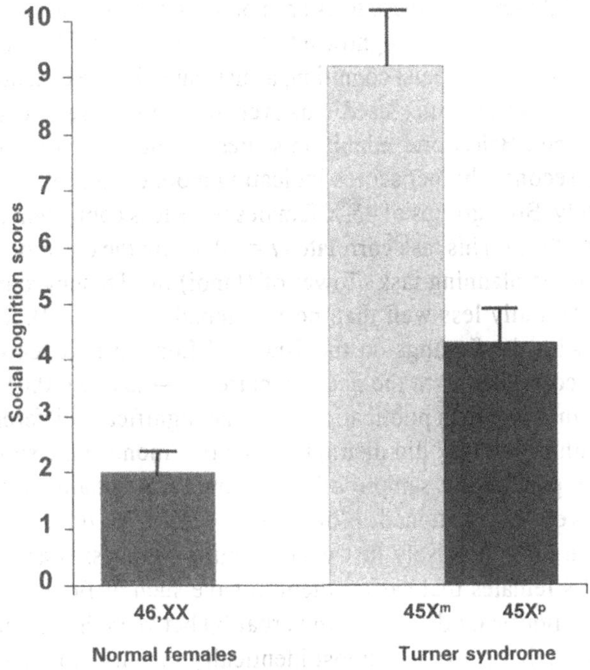

FIGURE 8.1. Subscale scores of questionnaire on social-cognitive impairment.

Table 8.2 shows that 45,Xp females have significantly higher verbal IQ than do 45,Xm subjects ($p < .02$), but neither Turner group differs significantly from the normal female comparisons. Nonverbal IQ was measured only in TS subjects and does not significantly distinguish the subgroups; it incorporates tests of visuospatial abilities which are known to be specifically impaired in this condition (10,20). In all analyses employing the executive function measures age, which has been covaried, because, unlike

TABLE 8.2. Neuropsychological test results.

	Turner syndrome		Normal females
	45,Xm mean ± SD	45,Xp mean ± SD	46,XX mean ± SD
IQ			
Verbal	95.2 ± 17.6	104.2 ± 20	97.8 ±18.4
Nonverbal	79.9 ± 19.0	80.2 ±16.9	—
Executive function tasks			
Behavioral inhibition	8.8 ± 7.1	7.4 ± 5.0	5.7 ± 4.1
Planning ability	5.8 ± 2.4	6.1 ± 2.9	6.4 ± 1.8

conventional IQ measures, these tests are not yet standardized for age. The hypothesis that there would be a significant correlation between the scores on these tasks and impairment in social cognition, as measured by the questionnaire, was supported. The two measures used, however, were not correlated significantly with one another. Behavioral inhibition scores (Same–Opposite World) were measured in seconds, higher scores indicating more difficulty completing the task accurately. Both groups of 45,X females were less competent than normal females ($p < .0001$). This task correlated $r = -0.3$ with the questionnaire scores ($p < .01$). On the planning task (Tower of Hanoi) the TS subgroups also performed substantially less well than normal females ($p < .002$). The result is compatible with the findings on the Tower of London task reported earlier (15). Scores correlated with the questionnaire $r = -0.31$ ($p < 0.01$). Although we reported in a previous publication (43) that significant differences on the behavioral inhibition task did distinguish the two monosomic subgroups, we have since expanded the sample of monosomic TS females tested and the differences were not sustained. More work needs to be done in order to be able to define more precisely just what cognitive processes are impaired in the 45,Xm TS females that causes them to have such difficulties interacting socially. The significant difference in verbal IQ between the groups is clearly a clue, as nonverbal skills are almost identically impaired to the same extent in all monosomic subjects. We are continuing our investigations into this conundrum. Some tantalizing clues are emerging, but no firm conclusions have yet been reached.

Conclusions

We undertook a cytogenetic, molecular, phenotypic, behavior and cognitive study of girls with TS and found evidence for X-linked genes that influence social-cognitive skills and behavior (43). We found that aspects of social adjustment, and verbal IQ, were significantly better in monosomic females in whom the single X chromosome was paternally derived (45,Xp) than in those with a single maternally derived X chromosome (45,Xm). Our findings suggested there may be an imprinted gene on the X chromosome that is responsible. This genetic locus would be active only on the paternally derived X chromosome, and would be preferentially inactivated on the maternally derived X chromosome.

The observation that there could be imprinting of genes on the X chromosome in the way we suggest has far-reaching implications for the understanding of gender differences in cognition, behavior, and susceptibility to both genetic and environmental influences on social development. One of the most striking, although not necessarily the most obvious, finding of our investigation is that the "phenotype" we investigated—within the monosomic

TS population—was an aspect of social cognition that would not have been measured sufficiently sensitively for us to have detected group differences by conventional "behavioral screening instruments." Neither scores on the CBCL, the YSR, nor the TRF subscales distinguished the two monosomic samples. The definition of phenotype is crucial to successful studies of genetic predispositions in so many areas, but especially so in psychiatry and psychology. Our screening instrument (the questionnaire we employed in the first phase of our study) was not pulled off the shelf, but was developed in consultation with girls with TS, their parents, their teachers, and pediatricians who were experienced in managing the disorder.

The same principle applies to our choice of measures of cognitive abilities. Even though we did use a comprehensive battery of cognitive tasks that have been employed in studies of Turner syndrome in the past, there were good theoretical reasons to add measures of executive skills. The vast majority of such assessment procedures were developed on adults, and a review of the literature on their use with children showed that the adult versions had often been used with little or no modification. In collaboration with colleagues we devised a set of executive function measures that were not only applicable to children, but which proved both reliable and which possessed good predictive validity. We would argue, therefore that the high-fidelity measurement of phenotype, whether in behavioral or cognitive terms, is crucial to the success of any endeavor aimed at clarifying the genetic underpinnings of cognitive and behavioral development in general, and neurodevelopmental disorders in particular. The implications of our findings for TS are important in both theoretical and practical terms. If we can refine our measures so that we can understand just what cognitive processes are impaired, particularly among girls who are monosomic for their maternal X chromosome, we should be able to devise focused interventions that could help affected children learn to overcome those difficulties.

Acknowledgments. The research was supported by the Wellcome Trust and the Child Growth Foundation. Compilation of the national register of TS was supported by the British Society for Paediatric Endocrinology and by Pharmacia Ltd. Specific assistance was given by Elinore Percy, Sarah Cave, Anne O'Herlihy, Rikki South, Jennifer Smith, Gina Aamodt-Leeper, Catharine Creswell, Rhona McGurk, Rowena James, Paola Dalton, Brian Coppin, Monique Bacarese-Hamilton, Monica Power, and David Robinson. Marcus Pembrey provided many valuable insights. We are grateful to all those pediatric consultants who assisted with the recruitment of patients, and to the schools who participated. The cytogenetic analyses were undertaken at the Wessex Regional Genetics Laboratories, Salisbury, Wiltshire under the direction of Professor P.A. Jacobs. Finally, we thank especially all the subjects of our investigation and their families for the time they generously gave to us.

References

1. Rovet JF, Ireland L. The behavioural phenotype in children with Turner syndrome. Ped Psychol 1994;19:779–90.
2. McCauley E, Kay T, Ito J, Trader R. The Turner syndrome: cognitive deficits, affective discrimination and behavior problems. Child Dev 1987;58:464–73.
3. McCauley E, Ross JL, Kushner H, Cutler G. Self-esteem and behavior in girls with Turner syndrome. Dev Behav Pediatr 1995;16:82–88.
4. Downey J, Elkin EJ, Erhardt AA, Meyer-Bahlburg M, Bell J, Morishima A. Cognitive ability and everyday functioning in women with Turner syndrome. J Learn Dis 1991;24:32–39.
5. Downey J, Ehrhardt AA, Gruen R, Morishima A, Bell J. Turner syndrome versus constitutional short stature: psychopathology and reactions to height. In: Stabler B, Underwood LE, eds. Slow grows the child: psychosocial aspects of growth delay. Hillsdale, NJ: Lawrence Erlbaum Associates, 1986:123–38.
6. McCauley E, Ito J, Kay T. Psychosocial functioning in girls with the Turner syndrome and short stature. J Am Acad Child Psychiatr 1986;25:105–12.
7. Shaffer J. A specific cognitive deficit observed in gonadal aplasia (Turner's syndrome). J Clin Psychol 1962;18:403–6.
8. Wechsler D. Wechsler Preschool and Primary Scales of Intelligence—revised. San Antonio: Psychological Corporation, 1989.
9. Wechsler D. Wechsler Intelligence Scale for Children—Third UK edition. Sidcup, Kent: Psychological Corporation, 1992.
10. Ross JL, Kushner H, Zinn AR. Discriminant analysis of the Ullrich-Turner syndrome neurocognitive profile. Am J Med Genet 1997;72:275–80.
11. Harris DB. Children's drawings as measures of intellectual maturity: a revision and extension of the Goodenough Draw-A-Man Test. New York: Harcourt, Brace and World, 1963.
12. Waber DP, Holmes JM. Assessing children's memory productions of the Rey-Osterrieth complex figure. J Clin Exp Neuropsychol 1986;8:563–80.
13. Stroop JR. Studies of interference in serial verbal reactions. J Exp Psychol 1935;18:643–62.
14. Welsh MC. Rule-guided behaviour and self-monitoring on the Tower of Hanoi disk transfer task. Cog Dev 1991;6:59–76.
15. Temple CM, Carney TA, Mullarkey S. Frontal lobe function and executive skills in children with Turner's syndrome. Dev Neuropsychol 1996;12:343–63.
16. Collins AL, Lockwell AE, Jacobs PA, Dennis NR. A comparison of the clinical and cytogenetic findings in 9 patients with a ring (X) cell line and 16 45,X patients. J Med Genet 1994;31:528–33.
17. Temple CM, Carney RA. Reading skills in children with Turner's syndrome: an analysis of hyperlexia. Cortex 1996;31:109–18.
18. Temple CM, Carney RA. Intellectual functioning in children with Turner's syndrome: a comparison of behavioral phenotypes. Dev Med Child Neurol 1993;35:691–98.
19. Salbenblatt JA, Meyers DC, Bender B, Linden M, Robinson A. Gross and fine motor development in 45,X and 47XXX girls. Pediatrics 1989;84:678–87.
20. Temple CM, Carney RA. Patterns of spatial functioning in Turner's syndrome. Cortex 1995;31:109–18.

21. Netley C, Rovet J. Atypical hemispheric lateralization in Turner syndrome subjects. Cortex 1982;18:377–84.
22. Jacobs PA, Betts PR, Cockwell AE, Crolla JA, Mackenzie MJ, Robinson DO, et al. A cytogenetic and molecular reappraisal of a series of patients with Turner's syndrome. Ann Hum Gen 1990;54:209–23.
23. Lyon MF. X-chromosome inactivation. Pinpointing the centre. Nature 1996;379:116–17.
24. Achenbach TM. Manual for the child behavior checklist/4–18 and 1991 profile. Burlington, VT: Department of Psychiatry, University of Vermont, 1991a.
25. Achenbach TM. Manual for the teacher's report form and 1991 profile. Burlington, VT: Department of Psychiatry, University of Vermont, 1991c.
26. Achenbach TM. Manual for the youth self-report form and 1991 profile. Burlington, VT: Department of Psychiatry, University of Vermont, 1991b.
27. Skuse D, Percy EL, Stevenson J. Psychosocial functioning in the Turner syndrome: a national survey. In: Stabler B, Underwood L. eds. Growth, stature, and adaptation. Behavioral, social, and cognitive aspects of growth delay. Chapel Hill: University of North Carolina Press, 1994:151–64.
28. Wechsler D. Wechsler Adult Intelligence Scales—revised. New York: Psychological Corporation, 1986.
29. Damasio AR. On some functions of the human prefrontal cortex. Proc New York Acad Sci 1995;769:241–51.
30. Pennington BF, Ozonoff S. Executive functions and developmental psychopathology. J Child Psychol Psychiatr 1996;37:51–87.
31. Manly T, Robertson IH, Anderson V, Nimmo-Smith I. The test of everyday attention for children (TEACh). Bury St. Edmunds, U.K.: Thames Valley Test Company, 1998.
32. Thurstone L. Primary mental abilities. Chicago: University of Chicago Press, 1938.
33. Grant DA, Berg EA. A behavioral analysis of degree of reinforcement and ease of shifting to new responses in Weigl-type card sorting problems. J Exp Psychol 1948; 38:404–11.
34. Shallice T. Specific impairments of planning. Phil Trans Roy Soc London, series B, 1982;298:199–209.
35. Borys SV, Spitz HH, Dorans BA. Tower of Hanoi performance of retarded young adults and nonretarded children as a function of solution length and goal state. J Exp Child Psychol 1982;33:87–110.
36. Rabbitt PMA. Introduction to methodologies and models in the study of executive function. In: Rabbitt P.M.A., ed. Methodologies of frontal and executive function. Hove: Psychology Press, 1997:1–38.
37. Jacobs PA, Dalton P, James R, Mosse K, Power M, Robinson D, et al. Turner syndrome: a cytogenetic and molecular study. Ann Hum Genet, 1997;61:471–83.
38. Tsuchiya K, Reijo R, Page DC, Disteche CM. Gonadoblastoma: molecular definition of the susceptibility region on the Y chromosome. Am J Hum Genet 1995;57:1400–7.
39. Freeman JV, Cole TJ, Chin S, Jones PRM, White EM, Preece MA. Cross-sectional stature and weight reference curves for the UK, 1990. Arch Dis Child 1995; 73:17–24.
40. Boyce L, Cole T. Castlemead Growth Program. Welwyn Garden City: Castlemead Publications, 1993.

41. Hassold T, Pettay D, Robinson A, Uchida I. Molecular studies of parental origin and mosaicism in 45,X conceptuses. Hum Genet 1992;89:647–52.
42. Pennington BF, Heaton RK, Karzmark P, Pendleton MG, Lehman R, Shucard DW. The neuropsychological phenotype in Turner syndrome. Cortex 1985;21:391–404.
43. Skuse DH, James RS, Bishop DVM, Coppins B, Dalton P, Aamodt-Leeper G, et al. Evidence from Turner's syndrome of an imprinted X-linked locus affecting cognitive function. Nature 1997;387:705–8.

9

Standards of Care Needed to Optimize Outcomes for Turner Syndrome

MARGARET H. MACGILLIVRAY AND TOM MAZUR

Comprehensive guidelines for optimizing the outcomes for girls with Turner syndrome (TS) have been proposed (1–8). Much credit is owed to the advocacy positions taken by the TS Societies and their strong endorsement of clinical studies carried out by pediatric endocrinologists, psychologists, and geneticists. These collaborative efforts have resulted in significant advances in our understanding of the scope of the problems that may be encountered by girls with TS. They have also, led to the development of effective new treatment strategies. Credit must also be given to the parents of these children without whom our knowledge base would be incomplete.

This chapter focuses on those standards of care that enhance outcomes in girls with TS. Three areas will be discussed: medical, educational, and psychosocial. All three have one thing in common (i.e., the requirements for early diagnosis using accurate cytogenetic analyses). Without this information, the guidelines would not be implemented and the opportunity would be lost to assist with growth augmenting therapies, educational guidance, and emotional support in the early childhood years. Diagnosis at a late age undermines the beneficial potential of the proposed guidelines. Although much progress has been made in developing treatment strategies, we must acknowledge that the proposals represent a "work in progress" since many outcome measures are still being analyzed.

Medical Guidelines

Early diagnosis of TS is most likely when obvious signs are present in infancy. Features such as lymphedema, web neck, low posterior hairline, cubitus valgus, and hypoplastic nails occur in more than 60% of girls with 45,X karyotype. A significant proportion of infant females with TS have subtle or negligible physical characteristics and are likely to be diagnosed later in life because of short stature or primary amenorrhea and absence of breast development. Often these girls have a different karyotype (X/XX, isochromosomes or deletions) but the genotype–phenotype correlations have not been fully elucidated.

Sex chromosome analysis should be performed on all short girls with unexplained growth failure and in girls with delayed adolescence and elevated gonadotropins. During infancy, karyotypes should be done in girls with lymphedema, nuchal folds, left sided cardiac anomalies (coarctation and hypoplastic left heart), and other characteristics of the syndrome (low posterior hairline, ptosis, small mandible, cubitus valgus). Peripheral blood karyotype is usually sufficient, but skin fibroblasts are occasionally needed for chromosome analysis if standard tests are noncontributory. Approximately 50% of girls with TS have 45,X karyotype; in 80% of these females, the X is derived from the mother. The remaining 50% of girls with TS have either mosaicism and/or X deletions, ring X, or fragments. Additional genetic tests to check for Y-specific DNA sequences are required if virilization or an unknown marker chromosome is present (9–13). These tests include DNA hybridization, polymerase chain reaction, or fluorescent in situ hybridization.

A majority of girls with TS have relatively good health with the exception that they are at increased risk for diseases that involve specific organs and tissues: mainly skeletal/orthopedic, ear, cardiac, renal, thyroid, vision and lymphedema.

The clinical characteristics of 45,X TS are outlined in Table 9.1. Cardiac and renal malformations, lymphedema, and web neck are less frequent in girls with TS and X/XX karyotype, X deletions, or isochromosomes (2). The frequency of TS is approximately 1 in 2,000 live born females, thus, it is similar to that of growth hormone (GH) deficiency (1 in 4,000 for males and females).

Growth/Skeletal

The most common consequence of TS is growth failure during childhood (98%) which if untreated, leads to adult heights that are 88% of the mean height for the country of origin. This translates to a 20 cm adult height deficit (14). In the United States, the mean adult height for untreated TS is 143–144 cm compared with control females whose mean adult height is 163.7 cm (15,16). The growth disorder starts in intrauterine life followed by a period of relatively normal growth velocity in the first 2–3 years; subsequently, there is gradual growth deceleration in childhood coupled with absence of the growth spurt during the adolescent years. Previous attempts with androgens or estrogens to augment heights resulted in short-term gains without any significant impact on final heights. Growth hormone treatment has been proven to be the only effective safe means of improving childhood as well as adult heights in TS (17–30). The height gains, however, have been variable

TABLE 9.1. Frequency of physical features in Turner syndrome with 45,X karyotype.

Growth/skeletal	Percentage
Short stature	98
Cubitus valgum	45–75
Short metacarpals	37–65
Webbed neck	25–65
Low posterior hairline	42–80
Short neck	44–80
Scoliosis	13
Abnormal upper-to-lower ratio	90
Lymphedema	20
Nail dysplasia	13
Gonadal dysgenesis/gonadal failure	86–94
infertility	99
Otitis media/hearing loss	50–80
conductive/sensorineural	45–70
Eye/ptosis/strabismus	30–40
Cardiovascular anomalies	20–30
hypertension	15–20
Renal anomalies	30–40
Autoimmune thyroiditis/hypothyroidism	10–30
Carbohydrate intolerance	40

Adapted from References 1, 2, and 3; higher percentage of ranges shown indicate incidence in 45,X TS.

with some girls showing greater responsivity than others. In addition, the beneficial effects of GH on adult heights have been shown to correlate positively with early onset and longer duration of treatment, larger doses of growth hormone and later introduction of estrogen replacement (see Chapter 7). The etiology of the height deficit in TS has been recently attributed to absence of the SHOX gene located in the pseudoautosomal region of the X chromosome (31).

Apart from slow skeletal growth, which is almost universally observed in girls with TS, there is also an increased risk of orthopedic problems that include congenital hip dislocation, hip dysplasia, scoliosis, kyphosis, dislocation of patella, arthritis (rheumatoid and other forms), and adult onset degenerative hip disease secondary to hip dysplasia/congenital hip dislocation (2).

The incidence and severity of osteoporosis in TS are not well defined. An increased prevalence of osteopenia and reduced bone mass have been reported in TS during childhood as well as adulthood (32–34). It is not clear, however, whether the bone findings are identical to those observed in estrogen-deficient postmenopausal women or whether they represent a bone dysplasia related to the chromosome abnormality. Most studies also did not adjust the measurement of bone mineral density (BMD) for height, and without incorporation of this variable, there is an underestimation of bone mass. Studies have documented improved BMD in GH treated girls with TS (36,37).

It is now reasonable to expect that early GH treatment and age-appropriate estrogen replacement will improve the chances of attaining normal peak bone mass in early adulthood measured by dual photon absorptiometry (DEXA) adjusted for height.

It is interesting that an increased risk of hip fractures and loss of height have not been reported in women with TS (2,33). The only exception is the report of increased frequency of wrist fractures in girls with TS who had normal BMD (35).

More extensive longitudinal research is needed in order to establish which treatment strategies during childhood and adulthood are most likely to result in the attainment and maintenance of normal BMD in TS. Current guidelines include regular clinical evaluation of joints and spine especially during treatment periods that accelerate growth, good nutrition, adequate daily intake of calcium (1000–1500 mg), and vitamin D (400 U/day), incorporation of at least 30 minutes of weight-bearing exercise daily, avoidance of smoking, maintenance of normal weight for height and compliance with estrogen replacement throughout adolescence and adulthood. We have yet to identify what is optimal estrogen therapy in TS (i.e., what dose, which estrogen, which delivery method—oral, transdermal—will prove to be the most effective and safe treatment?) The need exists for a multicenter study that addresses these questions and provides us with information not presently available.

Newer agents that are agonists to the estrogen receptor beta are likely to be additional therapies for maximizing bone mass and skeletal health. When should BMD be measured in TS? Because health insurance companies are unwilling to pay for DEXA studies, it is necessary to restrict their use until we have established guidelines. Baseline measurement at approximately 20 years of age will provide information concerning peak bone mass. The timing of subsequent measurements will depend on this reading. Girls with TS should be informed early in childhood that life-long estrogen replacement is necessary for sexual maturation as well as skeletal well being in order to improve compliance during adulthood.

Gonadal Dysgenesis

Ovarian failure, a dominant characteristic in TS, requires that decisions be made concerning the timing and doses of estrogen replacement in the second decade. Estrogen replacement is currently introduced between 13 and 15 years, depending on the patient's interest in starting breast development and the relative importance given to achieving maximal adult height (38). Estrogen therapy is seldom begun before the bone age reaches 11 years. Initiation of growth hormone treatment at an early age will ideally give these girls the opportunity to have sexual maturation at an age compatible with their peers. Opinions differ on the possible negative impact of low doses of estrogens on the pace of bone maturation and final height (30). The choices of estrogen treatment have mainly been conjugated estrogens (0.3 mg/day) or estradiol (100 ng/kg/day or less). Extremely low dose depot or transdermal estradiol have been proposed as alternatives that may facilitate improved growth without advancing bone maturation (39). Controlled studies using these newer strategies have not been performed. Introduction of cyclic estrogen–progesterone treatment will depend on which estrogen regimen is used initially; in general, cyclic treatment is begun soon after onset of first vaginal bleeding.

Spontaneous onset of puberty has been reported in 14% of 45,X girls and 32% of girls with cell lines containing more than one X (40). Uterine volume by ultrasound exam and gonadotropin levels are the most reliable predictors of duration of ovarian function (41). Over time, most girls with spontaneous puberty will develop ovarian failure and require estrogen and progesterone treatment for menses and protection from osteoporosis. TS girls with persistence of menses may have germ cells and be capable of reproduction. In one study of 84 girls with TS and spontaneous menarche, three patients (3.6%) became pregnant, and a chromosomal abnormality and congenital malformations were present in two of the three offspring (40). Hence, encouragement of oocyte preservation or spontaneous pregnancy is a debatable issue because of the increased risk for chromosomal abnormalities and congenital malformations in offspring. In vitro fertilization with donor oocytes or adoption are alternative ways in which women with TS have families. Although much has been written about the adverse effects of early estrogen treatment on adult height of TS girls receiving GH treatment, there is no convincing data that adult heights are compromised by spontaneous puberty.

Pelvic ultrasound and measurement of gonadotropin levels are most informative after approximately 10 years of age (41). TS girls with high gonadotropin and/or irregular menses should receive estrogen and progesterone replacement in order to avoid the risk of endometrial hyperplasia and the development of ovarian cysts and torsion. TS girls with Y chromosome material should have bilateral gonadectomy to protect them from gonadoblastoma (42,43).

Otitis Media/Hearing Loss

Hearing loss due to conductive or sensorineural problems is strongly associated with TS and may escape detection unless included as a routine component of overall medical care (44–46). During childhood, ear disease is the major cause of morbidity in TS; the problems include chronic or recurrent otitis media (80%), middle ear effusions (45%), myringotomy and tube placement (50%) and hearing loss (73%; 36% pure conductive, 14% pure sensorineural, and 14% mixed). Only 27% of girls in one study had normal hearing (45). Sclerotic mastoids were detected in 50% of girls in this study. Downward sloping of the external auditory canals were observed using coronal CT scans in some patients but ossicular malformations were not found. The factors responsible for the hearing loss are still largely unexplained. In general, ear infections occur most often during childhood but may persist into the second decade. Mastoiditis and/or cholesteatoma may develop. Vigorous medical treatment and annual objective hearing tests are recommended when indicated by physical examination or history in order to monitor for hearing loss throughout childhood and adolescence.

In adult women with TS, hearing impairment has been documented with remarkably high prevalence (50–80%). It is generally accepted that the conductive hearing loss in girls with TS results from chronic otitis media during childhood. Sensorineural hearing loss however, is also more common in women with TS compared to the general population and was not correlated with recurrent otitis media in one study. This prompted the author to speculate that sensorineural hearing loss might be due to the X chromosome abnormality, but this has not been confirmed. In 80 TS women, ages 15–69 years, Huetcrantz and Sylven reported that the main cause of hearing loss was a sensorineural defect (i.e., in 45% of those 15–34 years old and in 68% of those older than 35 years) (46). The severity of the sensorineural hearing loss increased each decade and indicated a premature aging of the ear. On average, Turner women, age 30–39 years, were observed to have the same hearing level as control women, age 60–69 years. The earliest predictor of future deafness was a typical sensorineural dip in the midfrequency range (1.5–2 kHz) that progressed over time to also include losses in the high frequency ranges. The latter resulted in severe social deafness. The mean magnitude of the hearing loss in the nadir of the sensorineural dip was 40 dB before 35 years and 50 dB after 35 years in TS women. Hearing disability was often not recognized by the patient, and, when finally identified, had already caused social problems. In this study, 27.3% of TS women older than 35 years required a hearing aid, compared with 3% of the control population. Prior to 35 years, the need for a hearing aid in TS women was still higher than the control population (6.3 vs. 3%, respectively). The message from this study is that identifying hearing loss early and providing a hearing aid when indicated are practical and essential components of health care that have a profound impact on the social life of women with TS (46).

Eye

Approximately 30–40% of girls with TS will have an ocular abnormality—mainly, strabismus, amblyopia, or ptosis. An ophthalmologist should evaluate vision at diagnosis, and the assessments subsequently should be repeated annually depending on the findings (8,47–49).

Cardiovascular

Congenital cardiovascular malformations have been observed in 26% of girls with TS; aortic valve abnormalities accounted for 18% (bicuspid, stenosed or incompetent aortic valve), and aortic coarctation occurred in 10%. Bicuspid aortic valve predisposes the TS patient to valvular stenosis, insufficiency, and aortic root dilation with advancing age. There is also an increased risk of infective endocarditis. Less common heart anomalies include pulmonic stenosis (in 45,X patients only) and partial anomalous pulmonary venous drainage. Sudden death from dissection of the aorta is a catastrophic rare cause of mortality in women with TS. The prevalence and severity of the heart malformations are closely linked to the karyotype; 38% of 45,X TS had cardiovascular abnormalities compared with only 11% in girls with mosaic TS (2,50,51).

Cardiac examination, including electrocardiogram and Doppler echocardiography, or MRI, to include evaluation of the aorta, are recommended for all girls with TS at diagnosis and subsequently at yearly intervals if an abnormality is identified. When no lesion is found, Doppler echocardiography should be done every 2 years to monitor the width of the aortic root. Increasing aortic root width may be an early predictor of aortic dissection. Prophylactic antibiotic treatment is necessary for protection against subacute bacterial endocarditis if a heart lesion is detected.

Kidney

Renal anomalies are present in approximately one-third of females with TS, including horseshoe kidney, duplicated renal pelvis, malrotation, renal ectopia, or vascular anomalies (3). Renal ultrasound should be performed at diagnosis and once or twice yearly if a horseshoe kidney is identified because of the increased risk of Wilm's tumor. Renal function tests and urine cultures should be periodically monitored if indicated. Blood pressure measurements should be made at each visit because hypertension may develop in the absence of cardiac or renal abnormalities (3,5).

Autoimmune and Inflammatory Disorders

The most common autoimmune disease in TS is Hashimoto's thyroiditis, which causes hypothyroidism in 10–30% of patients (52). The prevalence increases with age with peak incidence around 15 years, after which a plateau is seen. Most patients have no symptoms or signs. Antithyroid antibodies are positive in as many as 50–85% of girls with TS depending on the series; their presence is predictive of thyroid dysfunction after age 10 years but not earlier. Once thyroid antibodies are detected, there is no reason to repeat the tests. Hypothyroidism may develop in TS in the absence of thyroid antibodies. Thyroid function (T4, TSH, thyroid antibodies) should be monitored at diagnosis and every 1–2 years.

Less common autoimmune diseases are rheumatoid arthritis, myasthenia gravis, vitiligo, alopecia, hypoparathyroidism, and Addison's Disease.

Inflammatory bowel disease, giant cell hepatitis, intestinal telangiectasia, Crohn's disease, and ulcerative colitis appear to occur with higher frequency and severity in TS. Early diagnosis and treatment of bowel disease has been recommended because of the higher mortality when bowel surgery is done late in the course of inflammatory bowel disease.

Glucose Intolerance

Peripheral insulin resistance and hyperinsulinemia are defects in carbohydrate metabolism that develop during childhood in TS. With increasing age and/or excess weight gain, the prevalence of glucose intolerance increases (53–55). Treatment with GH and oxandrolone in higher doses aggravates the hyperinsulinemia seen in TS (55–56). The defect in glucose homeostasis resembles that seen in Type II diabetes mellitus in that there is no evidence of an immunologic disorder (i.e., islet cell antibodies or HLA linkage) nor any tendency to develop ketones. In adult women with TS, there is a high incidence of Type 2 diabetes mellitus (57,58). Maintaining normal body weight throughout life is an important goal because the tendency to hyperinsulinemia and insulin resistance are worsened by obesity. Newer therapies aimed at reducing the stress on the beta cell and improving the peripheral actions of insulin may help to reduce the incidence of Type 2 diabetes mellitus.

Lymphedema

Lymphedema over the dorsum of the hands and feet is seen in approximately 40% of girls with TS; it is most prevalent in the neonatal and infancy period and usually resolves (1–6). Lymphedema occasionally recurs during adolescence after introduction of estrogen treatment. Support hose may help; also, overly constricting shoes and kneesocks should be avoided. Diuretic therapy is not indicated. The problem is due to a congenital defect in lymphatic development. Recurrent sudden severe cellulitis has occasionally been observed in girls with TS. Aggressive use of intravenous antibiotic therapy may be necessary. Prophylaxis with once daily penicillin treatment in two girls prevented recurrence (Faden, MacGillivray, unpublished manuscript).

Skin, Keloids, Nevi

The tendency to develop keloid scars is high in girls with TS; if surgery is needed, the patient should be informed about this potential outcome. Also, women with TS may develop premature wrinkling (1–6).

Pigmented nevi are commonly observed in girls with TS and they increase during adolescence and adulthood. Melanoma is not more frequent in TS. Nevi seldom cause problems apart from cosmetic concerns, but if they are constantly being rubbed by clothing, removal is advised.

Educational Issues

Educational competence is influenced in many ways by the psychosocial/behavioral characteristics of TS. The behavioral difficulties include immaturity, inattention, inability to concentrate, hyperactivity, nervousness, tendency to daydreaming, and an inclination to act young and to seek younger friends. Memory and recall skills may be affected (60–63).

Learning difficulties are more prevalent in girls with TS because they tend to have impairment of nonverbal, cognitive abilities. They specifically may have disabilities relating to visual–perceptual, visual–motor, and visual–spatial tasks. They are also more likely to have impairments involving numerical computational skills, working memory, and executive functioning capabilities (60). Numerous studies confirm that even though verbal skills in TS are normal, nonverbal performance scores are lower. The impaired nonverbal cognitive skills have been attributed to a multifocal or diffuse right cerebral hemisphere dysfunction (62). As a group, girls with TS are more likely to have failed a grade in school.

Thorough educational assessment should be made in the preschool years or at diagnosis. Every effort should be made in the school environment to develop and strengthen visual–spatial and visual motor skills. Girls with TS should be tested for accuracy and speed of performance of computational tasks and increased time allotted when indicated. Remediation with self-cognitive modeling and cognitive behavior rehearsals have helped TS girls to improve interpersonal relationships and attention span. Rovet has recommended that during the performance of a task, the girl with TS should simultaneously verbalize the problem-solving strategy in order to incorporate the stronger verbal skills into the remediation process (60). For example, math teaching should be presented verbally to capitalize on the verbal strengths of TS girls. Intensive fact training should also be emphasized early in childhood until number facts become automatic and readily accessible.

Whether the visual–spatial cognitive defects seen in TS are due to hormonal deficiencies or to neuromaturational abnormalities is unknown; the latter seems to be the more likely cause. Ross and colleagues reported positive effects of estrogen replacement on psychological well-being in girls with TS and Rovet observed a beneficial influence of height gain during GH treatment (63,64).

Psychosocial Issues

Much has been written about the behavioral and psychosocial problems in girls with TS. It is important to emphasize that 24% of TS girls tested had no social problems and this figure may be higher given the nonparticipation of TS patients who may escape diagnosis because they have subtle or negligible features of the syndrome (60). In addition, 71% of a large group of girls with TS (60) were unaffected behaviorally. Taller stature in TS correlated with better social competence, but not with other behavioral problems. Chromosome complement predicted behavior problems in one study (i.e., greater risk of behavioral problems were observed in TS girls who had the presence of a ring X,Y chromosome material or an X deletion) (65).

The psychosocial problems identified in TS include less social competence, more immaturity, hyperactivity, difficulties processing facial affect, extreme shyness, lack of restraint, fewer activities, less time spent with friends, less ability to get along with friends, preference for acting younger and having younger friends, and an increased tendency to be nervous and highly strung (60,61).

In adulthood, women with TS are more likely to have delayed or infrequent dating, delayed initiation of sexual activities, and less likely to live independently, to be married, or to be sexually active. In the workplace, women with TS have been observed to be overqualified for the position held, and they ae characterized by limited emotional arousal, high tolerance for adversity, unassertive behavior, and a tendency for overcompliance (1–5).

Specific recommendations have been made concerning how best to enhance the lives of girls with TS. Earlier diagnosis is of critical importance. At diagnosis, an assessment must be made of psychosocial skills, intellectual strengths, motor abilities, and level of maturity. This preferably should be done before entering kindergarten. Intervention should be initiated early to improve social skills and interpersonal involvement. Parents should be educated about ways in which they can enhance their daughters' ability to socialize and mature. Parents may need help to curb a natural inclination to be overprotective, which worsens clinging behavior. Information about the potential learning problems associated with TS must be shared with parents at diagnosis.

Remedial treatment must be provided for learning disabilities if they exist because this can be a major reason for delaying independent living and achieving successful careers. Girls with TS need to be given information on all aspects of their condition at an early age, and sex education must be provided at an appropriate age. At present, it is a realistic goal to achieve sufficient height in the first decade in order to begin estrogen treatment at the usual age for puberty. It is likely that this achievement will have a significant beneficial impact on the psychosocial adjustment of girls with TS.

The most profound psychosocial benefits come from support groups that have been established through the TS Societies in different countries. In our own center, we have had a long-standing partnership with psychologists who work alongside us in our clinic. Together we have developed a program that provides a social as well as medical focus. This is accomplished by having a Turner clinic that provides medical care in the first 2 hours followed by a social program that allows the girls to meet in a nearby room while the parents get together in an adjacent area. The parents bring in snacks and arrange for fun activities in order for the children to develop friendships. For the first time, we have been told by our TS girls that they look forward to seeing their friends at the next clinic and some families have arranged for social outings for their children. The atmosphere is very interactive and cheerful. We hold these Turner clinics every 3 months and see about 30 girls each time. This arrangement has been a practical way to use clinic time to enhance social interchange and foster a family support network. The newsletter from our Children's Growth Foundation, a local parent support group, provides informational material on many of the medical and psychological issues of importance to families and girls with TS.

Pediatric endocrinologists and all primary care physicians can impact favorably on the self-esteem of girls with TS by providing positive reinforcement and by avoiding exposing them to stigmatizing experiences. The physical features of TS should not be pointed out to residents and students in the presence of the patient and family. Slides and photographs can be used as teaching aids, thereby protecting young girls from having their physical characteristics repeatedly discussed in the presence of unfamiliar physicians.

All families should be provided with the excellent monographs on TS and should be encouraged to join the TS Society and to participate in their annual meetings. The address is:

Turner's Syndrome Society of the United States
1313 SE Fifth Street, Suite 327
Minneapolis, MN 55414
(800/365-9944) http://www.turner-syndrome-us.org

Turner's Syndrome Society
814 Glencairn Avenue
North York, Ontario M6B 2A3
Canada
Phone: 416/781-2086
416/718-7245
800/465-6744

References

1. Nielsen J. What more can be done for girls and women with Turner's syndrome and their parents? Acta Paediatr Scand 1989;356(suppl):93–100.
2. Hall JG, Gilchrist DM. Turner syndrome and its variants. Pediatr Clin N Am 1990;37:1421–40.
3. Lippe B. Turner syndrome. Endocrinol Metab Clin N Am 1991;20:121–51.
4. Saenger P. The current status of diagnosis and therapeutic intervention in Turner syndrome. J Clin Endocrinol Metab 1993;77:297–301.
5. Rosenfeld R, Tesch L-G, Rodriguez-Rigau LJ, McCauley E, Albertsson-Wikland K, Asch R, et al. Recommendations for diagnosis, treatment, and management of individuals with Turner syndrome. Endocrinologist 1994;4:351–58.
6. Committee on Genetics, Academy of Pediatrics. Health supervision for children with Turner syndrome. Pediatrics 1995;96:1166–73.
7. Sybert VP. The adult patient with Turner syndrome. In: Albertsson-Wikland K, Ranke MB, eds. Turner syndrome in a life span perspective: research and clinical aspects. Amsterdam: Elsevier Science Publishers, 1995:205–18.
8. Doherty L, Brown DM, Ainslie M, Eugster E, Hirsch B, Kashtan C, et al. Turner syndrome practice guidelines. Endocrinologist 1997;7:443–47.

9. Page DC. Hypothesis: a Y-chromosome gene causes gonadoblastoma in dysgenetic gonads. Development 1987;101(suppl):151–55.
10. Page DC. Y chromosome sequences in Turner syndrome and risk of gonadoblastoma or virilization. Lancet 1994:343:240.
11. Kocova M, Siegel SF, Lee PA, Trucco M. Detection of Y chromosome sequences in Turner syndrome by Southern blot analyses of amplified DNA. Lancet 1993; 342:140–43.
12. Kocova M, Witchel SF, Nalesnik M, Lee PA, Dickman PS, MacGillivray MH, et al. Y chromosomal sequences identified in gonadal tissue of two 45,X patients with Turner syndrome. Endocrinol Pathol 1996;6:311–21.
13. Binder G, Koch A, Wajs E, Ranke MB. Evaluation of "hidden Y-chromosome" in Turner syndrome (TS): a review of screening results. In: Albertsson-Wikland K, Ranke MB, eds. Turner syndrome in a life span perspective: Research and clinical aspects. Amsterdam: Elsevier Science Publishers, 1995:25–32.
14. Rochiccioli P, David M, Malpuech G, Colle M, Limal JM, Battin J, et al. Study of final height in Turner syndrome: ethnic and genetic influences. Acta Pediatr 1994;83:305–8.
15. Hamill PVV, Drizd TA, Johnson CL, Reed RB, Roche AF, Moore WM. Physical growth: National Center for Health Statistics percentiles. Am J Clin Nutrition 1979;32:607–29.
16. Lippe BM, Plotnick LP, Attie KM, Frane J. Growth in Turner syndrome: updating the United States experience. In: Hibi I, Takano K, eds. Basic and clinical approach to Turner syndrome. Amsterdam: Elsevier Science Publishers, 1993:77–82.
17. Rosenfeld RG, Attie K, Frane J, Johanson A and the Genentech Study Group. Turner syndrome: optimizing treatment for short stature. In: Albertsson-Wikland K, Ranke MB, eds. Turner syndrome in a life span perspective: research and clinical aspects. Amsterdam: Elsevier Science Publishers, 1995:87–88.
18. Nilsson KO, Albertsson-Wikland K, Alm J, Aronson S, Gustafsson J, Hagenäs L, et al. Growth promoting treatment in girls with Turner syndrome: final height results according to three different Turner syndrome growth standards. In: Albertsson-Wikland K, Ranke MB, eds. Turner syndrome in a life span perspective: research and clinical aspects. Amsterdam: Elsevier Science Publishers, 1995:89–94.
19. Stahnke N, Attanasio A, van den Broeck J, Partsch CJ, Zeisel HJ. GH treatment studies to final height in girls with Turner syndrome—the German experience. In: Albertsson-Wikland K, Ranke MB, eds. Turner syndrome in a life span perspective: research and clinical aspects. Amsterdam: Elsevier Science Publishers, 1995:95–104.
20. Werther GA, Dietsch S. Multicentre trial of synthetic growth hormone and low dose oestrogen in Turner syndrome: analysis of final height. In: Albertsson-Wikland K, Ranke MB, eds. Turner syndrome in a life span perspective: research and clinical aspects. Amsterdam: Elsevier Science Publishers, 1995:105–12.
21. Takano K, Ogawa M, Okada Y, Tanaka T, Tachibana K, Hizuka N, et al. Final height and long-term effects after growth hormone therapy in Turner syndrome: results of a 6-year multicentre study in Japan. In: Albertsson-Wikland K, Ranke MB, eds. Turner syndrome in a life span perspective: research and clinical aspects. Amsterdam: Elsevier Science Publishers, 1995:113–22.
22. Rochiccioli P, Chaussain JL. Final height in patients with Turner syndrome treated with growth hormone (n = 117). In: Albertsson-Wikland K, Ranke MB, eds. Turner

syndrome in a life span perspective: research and clinical aspects. Amsterdam: Elsevier Science Publishers, 1995:123–28.

23. The Italian Study Group for Turner syndrome (ISGTS). Spontaneous growth and results of growth hormone therapy in patients with Turner syndrome. In: Albertsson-Wikland K, Ranke MB, eds. Turner syndrome in a life span perspective: research and clinical aspects. Amsterdam: Elsevier Science Publishers, 1995:129–36.
24. Heinrichs C, De Schepper J, Thomas M, Massa G, Craen M, Malvaux P, et al. Final height in 46 girls with Turner syndrome treated with growth hormone in Belgium: evaluation of height recovery and predictive factors. In: Albertsson-Wikland K, Ranke MB, eds. Turner syndrome in a life span perspective: research and clinical aspects. Amsterdam: Elsevier Science Publishers, 1995:137–48.
25. Tillmann V, Price DA, Bucknall JL, Clayton PE. Experience within the Manchester Growth Clinic of growth hormone treatment of girls with Turner syndrome: the influence of duration of treatment on final height. In: Albertsson-Wikland K, Ranke MB, eds. Turner syndrome in a life span perspective: research and clinical aspects. Amsterdam: Elsevier Science Publishers, 1995:149–54.
26. Massa G, van den Broeck, Attanasio A, Wit JM on behalf of the Lilly European Turner Study Group. In: Albertsson-Wikland K, Ranke MB, eds. Turner syndrome in a life span perspective: research and clinical aspects. Amsterdam: Elsevier Science Publishers, 1995:155–60.
27. Karlberg J, Albertsson-Wikland. Natural growth and aspects of growth standards in Turner syndrome. In: Albertsson-Wikland K, Ranke MB, eds. Turner syndrome in a life span perspective: research and clinical aspects. Amsterdam: Elsevier Science Publishers, 1995:75–86.
28. Ranke MB, Price DA, Maes M, Albertsson-Wikland K, Lindberg A. Factors influencing final height in Turner syndrome following GH treatment: results of the Kabi International Growth Study (KIGS). In: Albertsson-Wikland K, Ranke MB, eds. Turner syndrome in a life span perspective: research and clinical aspects. Amsterdam: Elsevier Science Publishers, 1995:161–66.
29. Hintz RL, Attie KM, Compton PG, Rosenfeld RG. Multifactorial studies of GH treatment of Turner syndrome: the Genentech national cooperative growth study. In: Albertsson-Wikland K, Ranke MB, eds. Turner syndrome in a life span perspective: research and clinical aspects. Amsterdam: Elsevier Science Publishers, 1995:167–74.
30. Attie KM, Chernausek S, Frane J, Rosenfeld RG for the Genentech Study Group. Growth hormone use in Turner syndrome; a preliminary report on the effect of early vs. delayed estrogen. In: Albertsson-Wikland K, Ranke MB, eds. Turner syndrome in a life span perspective: research and clinical aspects. Amsterdam: Elsevier Science Publishers, 1995:175–81.
31. Rao E, Weiss B, Fukami M, Rump A, Niesler B, Mertz A, et al. Pseudoautosomal deletions encompassing a novel homeobox gene cause growth failure in idiopathic short stature and Turner syndrome. Nat Genet 1997;16:54–63.
32. Rubin KR. Osteoporosis in Turner syndrome. In: Rosenfeld RG, Grumbach MM, eds. Turner Syndrome. New York: Marcel Dekker Publishers, 1990:301–17.
33. Bachrach LK. Osteopenis in Turner girls. In: Albertsson-Wikland K, Ranke MB, eds. Turner syndrome in a life span perspective: research and clinical aspects. Amsterdam: Elsevier Science Publishers, 1995:233–40.
34. Sylvén L, Hagenfeldt K, Ringertz H. Impact of hormonal replacement therapy on bone

mineral density in women with Turner syndrome. In: Albertsson-Wikland K, Ranke MB, eds. Turner syndrome in a life span perspective: research and clinical aspects. Amsterdam: Elsevier Science Publishers, 1995:241–48.
35. Ross JL, Meyerson LL, Feuillan P, Cassorla F, Cutler GB Jr. Normal bone density of the wrist and spine and increased wrist fractures in girls with Turner syndrome. J Clin Endocrinol Metab 1991;73:355–59.
36. Neely EK, Marcus R, Rosenfeld RG, Bachrach LK. Turner syndrome adolescents receiving growth hormone are not osteopenic. J Clin Endocrinol Metab 1993;76:861–66.
37. Kirkland RT, Lin T-H, LeBlanc AD, Kirkland JL. Effects of hormonal therapy on bone mineral density in Turner syndrome. In: Rosenfeld RG, Grumbach MM, eds. Turner syndrome. New York: Marcel Dekker Publishers, 1990:319–25.
38. Neely EK. Estrogen for feminization: a review. In: Albertsson-Wikland K, Ranke MB, eds. Turner syndrome in a life span perspective: research and clinical aspects. Amsterdam: Elsevier Science Publishers, 1995:219–26.
39. Rosenfield RL, Perovic N, Devine N, Mauras N, Moshang T, Root A, et al. Optimizing estrogen therapy for Turner syndrome. National Cooperative Growth Study Meeting abstract; 1997, p. 8, Sept. 25–28, Washington D.C.
40. Pasquino AM, Passeri F, Pucarelli I, Segni M, Municchi G on behalf of the Italian Study Group for Turner's Syndrome. Spontaneous pubertal development in Turner's syndrome. J Clin Endocrinol Metab 1997;82:1810–13.
41. Mezzanti L, Cacciari E, Bergamaschi R, Tassmari D, Magnani C, Perri A, et al. Pelvic ultrasonography in patients with Turner syndrome: age-related findings in different karyotypes. J Pediatr 1997;131:135–40.
42. Kocova M, Siegel SF, Wenger SL, Lee PA, Trucco M. Y chromosome sequences in Turner syndrome: detection by Southern blot analysis of amplified DNA. Lancet 1993;342:140–43.
43. Kocova K, Witchel S, Nalesnik M, Lee PA, Dickman PS, MacGillivray MH, et al. Y chromosomal sequences identified in gonadal tissue of two 45,X patients with Turner syndrome. Endocrine Pathol 1995;6:311–21.
44. Anderson H, Filipsson E, Fluur B. Hearing impairment in Turner's syndrome. Acta Otolaryngol 1969;247(suppl):1–26.
45. Sculerati N, Ledesma-Medina J, Finegold DN, Stool SE. Otitis media and hearing loss in Turner syndrome. Arch Otolaryngol Head Neck Surg 1990;116:704–7.
46. Hultcrantz M, Sylvén L. Hearing problems in women with Turner syndrome. In: Albertsson-Wikland K, Ranke MB, eds. Turner syndrome in a life span perspective: research and clinical aspects. Amsterdam: Elsevier Science Publishers, 1995:249–58.
47. Lessell S, Forbes AP. Eye signs in Turner's syndrome. Arch Ophthalmol 1966; 76:211–13.
48. Adhikary HP. Ocular manifestation of Turner's syndrome. Trans Ophthal Soc UK 1981;101:395–96.
49. Chrousos GA, Ross JL, Chrousos G, Chu F, Kenigsberg D, Cutler G, et al. Ocular findings in Turner syndrome: a prospective study. Ophthalmology 1984;91:926–28.
50. Mazzanti L, Prandstraller D, Tassinari D, Rubino I, Santucci S, Picchio M, et al. Heart disease in Turner's syndrome. Helv Paediat Acta 1988;43:25–31.
51. Krag-Olsen B, Gøtzsche C-O, Nielsen J, Sørensen KE, Kristensen BØ. Cardiovascular malformations in Turner syndrome. In: Albertsson-Wikland K, Ranke MB,

eds. Turner syndrome in a life span perspective: research and clinical aspects. Amsterdam: Elsevier Science Publishers, 1995:263–73.

52. Vanderscheuren-Lodeweyskx M. Autoimmunity problems in Turner syndrome. In: Albertsson-Wikland K, Ranke MB, eds. Turner syndrome in a life span perspective: research and clinical aspects. Amsterdam: Elsevier Science Publishers, 1995:267–74.
53. Neufeld ND, Lippe B, Sperling MA. Carbohydrate (CHO) intolerance in gonadal dysgenesis (GD): a new model of insulin resistance. Diabetes 1976;25(suppl):379.
54. Caprio S, Boulware S, Diamond M, Sherwin RS, Carpenter TO, Rubin K, et al. Insulin resistance: an early metabolic defect of Turner syndrome. J Clin Endocrinol Metab 1991;72:832–36.
55. Caprio S, Tamborlane WV. In vivo study on insulin action in children with Turner syndrome. In: Albertsson-Wikland K, Ranke MB, eds. Turner syndrome in a life span perspective: research and clinical aspects. Amsterdam: Elsevier Science Publishers, 1995:275–84.
56. Wilson DM, Frane JW, Sherman B, Johanson AJ, Hintz R, Rosenfeld RG, et al. Carbohydrate and lipid metabolism in Turner syndrome: effect of therapy with growth hormone, oxandrolone, and a combination of both. J Pediatr 1988; 112:210–17.
57. Forbes AP, Engel B. The high incidence of diabetes mellitus in 41 patients with gonadal dysgenesis and their close relatives. Metabolism 1963;12:420–36.
58. Nielson J, Johansen K, Yale H. The frequency of diabetes mellitus in patients with Turner syndrome and pure gonadal dysgenesis. Acta Endocrinol (Copenh) 1969; 62:251–58.
59. Rovet J, Netley C. Processing deficits in Turner syndrome. Dev Psychol 1982; 18:77–94.
60. Rovet JF. Behavioural manifestations of Turner syndrome in children: a unique phenotype? In: Albertsson-Wikland K, Ranke MB, eds. Turner syndrome in a life span perspective: research and clinical aspects. Amsterdam: Elsevier Science Publishers, 1995:285–96.
61. McCauley E, Kay T, Ito J, Trider R. The Turner syndrome: cognitive deficits, affective discrimination and behavior problems. Child Develop 1985;58:464–73.
62. Ross JL, Roeltgen D, Cutler GB Jr. The neurodevelopmental transition between childhood and adolescence in girls with Turner syndrome. In: Albertsson-Wikland K, Ranke MB, eds. Turner syndrome in a life span perspective: research and clinical aspects. Amsterdam: Elsevier Science Publishers, 1995:297–308.
63. Ross JL, McCauley E, Roeltgen D, Long L, Kushner H, Feuillan P, et al. Self-concept and behavior in adolescent girls with Turner syndrome: potential estrogen effects. J Clin Endocrinol Metab 1996;81:926–31.
64. Rovet J, Holland J. Psychological aspects of the Canadian randomized controlled trial if human growth hormone and low-dose enthinyl oestradiol in children with Turner syndrome. Horm Res 1993;39(suppl 2):60–64.
65. Stabler B, Clopper RR, Siegel PT, Stoppani CE, Compton PG. Behavior change in patients with Turner syndrome undergoing growth hormone therapy. In: Rovet JF, ed. Turner syndrome across the lifespan. Markham Ontario: Klein Graphics, 1994:81–90.

Part III

Treatment of Short, Non-Growth Hormone Deficiency: Efficacy, Innovation and Quality of Life

10

The Non-Growth Hormone-Deficient Child: Does Therapy with Growth Hormone Produce Benefit?

Louis E. Underwood and Brian Stabler

The availability of abundant supplies of recombinant human growth (GH) has made it possible to test the effects of GH treatment on short children with diagnoses other than GH deficiency. For example, treatment of girls with Turner Syndrome and children with chronic renal failure has been observed to accelerate rates of statural growth and to increase adult height (1,2). Despite improvement over the last 30–35 years in the tools used for determining the causes of short stature, no specific diagnosis is made in a large proportion of the short children who are brought to medical attention. These children are referred to as having "normal" short stature, idiopathic short stature, or are given one of a variety of other designations (Table 10.1). The number and nature of the mechanisms involved in the slow growth and short stature of these patients is not known.

This chapter focuses on those children whom we refer to here as having idiopathic short stature (ISS). They are more than two standard deviations (SD) below the mean for height: they may grow at a slow rate, they sometimes have relatively short parents; and they have no significant abnormalities in their medical history, physical examination, or laboratory tests that accounts for their shortness. The questions we will address are:

1. Do injections of exogenous growth hormone promote growth in these children?
2. Does prolonged GH therapy increase adult height?
3. Does prolonged treatment with GH produce psychological benefit?

TABLE 10.1. Designations applied to short children in whom the precise cause of the short stature is not known.

Non–GH-deficient short stature
Idiopathic short stature
Normal short stature
Normal-variant short stature
Familial short stature
Constitutional short stature
Constitutional growth delay

Do Injections of Exogenous Growth Hormone Promote Growth in Children with Idiopathic Short Stature?

Studies of the effects of exogenous GH in ISS children uniformly show that there is significant acceleration of statural growth in the short term (3–7). Starting with more than 200 children in the Kabi Pharmacia International Growth Study (KIGS), Albertsson-Wikland (7) reported that among 54 children with ISS completing 3 years of GH therapy, the median height SDS was raised from –2.5 to –1.5 (Fig. 10.1). This improvement in stature was judged to depend in part on the dose of

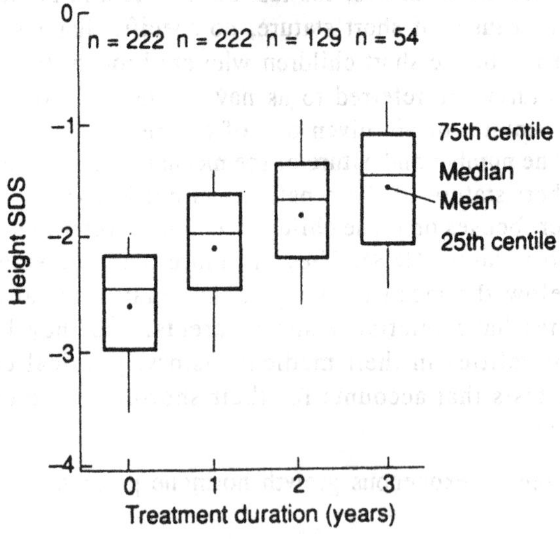

FIGURE 10.1. Stimulation of growth by growth hormone in children with idiopathic short stature. Data are from the Kabi Pharmacia International Growth Study (KIGS). The participants were given six or seven injections of recombinant GH per week. The figure shows that their median height standard deviation score (SDS) improved from –2.5 SD below the mean at the beginning of therapy to –1.5 after 3 years of therapy. From Albertsson-Wikland K., with permission (7).

GH used. On average, patients with ISS grow less rapidly with GH therapy than do children with documented GH deficiency.

Children with ISS have both accelerated growth during the interval of GH therapy, and they retain much of their gain in height for at least 2 years after the GH is stopped. Laron and colleagues (8) show that during 1–5 years of GH therapy, children with ISS gained 1.03 SDS over their pretreatment SDS (from group means of −2.7 ± 0.6 to −1.7 ± 0.6, SDS). In the 2 years after GH therapy was interrupted, the mean height SDS remained at −1.8 SDS. Another seemingly positive observation is the fact that as ISS children are treated with GH, their predicted adult height improves significantly (9). Most of this improvement in height prediction, however, occurs in the first 2 years of therapy and may tend to return toward the pretreatment prediction, as therapy is prolonged over several years (9).

Does Prolonged Therapy with GH Increase Adult Height of Individuals with ISS?

Our review of the literature in search of the answer to this question turned up eight reports of groups of ISS patients treated for sufficient periods of time and in sufficient numbers to provide meaningful data (Table 10.2) (6,9,10–15). The number of patients observed in these studies varies between 9 and 99; the mean ages at beginning of GH therapy is 8–12 years; the dose of GH ranges from the usual dose used in the United States for hypopituitary patients (0.3 mg/kg/wk) to about one half this dose; and therapy

TABLE 10.2. Adult height after growth hormone treatment. (Children not deficient in GH.)

Study	N	Age at beginning RX (Years)	Dose (mg/kg/wk)	Duration (Years)	Adult height minus predicted adult height
Kawai et al. (Ref. 10)	9	11.0 (5.5–12.3)	0.17	4.2 (3.0–4.8)	None (?negative effect)
Bierich et al. (Ref. 6)	15	8.0–14.3	≅ 0.3	3.0 (2.5–6.0)	None (mostly CGD)
Loche et al. (Ref. 11)	15	7.4–13.2	0.15, 7 pts. 0.3, 8 pts.	4–10	None
Wit et al. (Ref. 12)	12	11.2 ± 1.5	≅ 0.16 & 0.3	5.7	0.4 cm
Schmitt et al. (Ref. 9)	9	9.5 ± 2.6	0.2–0.3	4–5	2.4 cm
Hindmarsh and Brook (Ref. 13)	12	8.35 ± 1.88	0.13–0.23	Up to 8	2.8 cm (boys) 2.5 cm (girls)
Guyda (Ref. 14)	60 boys	12.11 ± 1.6			3.0cm
	39 girls	11.1 ± 1.5	≅ 0.3	≥3	2.6 cm
Hintz et al. (Ref. 15)	80	10.4	0.3	2–9	5.0 ± 5.1 cm (boys 5.9 ± 5.2 cm (girls)

ranges in duration from 2 to 9 years. Results vary, with four studies showing little or no change in adult height as a result of treatment (6,10–12), three studies reporting a 2.4–3.0 cm improvement (9,13,14), and one study showing a mean improvement of 5 cm in boys and 5.9 cm in girls (15). We conclude, therefore that GH treatment in doses at or slightly below those generally used to treat GH deficiency produce relatively small increments in adult height. Based on the evidence available, we believe that desire to produce a taller adult should not be the objective for treatment with GH of children with ISS.

One caveat that might slightly alter the interpretation of and conclusions from these results is that the Bayley-Pinneau height prediction method, which was used in most of these studies, tends to overstate what the adult height will be in these children. The height actually achieved by a GH-treated individual, therefore, might be slightly greater and closer to the predicted adult height than it would have been without treatment.

Does Prolonged Treatment of Children with ISS with GH Produce Psychological Benefit?

Even if one accepts that GH therapy does not increase adult height of individuals with ISS, there remains the need to determine whether the improvement in growth rate that occurs with such therapy provides psychological benefits in order to produce a more self-confident, better adjusted adult. Preliminary questions, however, are whether children with ISS suffer any psychological disadvantage that needs to be corrected, and, if so, is it correlated with short stature? There is a divergence of opinion on this question between pediatric endocrinologists and those who have done systematic psychological assessments of children with ISS. Cuttler et al. (16) have published the results of a detailed survey about short stature and GH therapy to which 434 pediatric endocrinologists provided replies. Two questions asked in this survey focused on the pediatric endocrinologist's perceptions and beliefs related to the emotional impact of short stature. First, these investigators asked how often height impairs the emotional well being of children whose height is third to fifth percentile? As indicated in Figure 10.2, more than 83% of the pediatric endocrinologists expressed the opinion that there were adverse emotional consequences sometimes, often, or always. When the question was rephrased to focus on children whose heights were below the third percentile, adverse emotional effects were felt to be present sometimes, often, or always in nearly 98% of the patients (Fig. 10.3).

Contrary to these findings, systematic, structured studies of the emotional status of children with ISS provide little evidence of handicap (17–20). Voss and Mulligan studied short children identified by screening more than 14,000 children in two school districts in the United Kingdom (17). Compared with controls, these investigators found no statistically significant deficits in in-

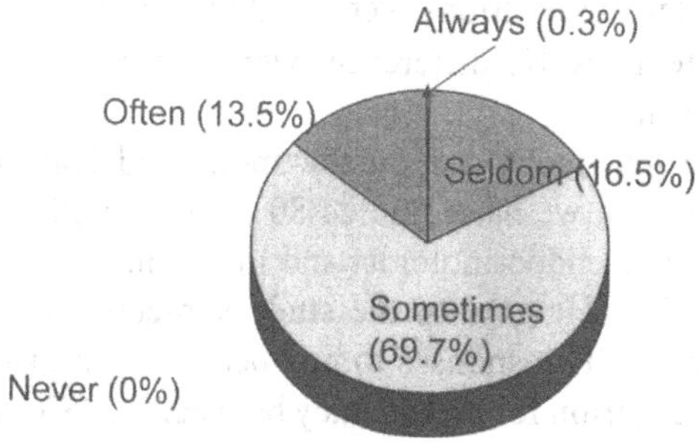

FIGURE 10.2. Responses of 434 pediatric endocrinologists to the question of how often they perceive that height impairs emotional well-being in children if the height is third to fifth percentile. Data from report of Cuttler L et al. (16).

telligence, school performance, self-esteem, or behavior, as rated by teachers. In follow-up, this group reported on the emotional effects of GH therapy, showing that treatment produced no psychological benefit (21). Sandberg and colleagues (18) compared short children (ages 6–10 years) referred to an endocrine clinic with children recruited from four elementary schools. They observed that the short boys had slightly lower (poorer adjustment) scores on the child behavior checklist for the scales dealing with activities and social and total competence. The short boys also exhibited higher social problems and thought problems scores. No differences were found between short and control girls. Furthermore, the differences observed in the boys were not robust and were the result of differences in very few items in the scales analyzed. Vance et al. (19) compared data on short and normal statured children from Cycle III of the National Health Examination Survey. They report that very tall males were better adjusted in school than were very

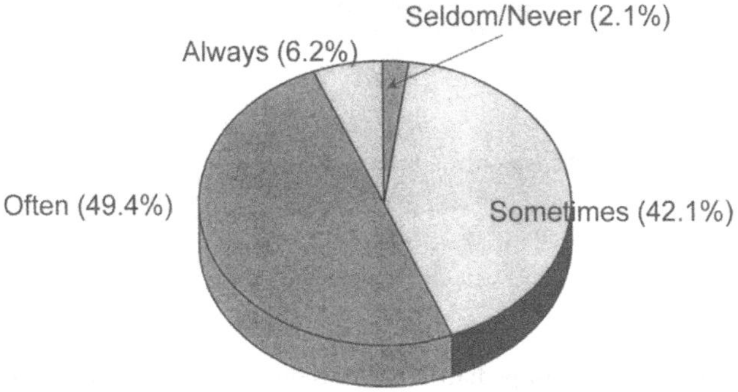

FIGURE 10.3. Responses of 434 pediatric endocrinologists to the question of how often they perceive that height impairs emotional well-being in children if the height is less than third percentile. Data from report of Cuttler L et al. (16).

short males. Similar observations were made when comparing very tall females with short females. No differences were observed that relate stature to anxiety or immaturity.

As part of the multicenter, industry-sponsored National Cooperative Growth Study (NCGS), we have studied 80 children with ISS who had been referred to a pediatric endocrinologist and in whom GH therapy was subsequently initiated (22). Heights of the study subjects were below the third percentile and serum GH responses to provocative stimuli were greater than 10 ng/ml. Using a criterion for discrepancy between IQ (Slosson) and achievement (WRAT-R) of 2 SD or more below the mean, 6, 8, and 11% of these children exhibited low achievement in reading, spelling, and arithmetic, respectively ($p < .05$ or greater, for each). Furthermore, significantly more than the expected 2% of ISS patients had elevated behavior problem scores on the child behavior checklist ($p < .001$). These included elevated rates both of internalizing (10%; e.g., anxiety and depression) and externalizing (8%; e.g., aggressive and hyperactive) types of problems.

In parallel with the diversity of findings and opinion of the psychological handicap of short stature, data on the benefits of GH therapy are varied. In general, it is not surprising that studies reporting that short stature presents no psychological handicap report that GH does not provide improvement in psychological state (21,23). At variance with these reports are the opinions of pediatric endocrinologists documented by Cuttler et al. (16). When asked their opinion on the likelihood that GH therapy would have a positive effect on the emotional well-being of the non-GH-deficient short child (even if there is no beneficial effect on adult height), 31.5% expressed the belief that improvement was likely or very likely (Fig. 10.4).

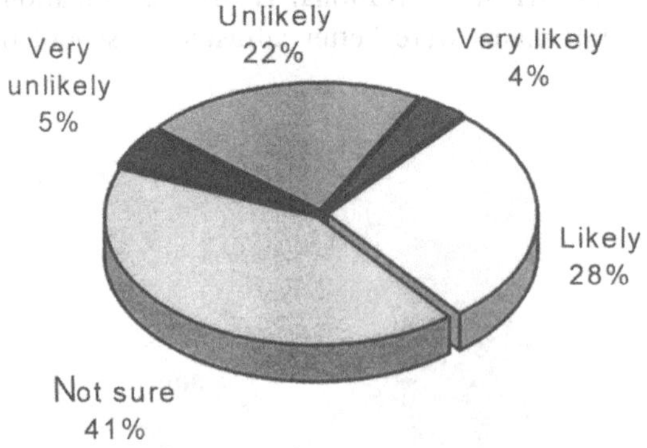

FIGURE 10.4. Responses of 434 pediatric endocrinologists to the question of what is the likelihood of GH having a positive impact on emotional well-being in short non–GH-deficient children, even if there is no impact on adult height? Data from report of Cuttler L et al. (16).

We have completed a study of the effects of GH therapy in children with ISS, as a continuation of the multicenter Genentech National Cooperative Growth Study (23). Fifty-nine ISS children have completed 3 years of GH treatment and psychometric testing. We observed no change in IQ or achievement test scores with treatment. The mean scores on the child behavior checklist, however, were improved with regard to total behavior problems ($p < .03$), the anxious/depressed component of the internalizing subscale ($p < .001$), and the social problems component of the ungrouped subscale ($p < .001$). These apparent improvements could result from the perceived benefit from the child's accelerated growth, the taller stature attained, a direct effect on the CNS of the added GH, an indirect effect derived from increased attention from parents and physicians, or a combination of these.

How Might One Account for Divergence of Findings on the Relative Handicap of Short Stature and the Effects of GH?

One possible answer for these diverse findings is that those investigating this question may be looking at different sets of subjects. For example, the studies initiated by psychologists that observe no handicap tend to begin with a large, unselected population-based sample. Within this sample, there are undoubtedly short children who are well adjusted and coping effectively. Inclusion of such children in the analysis of the "short child" group will inevitably dilute the study result. On the other hand, the individuals served by pediatric endocrinologists are highly selected. Among these latter patients, the family has become concerned about the height of the child and often have passed through one to several layers of the health care system. The point has been raised that among children reaching the pediatric endocrinologist the family may have concerns about behavior and adjustment that arise from problems other than short stature. Whereas this sometimes may be the case, the focus of the family is on the child's stature and growth, and on the negative effects of the child's physical condition on his/her psychological development and social adaptation. Even though there is no reliable means by which to predict whether a given child will accrue psychological benefit from GH therapy, the observations of pediatric endocrinologists on GH's beneficial psychological effects in thousands of short children indicate that the phenomena occurs. GH therapy should clearly not be used in isolation as the solution to the psychological/social problem of such patients. Family and patient counseling as adjunctive therapy is usually indicated. Such approaches have shown promise (25) and give an opportunity to provide optimal treatment programs incorporating GH and other forms of education or supportive therapy.

References

1. Rosenfeld RG, Frane J, Attie KM, Brazel JA, Burstein S, Cara JF, et al. Six year results of a randomized, prospective trial of human growth hormone and oxandrolone in Turner syndrome. J Pediatr 1992;121:49–55.
2. Fine RN, Kohut E, Brown D, Kuntze J, Attie KM. Long-term treatment of growth retarded children with chronic renal insufficiency, with recombinant human growth hormone. Kidney Internat 1996;49:781–85.
3. Hopwood NJ, Hintz RL, Gertner JM, Attie KM, Johanson AJ, Baptista J, et al. Growth response of children with non-growth hormone deficiency and marked short stature during 3 years of growth hormone therapy. J Pediatr1993;123:215–22.
4. Hindmarsh PC, Brook CGD. Effect of growth hormone on short normal children. Br Med J 1987;295:573–77.
5. Wit JM, Fokker MG, deMuinck Keizer-Schrama SMPH, et al. Effects of two years of methionyl growth hormone therapy in low-dosage regimens to prepubertal children with short stature, subnormal growth rate and normal growth hormone response to secretagogues. J Pediatr 1989;115:720–25.
6. Bierich JR, Nolte K, Drews K, Brugmann G. Constitutional delay of growth and adolescence. Results of short-term and long-term treatment with growth hormone. Acta Endocrinol 1992;127:392–96.
7. Albertsson-Wikland K. Characteristics of children with idiopathic short stature in the Kabi Pharmacia International Growth Study, and their response to growth hormone treatment. Acta Paediatr 1993;391(suppl):75–78.
8. Laron Z, Klinger B, Anin S, Pertzelan A, Lilos P. Growth during and 2 years after stopping GH treatment in prepubertal children with idiopathic short stature. J Ped Endocrinol Metab 1997;10:191–96.
9. Schmitt K, Blumel P, Waldhor T, Lassi M, Tulzer G, Frisch H. Short- and long-term (final height) data in children with normal variant short stature treated with growth hormone. Eur J Pediatr 1997;156:680–83.
10. Kawai M, Momio T, Yorfuji T, Yamanaka C, Sasaki H, Furusho K. Unfavorable effects of growth hormone therapy on the final height of boys with short stature not caused by growth hormone deficiency. J Pediatr 1997;130:205–9.
11. Loche S, Cambiaso P, Setzu S, Carta D, Marini R, Borrelli P, et al. Final height after growth hormone therapy in non-growth hormone deficient children with short stature. J Pediatr 1994;125:196–200.
12. Wit JM, Boersma B, deMuinch Keizer-Schrama SMPF, Nienhuis HE, Oostdijk W, et al. Long-term results of growth hormone therapy in children with short stature, subnormal growth rate and normal growth hormone response to secretagogues. Clin Endocrinol 1995;42:365–72.
13. Hindmarsh P, Brook CGD. Final height of short normal children treated with growth hormone. Lancet 1996;348:13–16.
14. Guyda HJ. Growth hormone treatment of non-growth hormone deficient subjects: the international task force report. Clin Pediatr Endocrinol 1996;5(suppl 7): 11–18.
15. Hintz RL, for U.S. Collaborative NCGS. Presented to the combined meeting of the European Society for Pediatric Endocrinology and the Lawson Wilkins Pediatric Endocrine Society. Stockholm, Sweden, June 1997.
16. Cuttler L, Silvers JB, Singh J, Marrero U, Finklestein B, Tannin G, et al. Short

stature and growth hormone therapy: a national study of physician recommendation patterns. JAMA 1996;276:531–37.
17. Voss LD, Mulligan J. The short normal child in school: Self-esteem, behavior, and attainment before puberty (The Wessex Growth Study). In: Stabler B, Underwood LE, eds. Growth, stature, and adaptation. Chapel Hill, NC: University of North Carolina, 1994.
18. Sandberg DE, Brook AE, Campos SP. Short stature in middle childhood: a survey of psychological functioning in a clinically referred sample. In: Stabler B, Underwood LE, eds. Growth, stature, and adaptation. Chapel Hill, NC: University of North Carolina, 1994.
19. Vance MD, Ingersoll GM, Golden MP. Short stature in a nonclinical sample: not a big problem. In Stabler B, Underwood LE eds. Growth, stature, and adaptation. Chapel Hill, NC: University of North Carolina 1994.
20. Skuse D, Gilmore J. Quality of life of children with normal short stature. Clin Pediatr Endocrinol 1997;6(suppl 9):29–37.
21. Downey AB, Mulligan J, McCaughey ES, Stratford RJ, Betts PR, Voss LD. Psychological response to growth hormone treatment in short normal children. Arch Dis Child 1996;75:32–35.
22. Lieberman E, Pilpel D, Carel CA, Levi E, Zadik Z. Coping and satisfaction with growth hormone treatment among short-stature children. Horm Res 1993;40: 128–33.
23. Stabler B, Clopper RR, Siegel PT, Stoppani C, Compton PG, Underwood LE. Academic achievement and psychological adjustment in short children. J Dev Behav Pediatr 1994;14:1–6.
24. Stabler B, Siegel PT, Clopper RR, Stoppani CE, Compton PG, Underwood LE. Behavior change after growth hormone treatment of children with short stature. J Pediatr 1998;133:366–73.
25. Eminson DM, Powell RP, Hollis S. Cognitive behavioral intervention with short statured boys: apilot study. In: Stabler B, Underwood LE eds.. Growth, stature, and adaptation. Chapel Hill, NC: University of North Carolina, 1994.

11

Impact of Short Stature on Quality of Life: Where Is the Evidence?

DENNIS DROTAR AND JANE R. ROBINSON

Advances in the medical diagnosis of endocrine-based growth disorders and the advent of biosynthetic growth hormone have altered the practice of treating only those individuals with "classic" growth hormone deficiency (GHD) and increased the number of children who can be treated with growth hormone (GH). There may be no clear indications for GH treatment in the case of a child who is short but otherwise normal other than the presence of short stature (SS). Clear empirical evidence that children's psychological adjustment is disrupted by short stature therefore has potential clinical relevance for decision making concerning GH treatment. For example, Cuttler and her colleagues' survey found that endocrinologists reported that they considered the psychological impact of short stature on their patients when making decisions about whether or not to treat with growth hormone (1). Physicians reported that individuals who were judged to have significant psychological problems related to their height were more likely to be treated with growth hormone (1).

How, then, does one judge the impact of SS on quality of life (QOL)? What is the empirical evidence that QOL is disrupted by short stature and GHD? A relatively large body of recent research has focused on the impact of short stature and GHD on the QOL of children and adolescents (2,3). There is, as a result, a continuing need to synthesize and critique this work and carefully articulate the clinical and research implications. The purpose of this chapter is to provide such a synthesis.

Method

Studies were selected for this review based on the following criteria: First, studies had to provide empirical data concerning one or more QOL outcomes of children, adolescents, and/or adults with SS and/or GHD. These included intellectual functioning/academic achievement, social behavior and functioning, emotional adjustment, and self-concept. Second, the study had to be published after 1960 in a journal or book. Data concerning individuals with Turner Syndrome were excluded because short stature is only one of many clinical features of this genetic disorder. Children with failure to thrive and/or psychosocial dwarfism were also excluded from this review because the QOL of these children is affected by family resource problems, stressors, and/or parent–child relationships that are associated with such problems (4).

Eligible studies were identified in several ways. Psych Lit and Med Line CD-ROMS were accessed (1960–1997) using the following terms and were entered either separately or in combination: short stature, growth retardation, psychological outcomes, psychosocial outcomes, intelligence, achievement, personality, behavior, cognition, emotional adjustment, and self-concept. The bibliographies of all identified reviews, articles, and book chapters were also referenced. A total of 40 studies were included in the present review.

Findings

Our review identified two types of descriptive studies: (1) single group descriptive studies in which the psychological or QOL outcomes of children with SS and/or GHD were compared with or clinical norms ($N = 21$); (2) descriptive studies in which individuals with SS and/or GHD were compared with a group of individuals with normal stature ($N = 19$). Studies that were reviewed included measures of the following four outcome domains based on Skuse et al. (5): cognition/achievement ($N = 32$); social behavior and adjustment ($N = 25$); emotional adjustment ($N = 31$); and self-esteem/body image ($N = 18$). Many assessed multiple outcomes in a single study.

Cognitive Functioning and Achievement

The empirical evidence for the impact of short stature on intelligence and achievement is inconsistent (2). Some studies have found that short children had more cognitive deficits than test norms or controls, whereas others have not; however, population-based studies in the United States and the United Kingdom, which provide the most representative data, have found minimal effects of stature on IQ, especially when the impact of socioeconomic status (SES) was controlled (6,7).

The evidence for the impact of SS on academic achievement was somewhat stronger than it was for intelligence. Several studies have found that children with short stature show more underachievement than controls (8,9). The preceding pattern of findings, however, is by no means consistent (10).

The evidence for the impact of GHD and SS on academic achievement was much stronger than for SS alone as shown by Stabler and colleagues (9) in the National Cooperative Growth Study, who found rates of discrepancies between children's achievement in reading, math, and spelling, and their intellectual abilities ranging from 6 to 14%. One fifth of this sample had evidence of achievement problems in one or more the preceding areas. These uncontrolled findings, however, could have been affected by clinical referral bias. These authors' interesting suggestion that there may be specific learning disabilities associated with GHD needs to be confirmed with more comprehensive assessments of information processing. Moreover, evidence for an association between GHD and learning disabilities from population-based samples is lacking.

Social Behavior and Competence

The hypothesis that children's social competence and peer interactions are affected by SS has received partial support, largely based on self-report measures. For example, Sandberg et al. (11) found that a large sample ($N = 258$) of clinically referred short children perceived themselves as less competent socially. They were also seen as less socially competent by their parents compared with norms for the instrument (Child Behavior Checklist) (12). Similar findings based on parent report were obtained in a controlled study by Siegel et al. (9) for both children with GHD and idiopathic SS. Children in these studies, however, were recruited from clinic samples. It is most important to note that the findings were based on limited measures of social competence that involved children's and parents' perceptions of children's social activities and participation rather than direct measures of social competencies or interactions based on other observers' (e.g., peer or teacher) reports that would provide more compelling evidence for how these children actually function in a social situation. Children's and parents' perceptions of their own social functioning would not be expected to correspond to the judgments of others.

To our knowledge, Skuse and colleagues (5) have conducted the only direct assessment of social competence based on peer and teacher reports. Peers reported that short children were well accepted within their class, and, if anything, were perceived by peers as better adjusted than controls with normal stature. Children with SS described themselves as equally well supported by parents, teachers, peers, and friends. In contrast, teachers and parents reported the behavior of children with short stature as being less mature. Differences in these findings underscores the need to carefully specify the precise construct of social competence and informant in evaluating the social outcomes of children with SS.

Emotional Adjustment

Synthesizing data concerning the impact of SS and/or GHD on children's emotional adjustment proved to be especially difficult given the multiple potential outcomes, in the domains of psychological symptoms and various personality dimensions, some of which were assessed with questionable measures. Consistent with definitions of health-related quality of life (HRQOL), which include psychological functioning and/or distress, our review focused primarily on assessment of general psychological adjustment, internalizing symptoms, and externalizing behavior based on teacher/parent or self-report. One issue that needs to be considered in evaluating these findings is that different informants have access to different types of information about the child's adjustment and hence may have different perspectives. In general, parents of children with SS have reported that this group, especially boys, have had more adjustment problems when compared with test norms. Few studies, however, have utilized self-report measures of psychological and/or behavioral symptoms.

Parents' evaluations of the adjustment of children with SS may be colored by their concern about the impact of stature. For this reason, children's impressions of their adjustment, as well as peer and teacher appraisals, are important. In Sandberg's (11) study, children and adolescents with short stature did not report more symptoms (i.e., depression, anxiety, etc.) than the normative sample. The Wessex Growth Study found no difference between 106 short normal children and 119 controls on psychological adjustment as reported by teachers (14). The evidence that the emotional adjustment of children with GHD and SS is disrupted is stronger than it is for SS alone (3,8,9). Even here, however, evidence from controlled studies is scarce.

Self-Concept/Body Image

In contrast to the long-standing assumption that SS disrupts self-esteem, findings of controlled studies indicate few differences in self-esteem among children with SS versus children of normal height. This finding is consistent across clinic-based and population-based studies. The data concerning body image for children with SS and/or GHD is difficult to evaluate because of variations in measures and constructs. At least one study (12) reported, however, that children with SS were more dissatisfied with their height than were controls.

Methodological Quality

We reviewed studies from the standpoint of methodological quality (i.e., sampling, study design, measurement, and data analysis) and will summarize this information here.

Sampling Considerations

Most of the studies received here involved relatively small, heterogenous samples (N = 20 or less) recruited from patient populations at one site. Although this research strategy has the advantage of describing these patients that are seen in practice, it limits inferences that can be drawn about the specific impact of SS and/or GHD on psychological outcomes and QOL, for several reasons. One issue concerns the heterogeneity of clinical samples and the potential for sampling bias. To the extent that factors associated with sampling characteristics can account for or contribute to differences that are obtained, investigators cannot conclude that SS and/or GHD is the primary factor that influences children's and/or adolescents' psychological status and QOL. This is a special problem because those children who are seen by pediatric endocrinologists for evaluation of SS are not necessarily representative of the broader population of children with such problems. In fact, one would expect that children who are referred to endocrinologists comprise a sample that is biased in some way (e.g., including parents who are more concerned and anxious about the child's problem and/or children who are having more adjustment problems because of their stature than nonreferred children of comparable stature). For these reasons, data from clinical samples may contribute to the description and characterization of children with short stature and GHD, but cannot provide a precise, let-alone definitive, answer to the question: What is the impact of GHD and short stature on QOL?

Other problems of inference are raised by the heterogenous samples that were employed. When differences between children with SS and controls were identified, it was not always clear what accounted for them. For the most part, samples were too small to clarify the impact of specific diagnostic subgroups on QOL. Moreover, most samples had variable age and gender composition. The impact of these factors was generally not assessed owing to small sample size.

Another sampling-related problem was that the family demographic characteristics (e.g., economic level and associated risk characteristics), which can clearly affect QOL outcomes, were not always described, making it difficult to know if and to what extent these important family factors affected QOL. For example, high levels of family resources would be expected to have a positive impact on many of the psychological outcomes that were assessed and might reduce or buffer the negative impact of SS or GHD. On the other hand, low economic resources and/or high levels of family stress (which is less likely given the nature of the clinical samples) could intensify the negative impact of SS and/or GHD on QOL. As a result, differences in SES family and characteristics between study versus comparison groups or test norms pose a threat to the validity of study findings. In this regard, another interesting but as yet uncharted set of family influences relates to how parents and family members from different socioeconomic and cultural groups perceive the child's SS and thus treat their children. Is SS accepted or seen as a significant problem by the primary caregivers in the child's life?

Design Problems

As noted earlier, the fact that control groups were not included in most descriptive studies poses interpretive problems. In the absence of controls, obtaining a positive finding (e.g., that SS is associated with a specific pattern of psychological outcome) does not mean that this can be directly attributed to short stature and/or GHD. Negative findings are also difficult to interpret and could reflect differences in the characteristics of the sample that were studied versus test standardization norms.

Measurement Considerations

The absence of gold standards for measurement of the outcomes utilized in studies reviewed here also pose difficulties. Most measures used with children with SS and/or GHD to describe their psychological status were neither designed nor validated for this population, but instead normed on psychiatrically ill or healthy populations [see Wiklund et al. (15)]. Moreover, even well-validated, standardized questionnaires that assess general maladjustment, which were frequently used in the studies reviewed here, are not sufficiently sensitive to detect more subtle effects such as distress related to short stature (e.g., embarrassment or frustration experienced in certain situations, e.g., peer relations). Available measures that assess the specific impact of stature on QOL unfortunately generally do not have extensive normative or validation data (Wiklund et al.).

Lack of Conceptual Frameworks to Guide Prediction

One of the most striking problems of the research that we reviewed concerned the limited use of conceptual frameworks to guide data analytic strategies and interpret findings. Many studies did not state hypotheses, let alone articulate a clear rationale for effects that were expected or obtained. Discussion sections of many studies had a decidedly post hoc flavor, and factors that accounted for patterns of differences (e.g., between children with SS and/or GHD versus controls) that were obtained on some measures but not on others, were not always clearly described. One would expect some differences by chance alone in studies that employed multiple outcome measures, each of which had several different subscales. Conceptually driven predictions of selective differences and/or correction for statistical significance, which were needed to counter this problem, were generally not utilized.

Despite the theoretical limitations of the studies that were reviewed, several interesting explanations have been proposed to account for the link between SS and/or GHD and QOL. For example, short stature has been assumed to affect children's psychological status indirectly by affecting family socialization practices and/or peer interaction and causing differences in how children were treated by parents and/or peers, eventually resulting in distress and/or maladjustment. An alternative potential mechanism postulates a direct impact of GHD on the brain and on key psychological functions. Investigators unfortunately did not assess variables that were assumed to influence the impact of stature and/or GHD on children's QOL. Moreover, researchers generally did not find a robust relationship between children's absolute level of height and a range of psychological outcomes, which would be expected if the key influence on these outcomes was stature.

Future Directions

Clinical Implications

Taken together, the findings indicate that there is little reason to assume that as a group children with SS have significant deficits in psychological status and QOL. The data are somewhat stronger for children with GHD, but even here they are not as especially robust, especially given methodological problems such as sampling bias, absence of controls, measurement problems, and an absence of predictive frameworks. Taken together, available data indicate a need for caution in treating children with SS with GH based on the presumed impact of stature on QOL. Moreover, the jury is still out concerning the extensiveness of the psychological impact of GHD.

Directions for Future Research

Our review suggests several directions for future research. One direction is to specify the variables that may interact with stature to influence psychological adjustment and QOL, especially in subgroups of children with GHD. Greater specification and testing of potential mechanisms of influence is critical. Why is it that we expect that stature and/or GHD are affecting QOL? Can these factors be observed and tested directly? Do we expect these effects in each and every child with SS and/or GHD? If not, can we specify which children and adolescents would be expected to show the greatest disruption of their QOL?

Moreover, individual differences in response to treatment with GHD on multiple outcomes of QOL should be carefully scrutinized. For example, do children who show a positive response in one domain (e.g., behavioral symptoms) show improvement in another domain (e.g., academic achievement)? Stabler and colleagues' data suggest that children's behavioral problems were much more responsive to treatment with GH than were their intelligence and achievement (9). Because of the potential for experimental designs and stronger inferences, studies of the impact of GH treatment on QOL measures are especially important. In evaluating such outcomes, measures that are more sensitive to specific stressful situations and the fabric of the QOL of children and adolescents with SS and GHD may be more productive than global outcomes (16).

A process-oriented approach that describes specific stressors that relate to SS and how children and families cope with them or which describe differential parental behavior toward children with SS and their siblings would provide useful information. Sandberg and Micheal (15) reported an interesting example of such research by identifying psychosocial stressors (e.g., teasing related to stature, reported by parents and children in a large sample).

Being treated as younger than their chronological age and teasing were commonly encountered among children with SS. Even though exposure to stature-related psychosocial stressors related to distress, however, clinically significant behavioral symptoms did not necessarily result. The fact that children were being teased, and potentially distressed by this problem, however, is nonetheless significant.

On the other hand, it is not as productive to design a study to assess global differences in social competence between children with SS and/or GHD and controls. More precise questions and measures are needed, such as: Do children with GHD show differences in how they process social information (e.g., how they read cues from others or in social skills), in their ability to engage peers in interaction, and in how distressed they are by their interactions with peers?

There is also a need for well-controlled studies with large sample sizes that focus on assessing the adjustment of children with SS and GHD during adolescence. We found some evidence that untreated short children showed a decline in self-esteem, social, and school competence in early adolescence (10) that was related to greater social isolation, fewer friendships, and decreased peer contacts.

The need for prospective studies that assess young adults who have GHD and/or SS and follow them through the transition to adulthood is compelling. On the one hand, we have provocative findings from some teams (e.g., Stabler and colleagues' (17,18) findings that a disproportionate number of adults who had been treated for GH deficiency during childhood had anxiety disorders, especially social phobia). When did these problems develop? Can they be prevented? On the other hand, Zimet and colleagues (19,20) found little evidence of an association of SS and disruption in psychological functioning within a sample of adults who were evaluated for SS as children.

It may also be useful for us to take our study designs to a new level and identify vulnerable subgroups of children with SS and GHD, or children, adolescents, or adults with these problems, who are resilient despite these problems. They have much to teach us. None of the foregoing recommendations will be easy to implement. High-quality science never is. The arduous multisite studies with carefully chosen controls and measures that are needed to advance knowledge in this area of scientific endeavor will require funders to see beyond the considerable resources that will be required for such research in order to appreciate the value of the product that can be achieved. Children, adolescents, adults, and families who seek help for problems of stature and GHD deserve nothing less.

References

1. Cuttler L, Silvers JB, Singh J, Marrero U, Finkelstein B, Tanin G, et al. Short stature and growth hormone therapy. JAMA 1996;276:531–37.
2. Voss LD. Short stature: does it matter? A review of the evidence. J Med Screen 1995:130–32.

3. Sandberg DE, Barrick C. Endocrine disorders in childhood: a selective survey of intellectual and educational sequelae. School Psychol Rev 1995;24:146–70.
4. Drotar D. Failure to thrive (growth deficiency). In: Roberts MC, ed. Handbook of pediatric psychology; New York: Guilford Press, 1995:516–35.
5. Skuse D, Gilmour J, Tian CS, Hindmarsh P. Psychosocial assessment of children with short stature: a preliminary report. Acta Paediatr Scand 1994;4406(suppl): 11–16.
6. Voss LD, Bailey BJR, Mulligan J, Witkin TJ, Betts PR. Short stature and school performance. The Wessex growth study. Acta Pediatr Scand 1991;377(suppl): 29–31.
7. Wilson DM, Hammer LD, Dunlan PM, Donnush SM, Ritter PC, Hintz RL, et al. Growth and intellectual development. Pediatrics 1986;78:646–50.
8. Siegel P, Clopper R, Stoppani C, Compton P, Stabler B. The psychological adjustment of short children and normal controls. In: Stabler B, Underwood L, eds. Growth, stature, and adaptation. Chapel Hill: University of North Carolina, 1994:123–34.
9. Stabler B, Clopper RR, Siegel PT, Stoppani C, Compton DG, Underwood LE. Academic and psychological adjustment in short children. J Dev Behav Pediatr 1994;15:1–6.
10. Holmes CS, Karlsson JA, Thompson RG. Social and school competencies in children with short stature: longitudinal patterns. J Dev Behav Pediatr 1985;6:263–67.
11. Sandberg D, Brook AE. Campos SP. Short stature: a psychosocial burden requiring growth hormone therapy? Pediatrics 1994;94:832–40.
12. Achenbach TM. Manual for the Child Behavior Check List. Burlington, VT: University of Vermont, 1991.
13. Drotar D, ed. Measuring health-related quality of life in children and adolescents. Hillsdale, NJ: Lawrence Erlbaum Associates, 1998.
14. Downie N, Mulligan J, Statford R, Betts P, Voss L. Are short normal children at a disadvantage? The Wessex growth study. Br Med J 1997;314:97–100.
15. Wiklund I, Erling A, Albertsson-Wikland. Critical review of measurement issues in quality of life assessment for children with growth problems. In: Drotar D, ed. Measuring health related quality of life in children and adolescents. Implications for research and practice. Hillsdale, NJ: Lawrence Erlbaum Associates, 1998.
16. Sandberg DE, Michael P. Psychosocial stresses related to short stature: Does their presence imply psychological dysfunction? In: Drotar D, ed. Measuring Health-related quality of life in children and adolescents. Implication for research and practice. Hillsdale, NJ: Lawrence Erlbaum Associates, 1998.
17. Stabler B, Clopper RR, Siegel PT, Nicholas LM, Silva SG, Tancer ME, et al. Links between growth hormone deficiency, adaptation and social phobia. Horm Res 1996;45:30–33.
18. Stabler B, Tancer ME, Ranc J, Underwood LE. Evidence for social phobia and other psychiatric disorders in adults who were growth hormone deficient during childhood. Anxiety 1996;2:86–89.
19. Zimet G, Cutler M, Litvene M, Owens R, Dahms W, Cuttler L. Psychosocial functioning of adults who were short as children. In: Stabler B, Underwood L, eds. Growth, stature and adaptation. Chapel Hill, NC: University of North Carolina, 1994;73–82.
20. Zimet G, Cutler M, Litvene M, Owens R, Dahms W, Cuttler L. Psychological adjustment of children evaluated for short stature: a preliminary report, J Dev Behav Pediatr 1995;16:264–70.

12

Mediators of Psychological Adjustment in Children and Adolescents with Short Stature

An Invited Contribution

Jessica C. Roberts, Martha U. Barnard, Michael C. Roberts, Wayne V. Moore, Eric M. Vernberg, Jerome A. Grunt, Campbell P. Howard, and I. David Schwartz

Introduction

Short stature is defined as growth below the fifth percentile for chronological age, or as height greater than 2 standard deviations (SDS) below the mean height for chronological age (1,2). Approximately 5 percent of all children (1.27 million) have significant short stature (SS) in the United States (2,3). Many posttreatment studies of children and adults treated for growth hormone deficiency (GHD) as children have shown these individuals to have poorer psychological and social adjustment than their normally developing peers (4–7). Higher unemployment rates (5), lower marriage rates (5), and increased incidents of psychiatric disorders and social phobia are reliably reported (7,8).

Some children with SS have poorer psychological adjustment than their normally developing peers (9–13). Parents reported four to six times the expected number of children with GHD displaying internalizing and externalizing problems on the child behavior checklist (CBCL) when compared with norms (12). Along these lines 48% of a sample of children with GHD had CBCL behavioral adjustment scores above the ninetieth percentile (9). A study that used the Weinberger Adjustment Inventory, however, found similar or better adjustment when comparing a sample of children with SS and the normative sample (14).

Behavioral characteristics of children with SS indicate inadequate social adjustment. They have been described as immature (10), less aggressive (13), and more withdrawn and socially isolated than peers (10,15–18). Parents and teachers describe children with SS as less socially competent than their peers on the CBCL (9,11,12,17). Elevated levels of problem behaviors (11,12) and lower involvement in activities are reported (15). The children with the greatest height discrepancies relative to peers were reported to have the poorest adjustment on the CBCL social competence subscale (9).

Children with SS report that they perceive themselves to be less popular than their peers (16,18). Fewer friends, limited contact with friends, and alienation from the peer group are common (10,11,15,17). Peer teasing also occurs and is hypothesized to lead to school and social adjustment difficulties (14,15,19–21). In one study, 66% of the parents and 60% of the children reported that the children were teased "sometimes" or "more frequently" (14). Finally, lack of adequate relationships with peers of the same sex and age and difficulties with heterosexual relationships were the two most commonly reported effects of SS in a retrospective study of adults treated for GHD as children (22). Little attention has been given to the role of peers in psychological adjustment. No studies have examined whether the friendships of children with GHD differ from those of children without the disorder, and it remains unclear whether these children experience comparatively more teasing than their normally developing peers or how peer teasing mediates social competence and psychological adjustment.

The impact of family functioning on the social and psychological adjustment of children with SS remains unclear. Parents of children with constitutional short stature (CSS) report a less strict approach to child rearing and less clear limits on behavior on the Maryland Parent Attitude Survey (16,18), and lower levels of cooperation and effective communication when compared with normal controls on the Family Life Survey (16,18). No differences were found, however, in level of family cohesion or adaptability for families of children with GHD when compared with families of children with idiopathic short stature (ISS) or the standardization sample using the Family Adaptability and Cohesion Scale III (11,12,23). More studies are needed that examine how family processes including parental attitudes, expectations, and support mediate adjustment in this group of children.

This study adapted the Wallander and Varni (1992) disability–stress–coping model of adaptation to a sample of children with SS, as a result of GHD, growth hormone neurosecretory deficiency (GHND), CSS, ISS, and constitutional delay (CD), in order to identify specific factors that contribute to risk and resistance in this population (24). Three disease/disability risk factors were hypothesized to affect adjustment: (1) the short stature diagnosis, (2) the relative height discrepancy of the child with respect to normally developing peers, and (3) the child's level of pubertal development. One psychosocial risk factor, peer rejection experiences, was hypothesized to affect adjustment. These risk factors were hypothesized to be mediated by resistance factors. Three social–ecological resistance factors—companionship with best friends, intimacy with best friends, and perceived social support–family—were hypothesized to act as buffers against adjustment difficulties (depression, anxiety, self-worth). The objective of the study was to identify variables that might differentiate those subjects with SS who were well-adjusted from those subjects with SS who were experiencing difficulties.

Hypotheses of the Present Study

It is unclear in the literature whether children with GHD/GHND and children with CSS/ISS/CD differ on measures of risk, resistance, and adjustment. No predictions were made, therefore, about potential differences between the two groups. It was also unclear whether children with SS would differ from normally developing children on measures of risk, resistance, and adjustment. No predictions were made, therefore, about potential differences between children with SS and normative information (available means and standard deviations).

In order to test Wallander and Varni's (1992) model, several hypotheses were made about the impact of risk factors, resistance factors, and the interaction of risk and resistance factors on adjustment (24). First, it was predicted that risk factors (e.g., diagnosis, degree of short stature, level of pubertal development, and rejection experiences with peers) would be negatively related to level of adjustment. Second, it was hypothesized that resistance factors (e.g., intimacy with best friends, companionship with best friends, and perceived social support–family) would be positively related to level of adjustment. Finally, it was hypothesized that significant interactions would occur between and among the risk and resistance factors in the model.

Methods

Participants and Procedures

The sample consisted of 51 subjects (37 male, 14 female), 26 subjects with GHD/GHND and 25 subjects with CSS, ISS, and/or constitutional delay (CD). Ages of the participants ranged between 9 and 18 years, with a mean of 13 years, 1 month (SD=2 years, 5 months). See Table 12.1 for additional characteristics of the sample. Participants were recruited during their routine visits to the pediatric endocrinology clinics of two hospitals in a large midwestern city. Written consent for participation in the study was obtained from the parent or guardian, and written assent was obtained from the participants at the time of initial contact. IRB approval was obtained from the participating institutions.

TABLE 12.1. Demographic characteristics of the sample.

Characteristics	N	%	Characteristics	N	%
Diagnosis			Ethnicity		
CSS/ISS/CD	25	49.0	Caucasian	47	92.2
GHD/GHND	26	51.0	African-American	1	2.0
			Hispanic	1	2.0
Receiving growth hormone			Repeated grade	6	11.8
Yes	38	74.5	Special education	10	19.6
No	13	25.5	Physical disability	10	19.6
			Chronic illness	7	13.7
Gender			Marital status-parent		
Male	37	72.5	Married/remarried	40	78.4
Female	14	27.5	Not married	9	17.6
Grade			Family income		
3	1	2.0	Under 10,000	3	5.9
4	3	5.9	10,001–20,000	4	7.8
5	7	13.7	20,001–30,000	6	11.8
6	6	11.8	30,001–40,000	4	7.8
7	6	11.8	40,001–50,000	5	9.8
8	8	15.7	50,001–60,000	9	17.6
9	7	13.7	60,001–70,000	0	0.0
10	5	9.8	70,001–80,000	5	9.8
11	4	7.8	80,001–90,000	2	3.9
12	4	7.8	90,001+	7	13.7

Measures

Diagnosis. Diagnosis of GHD was defined as peak stimulated growth hormone (GH) values less than 10 ng/ml in response to two or more secretagogue tests performed using insulin, levodopa, arginine, and clonidine. Diagnosis of GHND was defined as overnight pooled GH values of less than 3 ng/ml. The term *CSS* was applied to those subjects of normal height parents who were growing at a normal rate, but who were below the fifth percentile for height when compared with peers of the same age and gender. The term *ISS* was applied to those subjects below the fifth percentile for height for whom the cause of short stature remained undetermined. The term *CD* was applied to those children with CSS who had a bone age that lags approximately 1–4 years behind their chronological age. Diagnosis of CSS, ISS, and CD was determined by physician's report.

Height Discrepancy. Height discrepancy or height standard deviation score was calculated as the standard deviation below the mean for age and gender. It provided a means of comparing subjects with respect to the severity of their short stature.

Tanner Stage. The Tanner stage provided a measure of the child's degree of pubertal development. The Tanner scales rate the level of gonadal development (boys), breast development (girls), and pubic hair development (boys and girls) on a scale from 1 to 5, with 5 indicating complete pubertal development (25).

Family Information Form. This form requested information from the parent about the family, such as education, occupation, marital status, income, birth dates, and ages.

Hollingshead Four Factor Index. The Hollingshead Four Factor Index (26) was used to estimate the status positions occupied by the families in this study.

Perceived Social Support from Family. A 20-item self-report Perceived Social Support measure, family subscale, required the child to answer *Yes*, *No*, or *Don't Know* to a series of statements about the participants' perceived support within the family (27). A meta-analytic review of studies found that the internal consistency of the family scale ranged from $r = .88$ to $r = .91$ and test–retest reliabilities ranged from $r = .80$ to $r = .86$ (28).

The Friendship Interview. The questionnaire version of the Friendship Interview (29) asks the child to answer a set of 26 questions about the support provided by each of his or her three best friends. The measure evaluates six features of friendships in childhood: companionship, intimacy, prosocial intent, self-esteem, conflicts, and inequality. Internal consistencies range from .54 to .76 for this measure (30).

Rejection Experiences Questionnaire. The Rejection Experiences Questionnaire (31,32) was used to assess the child's experiences of being teased or picked on, threatened, hit or struck by another student, or excluded from peer activities during the last 3 months. High stability for this measure over a 6-month period ($r = .73$) (31) and adequate internal consistency for the measure ($a = .86$) was reported (33).

Social Anxiety Scale-Revised (Adolescent Version). The Social Anxiety Scale-Revised (SASC-R), is a 26-item self-report measure (34). The measure yielded three scores [i.e., Fear of Negative Evaluations (FNE), Social Anxiety, and Distress-New (SAD-N), which reflects social avoidance, distress, or inhibition related to new or unfamiliar peers, and Social Anxiety and Distress-Generalized (SAD-G), which reflects more generalized social avoidance, distress, or inhibition]. Subscales of the SASC-R have acceptable internal consistency, ranging from .86 for the FNE to .69 for SAD-G (35).

Children's Depression Inventory. The Children's Depression Inventory (CDI) is a 27-item self-report measure that discriminates depressed children and adolescents from nondepressed children. Internal consistency reliabilities for the measure range from .71 to .89 (36).

Harter Self-Perceptions Profile for children. The Harter Self-Perceptions Profile For Children is a 36-item self-report measure used to evaluate five specific domains of self-concept (i.e., scholastic competence, social acceptance, athletic competence, physical appearance, and behavioral conduct), as well as the child's overall self-concept, termed global self-worth. The six subscales have acceptable internal consistency reliabilities that range from .71 to .86 (37).

Results

Comparison of Diagnostic Groups

A MANOVA was performed to compare the subjects in the CSS and GHD groups on four dependent measures of adjustment: global self-worth, fear of negative evaluation, social anxiety and distress–generalized, and total depression. No significant effect for diagnostic group was obtained. As the two diagnostic groups did not differ significantly on measures of adjustment, they were combined for all future analyses.

Normative Comparisons

Independent sample *t*-tests were calculated, correcting for unequal sample sizes, to determine if differences exist between individuals with SS and normative information. Subjects' scores differed significantly from available normative information only on the global self-worth subscale of the Harter Self-Perception Profile. The SS individuals reported significantly higher self-worth scores ($p = .001$).

Correlational Analyses

See Table 12.2 for correlation coefficients and significance levels for the relationship among the risk, resistance, and adjustment measures. Of the risk factor measures, rejection experiences with peers was significantly negatively correlated with global self-worth ($r = -.312, p < .05$) and significantly

TABLE 12.2. Significant correlations among risk factors, resistance factors, and adjustment measures.

Scale	1	2	3	4	5	6
1. Rejection Experiences	1.000					
2. Companionship	−0.147	1.000				
3. Global Self-Worth	−0.312*	0.392**	1.000			
4. FNE	0.726**	−0.287*	−0.530**	1.000		
5. SAD–G	0.501**	−0.404**	0.626**	1.000		
6. Total Depression	0.505**	−0.160	−0.490**	0.595**	0.425**	1.00

FNE = Fear of Negative Evaluation, SAD–G = Social Anxiety and Distress–Generalized, *$p < .05$, **$p < .01$

positively correlated with fear of negative evaluation ($r = -.726$, $p < .01$), social anxiety and distress-generalized ($r = .501$, $p < .01$), and total depression ($r = .505$, $p < .01$). These correlations indicated that greater rejection experiences with peers was associated with lower self-worth, greater fear of negative evaluation, greater social anxiety in everday occurrences, and higher depression scores. Of the resistance factor measures, the significant negative correlation between companionship and fear of negative evaluations ($r = -.287$, $p < .05$) indicated that lower companionship was associated with greater fears of negative evaluation. The significant positive correlation between companionship and global self-worth ($r = .392$, $p < .01$) indicated that greater interaction with best friends was associated with higher self-worth scores. Finally, significant intercorrelations were found among the adjustment measures (i.e., global self-worth, fear of negative evaluations, social anxiety and distress–generalized, and total epression.

Contribution of Risk Factors to Adjustment

Linear regression analyses were performed to determine the contributions of three risk factors (i.e., height discrepancy, Tanner stage, and rejection experiences with peers), to the self-reported adjustment of subjects with SS. First, to test the contributions of the child's height discrepancy and rejection experiences with peers, these measures were hierarchically regressed on each adjustment measure. Second, to test the contributions of height discrepancy and Tanner Stage, these measures were hierarchically regressed on each adjustment measure. Finally, to test the contributions of Tanner Stage and rejection experiences, these measures were hierarchically regressed on each adjustment measure. No significant main effect was found for height discrepancy or Tanner Stage in the prediction of adjustment; however, rejection experiences with peers significantly predict overall adjustment in individuals with SS on all measures of adjustment. A main effect for rejection experiences with peers was found for total depression, F change $(2,41) = 14.05$, $p < .01$. Rejection experiences with peers accounted for 25.5% of the variance in total depression scores above that accounted for by the child's height discrepancy. a main effect for rejection experiences was also found for global self-worth, F change $(2,45) = 4.84$, $p = .033$, social anxiety and distress–generalized, F change $(2,46) = 15.45$, $p < .01$, and fear of negative evaluation, F change $(2,46) = 51.46$, $p < .01$. Rejection experiences with peers accounted for 9.7% of the variance in global self-worth scores, 25.1% of the variance in social anxiety and distress–generalized scores, and 52.6% of the variance in fear of negative evaluations scores, above that accounted for by the child's height discrepancy. Finally, a significant interaction was found for height discrepancy X rejection experiences with peers in the prediction of fear of negative evaluation, F change $(3,45) = 7.21$, $p < .01$. This interaction accounted for 6.5% of the variance in fear of negative evaluation with both height discrepancy and rejection experiences in the equation. The shorter subjects in our sample who experienced many rejection experiences with peers reported the greatest fear of negative evaluation by peers.

Contribution of Resistance Factors to Adjustment

Linear regression analyses were performed to determine the contributions of three resistance factors (i.e., perceived social support from family, companionship in best friendships, and intimacy in best friendships) to the prediction of adjustment. First, to test the contributions of perceived social support–family and companionship in best friendships, these measures were hierarchically regressed on each adjustment measure. A significant main effect was found for companionship in the prediction of global self-worth, F change (2,45) = 7.27, $p < .01$. Furthermore, companionship approached significance in the prediction of fear of negative evaluations, F change (2,46) = 3.87, $p < .06$. Companionship accounted for 13.5% of the variance in global self-worth scores and 7.7% of the variance in fear of negative evaluation scores above that accounted for by perceived social support–family. A significant interaction between perceived social support–family and companionship, F change (3,40) = 4.50, $p = .04$ was obtained for the prediction of total depression scores. This interaction accounted for 9.1% of the variance in total depression scores with both perceived social support–family and companionship in the equation. Those subjects who reported little companionship with peers and low perceived family support reported the highest depression scores.

Second, to test the contributions of perceived social support-family and intimacy in best friendships, these measures were hierarchically regressed on each adjustment measure. No main effect for intimacy in best friendships was found, and no main effect for perceived social support–family was found in the prediction of global self-worth, fear of negative evaluations, or SAD-G. Perceived social support-family, however, approached significance in the prediction of total depression scores, F change (1,42) = 3.60, $p < .07$). Perceived social support–family accounted for 7.9% of the variance in total depression scores.

Interaction of Risk and Resistance Factors in the Prediction of Adjustment

Finally, analyses were performed to determine the interaction between risk and resistance factors. Height discrepancy did not significantly interact with intimacy, companionship, or perceived social support–family in the prediction of adjustment. A second set of regression analyses were performed to determine whether a significant interaction existed between rejection experiences with peers (risk factor) and either intimacy with peers, companionship with peers, or perceived social support–family (resistance factors). No significant interaction was found between rejection experiences with peers and intimacy or companionship in the prediction of adjustment. Significant interactions between rejection experiences with peers and perceived social support–family were found in the prediction of fear of negative evaluation, F change (3,45) = 5.73, $p < .02$ and global self-worth, F change (3,44) = 7.45, $p < .01$. The interaction accounted for 4.9% of the variance in fear of negative evaluation scores, and 12.3% of the variance in global self-worth with rejection experiences and perceived social support–family in the equation.

Discussion

Overall, the results of this study suggests that subjects with CSS/ISS/CD and GHD/GHND are similar to each other and normally developing children on measures of anxiety and depression. The finding of significantly higher self-worth scores in subjects with SS is consistent with other studies (9,14,38,39). Disease variables, including diagnosis, height discrepancy, and level of pubertal development, were not good predictors of adjustment in this sample of children with SS. A large proportion of our sample, however, was receiving GH treatment at the time of the study. Rejection experiences with peers was found to be a good predictor of all adjustment measures. The significant interaction between height discrepancy and rejection experiences with peers in the prediction of fear of negative evaluation suggests that short children who have many negative experiences with peers will have the greatest worries about being liked by peers. Companionship with best friends was found to be a good predictor of self-worth for children with SS. When this was combined with family support it was related to lower depression scores. These findings suggest that peer interactions make important contributions to the adjustment of children with SS. In addition, under conditions of high rejection experiences, family support appears to act as a buffer. Children with high rejection experiences and high family support demonstrated fewer worries about being liked by peers and higher feelings of self-worth than did children with high rejection experiences and low family support. This study suggests that those children with SS who report high levels of peer rejection or low levels of companionship may benefit from social skills training as a means of increasing positive interactions in their relationships with peers. In addition, efforts by teachers and families to facilitate positive peer experiences and to intervene in instances of negative interactions with peers may promote more positive adjustment. Finally, the role of family support as a mediator of adjustment should be further explored in this group of children. Intervention studies that focus on increasing family support and teaching social skills to those short children demonstrating difficulties would be beneficial.

References

1. Lee P, Rosenfeld R. Psychosocial correlates of short stature and delayed puberty. Pediatr Adol Endocrinol 1987;34:851–63.
2. Rosenfeld R. Treatment of non-growth hormone deficient short stature. In: Hintz RL, Rosenfeld RG., eds. Contemporary issues in endocrinology and metabolism, vol. 4, growth abnormalities. New York: Churchill Livingstone, 1987:109–28.
3. Reiser P, Underwood LE. Growing children: a parent's guide. third ed. [brochure]. San Francisco: Genentech, Inc., 1997.
4. Bjork S, Jonsson B, Westphal O, Levin J. Quality of life of adults with growth hormone deficiency: a controlled study. Acta Paediatr Scand 1989;356(suppl):55–59.
5. Dean H, McTaggart T, Fish D, Friesen H. The educational, vocational, and marital status of growth hormone deficient adults treated with growth hormone during childhood. Am J Dis Child 1985;139:1105–10.
6. Rotnem D, Cohen D, Hintz R, Genel M. Psychological sequelae of relative "treatment failure" for children receiving human growth hormone replacement. J Am Acad Child Psychiatr 1979;3:505–20.
7. Stabler B, Tancer M, Ranc J, Underwood L. Psychiatric symptoms in young adults treated for growth hormone deficiency in childhood. In: Stabler B, Underwood L, eds. Growth, stature, and adaptation: behavioral, social, and cognitive aspects of growth delay. Chapel Hill: The University of North Carolina, 1994:99–106.
8. Downey J, Ehrardt A, Gruen R, Morishima A, Bell J. Turner syndrome versus constitutional short stature: psychopathology and reactions to height. In: Stabler B, Underwood L, eds. Slow grows the child. Hillsdale, NJ: Erlbaum Associates, 1986:123–38.
9. Allen KD, Warzak WJ, Greger NG, Bernotas TD, Huseman CA. Psychosocial adjustment of children with isolated growth hormone deficiency. Child Health Care 1993;22:61–72.
10. Rotnem D, Genel M, Hintz R, Cohen D. Personality development in children with growth hormone deficiency. J Am Acad Child Psychiatr 1977;16:412–26.
11. Siegel P, Clopper R, Stoppani C, Stabler B. The psychological adjustment of short children and normal controls. In: Stabler B, Underwood L, eds. Growth, stature, and adaptation; Behavioral, social, and cognitive aspects of growth delay. Chapel Hill: The University of North Carolina, 1994:123–34.
12. Stabler B, Clopper R, Siegel PT, Stoppani C, Compton PG, Underwood LE. Academic achievement and psychological adjustment in short children. Devel Behav Pediatr 1994;15:1–6.
13. Steinhausen H, Stahnke N. Psychoendocrinological studies in dwarfed children and adolescents. Arch Dis Child 1976;51:778–83.
14. Zimet GD, Cutler M, Litvene M, Dahms W, Owens R, Cuttler L. Psychological adjustment of children evaluated for short stature: a preliminary report. Dev Behav Pediatr 1995;16:264–70.
15. Sandberg D, Brook A, Campos S. Short stature in middle childhood: a survey of psychosocial functioning in a clinic-referred sample. In: Stabler B, Underwood L, eds. Growth, stature, and adaptation: behavioral, social, and cognitive aspects of growth delay. Chapel Hill: The University of North Carolina, 1994:19–33.
16. Gordon M, Crouthamel M, Post E, Richman R. Psychosocial aspects of constitutional short stature: Social competence, behavior problems, self-esteem, and family functioning. J Pediatr 1982;101:477–80.

17. Holmes C, Karlsson M, Thompson R. Social and school competencies in children with short stature: longitudinal patterns. Devel Behav Pediatr 1985;6:263–67.
18. Richman R, Gordon M, Tegtmeyer P, Crouthamel C, Post E. Academic and emotional difficulties associated with constitutional short stature. In: Stabler B, Underwood L, ed. Slow grows the child. Hillsdale, NJ: Erlbaum Associates, 1986:13–26.
19. Brust J, Ford C, Rimoin D. Psychiatric aspects of dwarfism. Am J Psychiatr 1976;133:160–64.
20. Eminson D, Powell R, Hollis S. Cognitive behavioral interventions with short statured boys: a pilot study. In: Stabler B, Underwood L, eds. Growth, stature, and adaptation: behavioral, social, and cognitive aspects of growth delay. Chapel Hill: The University of North Carolina, 1994:135–50.
21. Holmes C, Hayford J, Thompson R. Personality and behavioral differences in groups of boys with short stature. Child Health Care 1982;11:61–64.
22. Mitchell C, Johanson A, Joyce S, Libber S, Plotnik L, Migeon C, et al. Psychosocial impact of long-term growth hormone therapy. In: Stabler B, Underwood L, eds. Slow grows the child. Hillsdale, NJ: Erlbaum Associates, 1986:97–109.
23. Fung CM, Sandberg DE, Shine B, Grundner W. Influence of growth hormone therapy on aspects of family functioning. Proceedings of the Fifth Florida Conference on Child Health Psychology; April 20–22, 1995; Gainesville.
24. Wallander JL, Varni JW. Adjustment in children with chronic physical disorders: Programmatic research on a disability-stress-coping model. In: La Greca AM, Siegel, LT, Wallander JL, Walker CE, eds. Advances in pediatric psychology: stress and coping in child health. New York: Guilford Press, 1992:279–98.
25. Tanner JM. Growth at adolescence, Second ed. Oxford: Blackwell Scientific, 1962.
26. Hollingshead AB. Four factor index of social status. Unpublished manuscript, Yale University, Department of Sociology, 1975.
27. Procidano ME, Heller K. Measures of perceived social support from friends and from family: three validation studies. Am J Commun Psychol 1983;11:1–24.
28. Procidano ME. The nature of perceived social support: findings of meta-analytic studies. In: Spielberger CD, Butcher JN, eds. Advances in personality assessment, vol. 9. Hillsdale, NJ: Erlbaum Associates, 1992:1–26.
29. Berndt TJ, Hawkins J. Friendship interview. Unpublished manuscript, Purdue University, 1984.
30. Berndt TJ, Perry TB. Children's perceptions of friendships as supportive relationships. Devel Psychol 1986;22:640–48.
31. Vernberg EM. Psychological adjustment and experiences with peers during early adolescence: reciprocal, incidental, or unidirectional relationships? J Abnorm Child Psychol 1990;18:187–98.
32. Vernberg EM, Jacobs AK, Hershberger S. Peer victimization and attitudes about violence during early adolescence. J Clin Child Psychol 1990;28:386–95.
33. Zerger AK, Vernberg EM. Bystanders and attitudes towards peer victimization in early adolescence. Unpublished manuscript, University of Kansas, Lawrence, 1997.
34. La Greca AM. Social anxiety scale for children–revised. University of Miami, FL: Author, 1992.
35. La Greca AM, Stone WL. Social anxiety scale for children-revised: factor structure and concurrent validity. J Clin Child Psychol 1993;22:17–27.
36. Kovacs M. Children's depression inventory manual. Canada: Multi-Health Systems, Inc., 1992.

37. Harter S. Manual for the self-perception profile for children. University of Denver, CO: Author, 1985.
38. Young-Hyman D. Effects of short stature on social competence. In: Stabler B, Underwood L, eds. Slow grows the child. Hillsdale, NJ: Erlbaum Associates, 1986:27–45.
39. Siegel P, Hopwood N. The relationship of academic achievement and the intellectual functioning and affective conditions of hypopituitary children. In: Stabler B, Underwood L, eds. Slow grows the child. Hillsdale, NJ: Erlbaum Associates, 1986:57–72.

13

Turner Syndrome: Psychological Functioning Rated by Parents and by the Girls Themselves

An Invited Contribution

Ulla Wide Boman, Kerstin Albertsson-Wikland, and Anders Möller

Introduction

An improved understanding of the psychological aspects of Turner syndrome (TS) is important in order to optimize treatment and counseling. There is also a theoretical interest in a description of the psychosocial functioning associated with TS because this patient group could be considered as a model for the genetic and endocrine influences on human behavior. Knowledge of how patients cope with the impairments of TS may also contribute to our general understanding of psychological aspects of the functional impairment, and how people cope with chronic disorders. One question underlying the investigation of the psychological aspects of TS is whether there are specific difficulties and characteristics that are common to such individuals. Other questions relate to which effects are caused directly by the chromosome disorder (e.g., by genetic and endocrine factors), which are due to the psychological adaptation to such factors, and how the interplay between these factors can be understood.

It has been reported that although the frequency of psychopathologies is not increased in TS, there is an increased frequency of psychological difficulties. Hyperactivity has been described in preschool children and during the first years at school (1). From the age at which the children start school, there are reports of poor peer relationships and behavioral problems (2–4), as well as of impaired self-esteem, which may worsen during adolescence (1,5). There is often a large variability and the group is heterogenous. The large variability in psychological functioning among individuals with TS, although not yet convincingly correlated with the degree of genetic or physical abnormalities, is an argument for further studies on the psychological effects of TS, of the coping strategies and abilities shown by these individuals, and by the experience of living with TS.

Method

Results are presented from an ongoing multidisciplinary cross-sectional study of all girls diagnosed as having TS in the western part of Sweden, an area with a population of 1.5 million. In total, 43 girls, aged 6–17 years, were studied. Of these, 39 were on growth hormone (GH) treatment, and 4 had completed GH treatment; 21 were receiving oxandrolone, 17 were receiving ethinyl-oestradiol. The socioeconomic status of the patients' families did not differ from that of a reference population.

This chapter will give data from the first examination in the ongoing prospective study. The psychological examination was made when the subjects visited the pediatric clinic for their medical examination. The diagnosis of TS was confirmed by leucocyte karyotyping. The majority of the girls had a 45,X karyotype; however, 15% had a mosaicism, and the remaining 30% had a nonmosaic, partial deletion of the second X chromosome.

Psychological function was assessed using two generic measures: the self-perception scale "I think I am" (6), and the Child Behavior Checklist (CBCL) (7).

The "I think I am" is a Swedish self-perception scale (6). There is a theoretical relationship between psychological health and self-perception. Children with a good psychological health are thought to have a positive attitude to themselves, whereas children with impaired psychological health have a negative attitude to themselves. The "I think I am" scale gives a total value of the individual's self-perception, describing how the child perceives its physical abilities, talents, psychological well-being, and relationships with family and others. A high score reflects a high self-perception. The reference values, which are specific for gender and age, are expressed in a stanine form (normally distributed within a range of 1–9; mean = 5; 1 SD = 2), which allows comparison of children of different ages.

The Child Behavior Checklist parent version (CBCL-P) is a screening method developed by Achenbach (7). The CBCL-P gives a global picture of the problems and competencies of the child, as assessed by the respondent. It is a standardized questionnaire in which the parents answer questions about the child's social situation, activities, and school performance, as well as queries about the presence of different behavioral and emotional problems, such as aggressive behavior and anxiety, which are summarized as externalizing or internalizing. The result is presented in two total scores: total social competence (where a high score reflects a good social competence) and total behavior and emotional problems (where a high score reflects more problems). The study group was compared with a control group matched on sex and age, using a nonparametric statistical test, Mann-Whitney U–Wilcoxon Rank sum test.

Results

On the self-perception scale, the girls with TS on average did not deviate from the reference values. Expressed in the stanine score, the TS group had the mean score = 5.02, 1 SD = 2.02, and the reference is mean score = 5, 1 SD = 2. Most of the girls with TS described themselves as well functioning, with a normal psychological well being. The scores were distributed similarly to those of the reference group (i.e., there was a considerable variability). Some individuals scored low on self-perception, indicating the presence of a subgroup that is important to identify in clinical practice.

On the CBCL-P, parents rated their children as having significantly lower social competence and more behavioral problems than did parents of a matched control group. On the total competence scale, the TS group had median score = 14.5, range = 7.5–21.5; the control group had median score = 16.75, range = 11.0–25.0 ($p < .001$). On the total problem behavior scale, the TS group had median score = 17, range = 2–73; the control group had median score = 11, range = 0–65 ($p < .01$). As in the reference group, there was a large variability in scores. Behavior problem scores for this group were of the same magnitude as it was in other groups of children with chronic disorders. The scores of the TS group, however, average below the level of clinically referred children.

There was a lack of agreement between the ratings of the girls and their parents. On average the girls had a normal self-perception, whereas the parents rated their daughters as having more behavior and emotional problems and a lower social competence, than did parents of normal children.

Discussion

The possible interpretations of the preceding results will be discussed in relation to personality traits, handicap in general, and social psychology.

Personality Traits

The girls with TS in the present sample rated their self-perception as normal, on average. This is perhaps surprising as it could be expected to be impaired considering the difficulties associated with TS, and in the view of the ratings made by the parents. One interpretation could be that these girls have a typical personality style, which is a direct effect of the chromosome disorder. This personality style has previously been characterized as "inertia of emotional arousal," making females with TS compliant, phlegmatic, and tolerant of personal adversity (8). This personality type could protect against stress secondary to the disabilities associated with the condition. Women with TS have been reported to have low scores on a neuroticism scale, and a high tolerance for stress (9,10). The absence of an increased risk of psychopathology in females with TS could also be an argument for the existence of a typical TS personality type. This personality type may explain the discrepancy between the ratings of the girls and their parents.

The large variability in the results, however, is not easily explained this way. The variability in the girls self-perception scores was similar to that of the reference group. Whereas most of the girls score in the middle of the scale, some girls with TS had low scores, which indicates a low self-perception and a poor psychological well-being. This distribution is not in accordance with the typical personality style described earlier. In the literature, a similar variability has been described, with subgroups of females with TS reporting subjective psychological suffering, such as feelings of depression (11,12). Although there is some evidence of a TS personality type, at a group level this model cannot explain the variation in our sample.

Handicap

Is it possible to learn something about TS from studies of other groups of people with chronic disorders and handicaps? A general finding in individuals with chronic disorders is that their subjective well-being is better when rated by themselves than it is when rated by others. This may be one factor explaining why the girls in our sample rated their well-being as normal. From their point of view, it is normal.

The parents' rating of psychological functioning shows that many parents experience difficulties with their child. There can be direct problems with the girls' behavior and disabilities. Learning disabilities are common, and they represent additional problems for the parents. Social problems also make the child more dependent on her family. Parents may also have indirect problems concerning their own experiences of and reactions to having a child with a chronic disorder. These experiences and reactions are similar to those of other parents of children with chronic disorders. If the crisis reactions of the parents are not handled well, it may lead to a distorted perception of the child, resulting in over- or underestimation of problems. Parents may compare their child with other "normal" children, even with their imaginary ideal child. They might also suffer from anticipatory grief because they are worried about their child's future.

This handicap perspective may add to our understanding of the results of this study, and it may help to explain the normal ratings of the girls as well as the difficulties described by the parents.

Social Psychology

Our understanding and knowledge about other individuals influence the way we interact with them. Individuals with a label (e.g., a diagnosis of a chronic disorder) are at risk of being stigmatized. Social interaction may thus become a problem because others often tend to see the label rather than to consider the person as an individual.

According to social psychology, one part of our development of an identity is influenced by the way other people react to us. The process of developing an identity is particularly delicate for children with chronic disorders. The way in which other people relate to girls with TS is of utmost importance for their psychological development. In clinical practice, girls with TS and their parents should be given the message that although they have certain difficulties to handle throughout life, the chances are good that they will live a satisfactory life. Many of the girls and women in the project are satisfied with the way they live their lives. This satisfactory quality of life can be achieved by more girls and women with TS if we can optimize the care given to this group, and provide each of them with a more individual and hopeful "treatment."

Acknowledgments. The authors wish to thank Greta and Einar Askers foundation, First May Foundation, Swedish Medical Research Council No. 7509, Freemason's lodge, The Swedish Foundation for Health Care Sciences and Allergy Research, The Swedish National Board of Health and Welfare, and Bo Larsson for support.

References

1. Swillen A, Fryns J, Kleczkowska A, Massa G, Vanderschueren-Lodeweyckx M, Van den Berghe H. Intelligence, behaviour and psychological development in Turner syndrome. Genet Couns 1993;4:7–18.
2. Rovet J. The psychoeducational characteristics of children with Turner syndrome. J Learn Dis 1993;26:333–41.
3. McCauley E, Ito J, Kay T. Psychosocial functioning in girls with Turner's syndrome and short stature: social skills, behavior problems, and self concept. J Am Acad Child Psychiatr 1986;25:105–12.
4. Skuse D, Percy E, Stevenson J. Psychosocial functioning in the Turner syndrome: a national survey. In: Stabler B, Underwood L, eds. Growth, stature, and adaptation. Behavioral, social and cognitive aspects of growth delay. Chapel Hill: The University of North Carolina, 1994:151–64.
5. McCauley E, Ross J, Kushner H, Cutler G. Self-esteem and behavior in girls with Turner syndrome. J Dev Behav Pediatr 1995;16:82–88.
6. Ouvinen-Birgerstam P. Jag tycker jag är. Manual. Stockholm: Psykologiförlaget AB, 1985.
7. Achenbach T. Manual for the child behavior checklist/4–18 and 1991 profile. Burlington, VT: University of Vermont, Department of Psychiatry, 1991.

8. Money J, Mittenthal S. Lack of personality pathology in Turners syndrome: relation to cytogenetics, hormones and physique. Behav Genet 1970;1:43–56.
9. Baekgaard W, Nyborg H, Nielsen J. Neuroticism and extroversion in Turner's syndrome. J Abnorm Psychol 1978;87:583–86.
10. Raboch J, Kobilková J, Horejsí J, Stárka L, Raboch J. Sexual development and life of women with gonadal dysgenesis. J Sex Marital Ther 1987;13:117–27.
11. Sylvén L, Magnusson C, Hagenfeldt K, von Schoultz B. Life with Turner's syndrome—a psychosocial report from 22 middle-aged women. Acta Endocrinol (Copenh) 1993;129:188–94.
12. McCauley E, Sybert V, Ehrhardt A. Psychosocial adjustment of adult women with Turner syndrome. Clin Genet 1986;29:284–90.

Part IV

Treatment of Diabetes: Efficacy, Innovation and Quality of Life

14

Evaluating Quality of Life in Diabetes: Methods and Findings

ALAN M. JACOBSON

Introduction

Diabetes mellitus refers to a group of chronic illnesses, which manifest themselves because of a relative paucity of insulin compared with the metabolic needs of the person. Insulin dependent diabetes mellitus (IDDM) or Type 1 diabetes, is most commonly caused by an autoimmune process that leads to the destruction of the pancreatic beta cell so that insulin production capacity is eradicated. Noninsulin dependent diabetes (NIDDM), or Type 2 diabetes, is apparently caused by a gradual increase in cellular resistance to the effects of insulin, loss of beta cell mass, and subsequent reduction in insulin production. Obesity is a common precursor of Type 2 diabetes. The precise cause and sequence of events leading to Type 2 diabetes are not well understood. The clinical course of treatment varies from Type 1 diabetes, with its sudden onset and requirement for immediate insulin replacement. Type 2 patients can often be treated for many years with diet alone or combined with oral agents that improve insulin sensitivity and/or increase insulin release before insulin replacement is needed. Type 2 diabetes is approximately 10 times more common than Type 1 diabetes, and it occurs later in life. It is increasing in prevalence in developing nations as they adopt western eating and activity patterns. In the United States, Hispanic, African-American, and Indian populations are at especially high risk for Type 2 diabetes. Because Type 1 diabetes typically has its onset in childhood, it has a longer and possibly more profound personal impact on the individual patient and family. Its sudden onset, its requirement for insulin replacement, its threat of future complications, and its demand for extensive education have led to a large body of psychological research on the quality of life of patients and family members. In this chapter we will discuss the principal findings from this psychosocial literature. Because there are relatively few psychosocial studies of patients with Type 2 diabetes we will primarily focus on Type 1 diabetes.

Defining Quality of Life

Health-related quality of life may be defined as the individual's subjective perception of well-being as it relates to health status. Health-related quality of life (HRQOL) assessment is best thought of as being multidimensional, including such areas as physical functioning, role functioning, pain, emotional well-being, side effects from treatment, and concerns about the future (1). Studies addressing the psychosocial impact of diabetes address important dimensions of HRQOL (2,3). Many of these studies predate the conceptualization of quality of life. Thus, they serve as a useful backdrop for understanding studies that have been undertaken more recently and designed with the concept of quality of life in mind. Moreover, the findings from the earlier psychosocial literature have influenced the development of HRQOL measures for use with diabetic patients (2–4).

Two general approaches to HRQOL assessment have evolved over time: generic versus illness specific measurement. Generic or nonspecific assessments of HRQOL are best exemplified by measures such as the medical outcome survey (5), the quality of well-being instrument (6), and the sickness impact profile (7). Some of these tools are multidimensional assessments designed to evaluate a broad range of functioning applicable to patients with all illnesses (e.g., SF36).

However, even these cross-disease, multidimensional measures can differ in specific areas of function evaluated. Other measures were designed to provide a single utility index of overall quality of life (6). Such utility indexes have been used to compare costs versus the benefits of treatments. Generic measures are particularly useful for cross-illness comparisons and economic analyses of treatment. There have been some suggestions that generic measures may be less sensitive to change in functioning than illness specific measures (8). Their value may also depend on the stage and type of illness. For example, patients with Type I diabetes before the onset of complications may experience virtually no changes in physical functioning. Thus, measures like sickness impact profile (7), which emphasize assessment of physical capacity, may not be useful in detecting the HRQOL effects of diabetes until late in the course of this illness after complications have occurred. Indeed, studies of Type I diabetes in children, adolescents, and young adults suggest that the HRQOL impact may be most sensitively detected with measurement strategies that address psychological and social domains rather than the physical functioning (2,3). Even when Type 1 diabetes leads to early complications, such as episodic glycemic dysregulation causing severe hypoglycemia and/or repeated ketoacidosis, delayed puberty and/or short stature, measures of physical capacity may be less likely than psychosocial indexes to differentiate such patients from modal patients. Inquiries about fear of hypoglycemia and its impact on social, work, and school functioning may be especially important for detection of effects of diabetes treatment (9).

Illness-specific measures may be especially useful for addressing unique aspects of illness experience and areas of physical function affected by the particular disease. Even illness-specific quality of life assessment may not be sufficiently precise for addressing the concerns of specific clinical trials and programs. Thus, we have suggested a three-level approach that incorporates generic measures, illness-specific measures, and, finally, study-specific measures for use in clinical studies and trials (1–3).

Impact of Diabetes on HRQOL in Children, Adolescents, and Young Adults

As noted, the largest number of studies are those that were primarily focused on understanding the psychological impact of Type 1 diabetes (10). Over the past two decades a large number of such studies have been carried out. It is beyond the scope of this chapter to provide an extensive review of these studie; therefore, the reader is directed to other reviews that provide more extensive discussion of these issues (10–14).

Because Type 1 diabetes is inevitably associated with hypoglycemia that can lead to unconsciousness, coma, and/or seizures, questions have been raised about the impact of these severe events on neuropsychological function. A series of studies now suggests that very early onset of disease (prior to age 6) is associated with later alterations in neuropsychological functioning that are particularly manifested in areas of attention, concentration, and motor speed, and may result in subtle decrements in IQ (15–17). These studies also suggest that within this early onset group, patients with a history of serious hypoglycemia have the greatest likelihood of subsequent cognitive impairment (16,17).

It is unresolved whether serious hypoglycemia in older children and adults leads to similar deficits in cognitive function. Langnan et al (18) found that severe hypoglycemia in adults was associated with development of cognitive deficits. The Diabetes Control and Complications Trial (DCCT), however, failed to demonstrate an impact of severe hypoglycemia on neuropsychological functioning (19–21). In the DCCT, Type 1 patients, ages 13–39, were randomized to conventional or intensive therapy (19). The goal of conventional therapy was avoidance of symptomatic hypo- or hyperglycemia. The intensive regimen goal was improved glycemic regulation as close to the nondiabetic range as safely possible (19). The intensive treatment led to a 50–75% decrease in risk of microvascular complications over the follow-up (mean follow-up = 6.5 years) (19). It was also associated with a threefold risk of severe hypoglycemia (19,22). Because of the anticipated increase in severe hypoglycemia in the intensive therapy group serial neuropsychological assessments were incorporated in the study design (20,21). The study did not identify an effect of treatment group status or severe hypoglycemia on cognitive dysfunction (20,21). Because the trial randomized patients whose hypoglycemia was well characterized before and during the study, this study provides strong support for the contention that the severe hypoglycemia does not lead to cognitive impairment from adolescence through adulthood. To date, the DCCT cohort has been studied using neuropsychological assessments for a maximum of 10 years through a maximum age of approximately 49 years and duration of diabetes of 25 years. Cognitive impairment could develop as patients age and/or experience even longer-term diabetes. Follow-up of this cohort over a longer period into later adulthood would provide valuable information about the natural history of cognitive dysfunction related to the course of Type 1 diabetes and its associated microvascular and macrovascular complications. Because a 10-year follow-up study of the DCCT cohort is now underway, it will be possible to implement such an evaluation.

Because of the potential effects of Type 1 diabetes on cognitive functioning, some investigators have examined school performance of children and adolescents. One such study indicates that school performance problems may be more likely in boys compared with girls (23); however, there is no clear effect of diabetes in school performance overall.

Other researchers have examined the effects of diabetes on psychological dimensions such as: ego development (24) self-esteem, (25) psychiatric and behavioral problems (25,26) and social functioning (27). These studies have typically been cross-sectional in nature. Most of these studies indicate that child and early to mid adolescent patients do not differ from healthy controls along these dimensions (24,25,28).

There are indications that older adolescents and young adults may develop lowered self-esteem that is related to social functioning and may not experience as close relationships as individuals without diabetes (27,28). There are conflicting data finds regarding the effects of diabetes on work success in young adults (27,29). One longitudinal study examining depression and other psychiatric problems in an onset cohort of diabetic children followed over several years suggests that there may be an increase in depression in older adolescent and young adult patients of life (26). The study also shows that a substantial minority of patients develop situational reactions to diagnosis and that patients diagnosed with these conditions are most likely to develop other psychiatric problems later in the course of diabetes. This study unfortunately did not utilize a control group; thus it is difficult to interpret the impact of the repeated measurements on the findings. Because the principal comparison populations are derived from cross-sectional studies, it is possible that repeated interviewing leads to greater openness, which leads to overdiagnosis compared with individuals who are evaluated on one occasion.

Other cross-sectional studies of older adolescents and adults with type 1 diabetes, however, have also found an increased frequency of depressive disorders in patients with Type 1 diabetes (11,30,31). Taken together, these studies appear to support the hypothesis that Type 1 diabetes poses an increased risk for the depressive disorder, and also that the increase occurs before the development of serious complications. The mechanism for this relationship is not understood. It is possible that the increased risk reflects the psychological distress brought on by a complex chronic illness and may be understood through the learned "helplessness" model of depression. On the other hand, recurrent hypoglycemia or other hormonal and metabolic alterations of diabetes could predispose patients to affective disorder. No studies have examined these mechanisms to date. The evolving field of functional imaging may provide a useful methodology for evaluating the biological hypothesis. Relevant to this reasoning, one unpublished study suggests that patients with onset of Type 1 diabetes before age 10 years may be at special risk for depression as young adults (personal communication, Samson, Jacobson, and deGroot). This finding is interesting because patients with early onset of diabetes and severe hypoglycemia have also shown decrements in cognitive functioning. It is possible that early hypoglycemia may also be a risk factor for later depression.

There has also been considerable interest in the possibility that type 1 diabetes increases the risk of eating disorders particularly bulimia in young women. The findings from studies examining this issue are not entirely supportive (12). Polonsky et al. (32) found that insulin omission is a common occurrence in women with Type 1 diabetes ages 15–30, with 30% of women acknowledging at least occasional insulin omission and 16% acknowledging frequent insulin omission. Most of these patients did not meet diagnostic criteria for bulimia. The main reason for purposeful insulin omission appears to be that of weight control so that manipulation of insulin dose may be a common feature of eating problems in patients with diabetes. Although diabetes may not place women at greater risk for bulimia, bulimia leads to glycemic control problems (32) and increases the risk for diabetic retinopathy (33).

A few systematic studies have used HRQOL measures to study adults with diabetes in comparison to other chronic illness populations (34). Patients with diabetes appear to have HRQOL levels that are lower than the general population and similar to patients with other chronic illnesses, such as rheumatoid arthritis (34). The comparison across populations is complex to interpret without information about the severity of medical complications within each disease group. Because Type 2 diabetes is 10 times more common than Type 1 diabetes, and most of these patients are on oral agents or diet alone, quality of life scores should reflect the treatment regimen and the relative lack of complications. Indeed, Jacobson et al. found HRQOL decreases as the number of complications increases (1) (see Fig. 14.1). Furthermore, psychiatric disorders play an important role in determining HRQOL in patients with chronic illness (35). Thus, understanding the psychiatric status of patient populations can help tease out the effects of medical illness on HRQOL from co-occurring psychiatric disorders.

Diabetes Treatment and Quality of Life

Studies examining HRQOL effects of treatment have suggested that patients with Type 2 diabetes may experience worse quality of life on oral agents compared to diet (1,36). A more complex set of findings have been uncov-

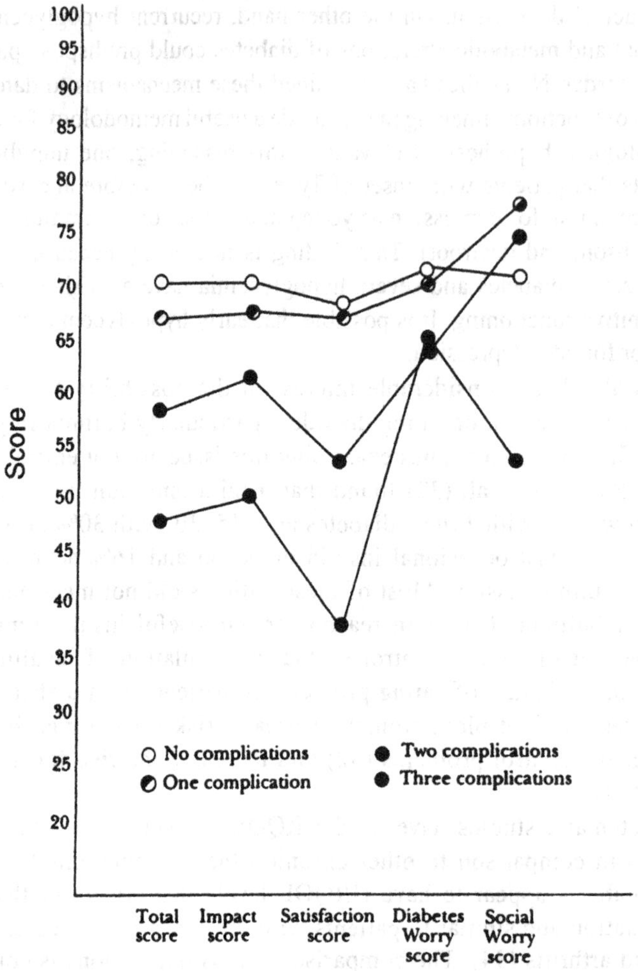

FIGURE 14.1. The effect of microvascular complications (neuropathy, nephropathy, retinopathy) on DQOL scores among patients with IDDM. Reproduced with permission (1).

ered with regard to the transition from oral agents to insulin. Jacobson et al. found that satisfaction, impact, and social worry scales of the Diabetes Quality of Life Measure (DQOL) were lower in patients on insulin compared with oral agents, but diabetes worries were lower in patients on insulin than they were patients on oral agents (1). This suggested that patients on oral agents anticipated worsening of the condition, and once insulin treatment was undertaken fears of the future waned. Welch et al. (36) found that patients who were on a combination of oral agents plus insulin had worse quality of life than did patients on either insulin alone or oral agents. This provided further evidence that the transition from oral agents to insulin was likely to be one of increased concern and distress; however, no studies have longitudinally followed patients with Type 2 diabetes over time to study the transition across therapies.

Among patients with Type 1 diabetes the major treatment issue has been whether intensified diabetes therapy with the goal of improving glycemic control to the nondiabetic range would be associated with decreased HRQOL. The DCCT Research Group therefore developed the DQOL, a diabetes-oriented quality of life measure, and also assessed psychiatric symptoms using the SCL 90 (4,37). At study end the SF-36 was also added to the assessment battery. The study showed that the intensive treatment group had HRQOL levels identical to the patients in the conventionally treated group over the entire length of other study (37). An ancillary study, examining in greater depth a subsample of patients in the DCCT, suggested that patients undergoing intensive treatment had a more positive view of their diabetes therapy than did patients on the conventional treatment (38). Thus, intensified treatment implemented in a carefully selected and followed population appears to be associated with maintained or even enhanced well-being.

Methods for Assessment of HRQOL in Diabetic Samples

Over the past 10 years there has been considerable interest in the development of measures that assess diabetes-related psychosocial issues, including treatment satisfaction, quality of life, distress, fear of hypoglycemia, family functioning, and barriers to adherence (39). Measures particularly relevant for the assessment of HRQOL include DQOL, Problem Areas in Diabetes Scale (PAID) and Hypoglycemia Fear Survey.

DQOL

DQOL was developed for specific use in the DCCT (1–4). It was designed, however, so that it would be applicable to a broad range of Type 1 and Type 2 diabetic patients. It has four subscales (treatment satisfaction, impact, diabetes worry, social worry), a single general well-being question, and several additional items of relevance to adolescents and young adults. The measure has also been modified for use with children and younger adolescents (40). The measure has been found to have favorable internal consistency, test–retest reliability, and convergent and discriminant validity. Its discriminant validity is supported by studies comparing patients with different levels of complications and treatments (1–4). It has now been applied in both Type 1 and Type 2 patient populations (1,36). The impact and satisfaction scales are especially applicable to Type 2 patients (1,36). The worry scales were incorporated into the original instrument because recognition that youngsters with diabetes often fretted about their futures. These scales may be less applicable for older Type 2 patients (1–3). Table 14.1 shows selected items of the DQOL.

TABLE 14.1. Diabetes quality of life measure (DQOL), selected items.

Satisfaction	
	How satisfied are you with the amount of time it takes to manage your diabetes?
	How satisfied are you with the flexibility you have in your diet?
Impact	
	How often are you embarrassed by having to deal with your diabetes in public?
	How often do you find your diabetes limiting your social relationships and friendships?
Social worry	
	How often do your worry about whether you will have children?
	How often do you worry about whether you will not get a job you want?
Diabetes worry	
	How often do you worry about whether you will pass out?
	How often do you worry that you will get complications from your diabetes?

Based on References 1, 3, and 4.

PAID

The PAID was designed initially for use with patients with Type 1 diabetes, but it has now also been evaluated in Type 2 populations (41,42). It is designed for two uses: (1) as a screen for diabetes-related distress and (2) to identify particular problem areas that could be the focus of education and psychological intervention. This scale has shown favorable internal consistency and test–retest reliability. It has also been shown to be sensitive to variation in the course of diabetes treatment (41,42). In one study of patients with Type 2 diabetes, who were evaluated on a battery of HRQOL related measures, the PAID was found to be the most sensitive measure of patient well-being (36). Table 14.2 shows selected items of the PAID.

TABLE 14.2. Problem areas in diabetes (PAID), selected items.

From your perspective, to what degree are the following diabetes-related issued currently a problem for you? Please circle the best answer for you for each question.

	A serious problem			Not a problem		
1. Not having clear and concrete goals for your diabetes care?	1	2	3	4	5	6
2. Poor blood sugar control?	1	2	3	4	5	6
3. Feeling discouraged with your diabetes treatment plan?	1	2	3	4	5	6
4. Feeling scared when you think about living with diabetes?	1	2	3	4	4	6

Based on References 41 and 42.

TABLE 14.3. Hypoglycemia fear survey, selected items.

I worry about . . .	Never	Rarely	Sometimes	Often	Always
1. Embarrassing myself or my friends in a social situation	0	1	2	3	4
2. Appearing stupid or drunk	0	1	2	3	4
3. Having a reaction while driving	0	1	2	3	4
4. Passing out in public	0	1	2	3	4

Based on Reference 43.

Hypoglycemia Fear Survey

The Hypoglycemia Fear Survey developed by Cox et al. (9,43) consists of two subscales, a behavior and a worry subscale. The behavior subscale depicts patient actions in response to hypoglycemia; the worry scale focuses on the emotional response to hypoglycemia. A new version of this scale has been developed. It may also be applicable for Type 2 patients on oral agents especially for comparison a cross treatment group, where oral agents pose different levels of risk for hypoglycemia. Like the PAID, it may be quite useful in the process of identifying issues for educational intervention. Table 14.3 shows selected items of the PAID.

Future Directions

Past psychosocial studies, the development of measures for assessing diabetes-specific psychosocial issues, and the increasing use of well-validated HRQOL measures provide a foundation for future research. The provocative findings about the relationship of deficits in cognitive functioning to early onset of diabetes and concomitant severe hypoglycemia leads to questions about appropriate treatment strategies in this age group. Studies of psychosocial and educational interventions in children and adolescents with diabetes will be quite useful in evaluating whether the risk for depression in adulthood is preventable. Because there is still a controversy about the effect of hypoglycemia on cognitive functioning among patients with onset in adolescence and adulthood, further study of these age groups is required. It would be especially useful to follow up the DCCT cohort to see whether longer duration of disease in an older population might show effects of cognitive deterioration associated with prior hypoglycemia. The expected increase in prevalence of Type 2 diabetes world-wide should lead to greater attention of the HRQOL aspects of this disease across cultures and in high-risk ethnic groups in the United States. Finally, HRQOL measures may be valuable for clinical practice. The complex nature of diabetes, its chronicity, course and demanding treatment all make it likely that understanding quality of life issues of individual patients and their families may assist clinical decision making and treatment planning.

References

1. Jacobson AM, deGroot M, Samson J. Quality of life in patients with type 1 and type 2 diabetes mellitus. Diabetes Care, 1994;17:167–274.
2. Jacobson A, deGroot M, Samson J. Quality of life research in patients with diabetes mellitus. In: Dimsdale JE, Baum A, eds. Underlying perspectives on behavioral medicine. NJ: Lawrence Erlbaum Associates, 1994.
3. Jacobson AM. The DCCT Research Group. The diabetes quality of life measure. In: Bradley CS, ed. Handbook of Psychology and Diabetes. Switzerland: Harwood Academic Publishers, 1996.
4. DCCT Research Group. Reliability and validity of a diabetes quality of life measure for the diabetes control and complication trial (DCCT). Diabetes Care 11: 725–32.
5. Ware JH, Sherbourne CD. The MOS 36-item short form health survey (SF36). I. Conceptual framework and core item selection. Med Care 1992;30:473–83.
6. Bush JM, Kaplan RM. Health-related quality of life measurement. Health Psychol 1982;1:61–80.
7. Bergner M, Bobbitt RA, Carter WB, Gibson BS. The sickness impact profile: development and final revision of a health status measure. Medical Care 1981;19: 787–805.
8. Guyatt G, Bombardier C, Tugwell P. Measuring disease-specific quality of life in clinical trials. Can Med Assoc J 1986;134:889–95.
9. Cox D, Irvine A, Gonder-Frederick L, Nowacek G, Butterfield J. Fear of hypoglycemia: quantification, validation, and utilization, Diabetes Care 1987;10:617–21.
10. Jacobson AM. Psychological care of patients with IDDM. N Eng J Med 1996; 334:1249–53.
11. Lustman PJ, Griffith LS, Gavard JA, Clouse RE. Depression in adults with diabetes. Diabetes Care 1992;15:1631–39.
12. Rodin GM, Daneman D. Eating disorders and insulin-dependent diabetes mellitus: a problematic association. Diabetes Care 1992;15:1402–12.
13. Rubin RR, Peyrot M. Psychosocial problems and interventions in diabetes: a review of the literature. Diabetes Care 1992;15:1640–57.
14. Surwit RS, Schneider MS, Feinglos MN. Stress and diabetes mellitus. Diabetes Care 1992;15:1413–22.
15. Ryan CM, Vega A, Drash A. Cognitive deficits in adolescents who developed diabetes early in life. Pediatrics 1985;75:921–27.
16. Rovet JF, Ehrlich RM, Hoppe M. Intellectual deficits associated with early onset of insulin-dependent diabetes mellitus in children. Diabetes Care 1997;10:510–16.
17. Bjorgaas M, Gimse R, Vik T, Sand T. Cognitive function in Type I diabetic children with and without episodes of severe hypoglycaemia. Acta Paediatr 1987;86: 148–53.
18. Langan SJ, Deary IJ, Hepburn DA, Frier BM. Cumulative cognitive impairment following recurrent severe hypoglycemia in adult patients with insulin-treated diabetes mellitus. Diabetologia 1991;34:337–44.

19. DCCT Research Group. The effect of intensive treatment of diabetes on the development and progress of long-term complications in insulin-dependent diabetes mellitus. N Engl J Med 1993;329:977–86.
20. DCCT Research Group. Prepared by Lan SP, Ryan CM, Adams KM, Grant I, Heaton RK, Rand LI, et al. A screening algorithm to identify clinically significant changes in neuropsychological function diabetes control and complications trial. J Clin Exp Neuropsychol 1994;16:303–16.
21. DCCT Research Group. The effects of intensive treatment on neuropsychological function in adults in the DCCT. Ann Intern Med 1996;124:379–88.
22. DCCT Research Group. Epidemiology of severe hypoglycemia in the diabetes control and complications trial. Am J Med 1991;90:450–59.
23. Holmes CS, Dunlap WP, Chen RS, Cornwall JM. Gender differences in the learning status of diabetic children. J Consult Clin Psychol 1992;60:698–704.
24. Hauser ST, Jacobson AM, Noam G, Powers S. Ego development and self-image in early adolescence: longitudinal studies of psychiatric and diabetic patients. Arch Gen Psychiatr 1983;40:325–32.
25. Jacobson AM, Hauser S, Willett J, Wolfsdorf J, Dvorak R, Herman, et al. Psychological adjustment to insulin-dependent diabetes mellitus: Ten-year follow-up of onset cohort of child and adolescent patients. Diabetes Care 1997;20:811–15.
26. Kovacs MHV, Pollock MH. Criterion and predictive validity of the diagnosis of adjustment disorder: a prospective study of youths with new-onset insulin-dependent diabetes mellitus. Am J Psychiatr 1995;152:523–28.
27. Jacobson AM, Hauser S, Willett J, Wolfsdorf J, Dvorak R, Wolpert H, et al. Social relationships among young adults with insulin-dependent diabetes mellitus: ten-year follow-up of an onset cohort. Diabetic Med 1997;14:73–79.
28. Lloyd CE, Robinson N, Andrews B, Elston MA, Fuller JH. Are the social relationships of young insulin-dependent diabetic patients affected by their condition? Diabetic Med 1993:10:481–85.
29. Lloyd C, Robinson N, Fuller J. Education and employment experiences in young adults with Type 1 diabetes mellitus. Diabetic Med 1992;9:661–66.
30. Lustman PJ, Griffith LS, Clouse RE, Cryer PE. Psychiatric illness in diabetes mellitus. J Nerv Mental Dis 1986;174:736–42.
31. Robinson N, Fuller JH, Edmeades SP. Depression and diabetes. Diabetic Med 1988;5:268–74.
32. Polonsky W, Anderson B, Lohrer P, Aponte J, Jacobson A, Cole C. Insulin omission in women with IDDM. Diabetes Care 1994;17:1178–85.
33. Rydall AC, Robin GM, Olmsted MP, Devenyi RG, Daneman D. Disordered eating behavior and microvascular complications in young women with insulin-dependent diabetes mellitus. N Engl J Med 1997;336:1846–54.
34. Stewart AL, Greenfield S, Hays RD. Functional status and well-being of patients with chronic conditions. JAMA 1989;262:907–13.
35. Jacobson AM, DeGroot M, Samson J. The effects of psychiatric disorders and symptoms on quality of life in patients with type 1 and type 2 diabetes mellitus. J Qual Life Res 1997;6:11–22.
36. Welch G, Bakst A, Revicki D, Marquis P. Psychological adjustment among NIDDM patients in transition from tablet to insulin therapy. Diabetes 1997;46A:1025.
37. DCCT Research Group. The effect of intensive treatment on quality of life outcomes in the diabetes control and complications trial. Diabetes Care 1996;9: 195–203.

38. Young-Hyman D, Peyrot M, Jacobson AM, Schlundt D, Drotar D. Impact of intensive treatment on diabetes-related attitudes and behaviors in the DCCT. Diabetes 1994;43A.
39. Bradley C. Handbook of psychology and diabetes. Langhorne, PA: Harwood Academic Publishers, 1994.
40. Ingersoll GM, Marrero DG. A modified quality of life measure for youths: psychometric properties. Diabetes Ed 1991;17:114–18.
41. Polonsky W, Anderson B, Welch G, Jacobson AM. Assessment of diabetes-specific distress. Diabetes Care 1995;18:754–60.
42. Welch G, Jacobson A, Polonsky W. The problem areas in diabetes (PAID) scale. An examination of its clinical utility. Diabetes Care 1997;20:760–66.
43. Irvine A, Cox D, Gonder-Frederick L. The fear of hypoglycemia scale. In: Bradley C, ed. Handbook of psychology and diabetes. Langhorne, PA: Harwood Academic Publishers, 1994.

15

Effective Utilization of Self-Monitored Blood Glucose Data: Cognitive and Behavioral Prerequisites

TIM WYSOCKI

Introduction

American Diabetes Association consensus statements have affirmed the crucial role of self-monitoring of blood glucose (SMBG) in modern therapy for diabetes mellitus (1,2). The 1987 statement emphasized the use of SMBG data by health care providers for evaluating and modifying the treatment regimen, whereas the 1994 statement gave greater emphasis to patients' use of SMBG data to guide day-to-day treatment adjustments. Among the key functions of SMBG identified in the 1994 consensus statement were that patients should learn to use SMBG for self-adjustment of diet, exercise and/or medication, identifying and properly treating hypo- and hyperglycemia, and improving diabetes decision making and problem solving. The American Diabetes Association's standards for patient education programs similarly include training in the use of SMBG data as a required content area, and its clinical practice recommendations also encourage this (3,4). As a result, the American Diabetes Association has sanctioned efforts to teach patients how to use SMBG data actively as part of a patient-centered diabetes self-management regimen.

Since the Diabetes Control and Complications Trial (DCCT), it has become clear that maintenance of near-normoglycemia depends very heavily on the extent to which patients can be helped to develop sophisticated skills in the use of SMBG data (5–7). This chapter will review the literature on patients' active and proactive use of SMBG data for treatment adjustments. As we shall see, this limited literature suggests that underutilization of SMBG data by patients was common in the years prior to the DCCT. Next, the chapter will analyze the complex psychological context that surrounds

SMBG, which illustrates why our attempts to promote patients' skills in these domains must acknowledge and address this complexity. The chapter will conclude with a conceptual framework for developing pertinent instructional objectives at several levels of cognitive sophistication. Such a strategy could guide the selection of patients for training in aggressive diabetes self-management and enhance the capacity to help more patients to achieve that level of sophistication.

Active Self-Management Based on SMBG Data

As SMBG came into use in the early 1980s, test results were used primarily by health care providers to evaluate and modify the diabetes regimen during clinical encounters. Few could have envisioned that today there would be a much greater emphasis on encouraging patients and their families to play a central role in evaluating and modifying the diabetes regimen in response to SMBG results, dietary intake, and physical activity. Multiple factors probably account for this shift in emphasis over the past 15 years:

- Increasing experience and improved comfort in reacting to SMBG data by health care providers.
- Realization that many patients could and would perform SMBG accurately enough and frequently enough to justify its clinical application.
- Growth and proliferation of the "patient empowerment" movement.
- Expansion of managed care and its encouragement of reliance on physician-extenders, and encouragement of prevention of hospitalizations.
- The DCCT has resulted in an evolution of diabetes treatment toward more intensive treatment aimed at maintaining near-normoglycemia in as many patients as possible and in improving glycemic control in all patients.
- Recognition that prevention of severe hypoglycemia must be a priority of intensified diabetes management and that this requires timely response to SMBG data.

The DCCT did not include efforts to demonstrate the specific mechanisms responsible for successful maintenance of near-normoglycemia in that trial. Experienced clinicians who were involved in that trial, however, pointed to patients' acquisition and mastery of flexible diabetes problem solving based on SMBG data as a critical ingredient of intensive therapy (6,7). In view of the importance of active and proactive use of SMBG data to successful self-management of diabetes, it is surprising that there has been relatively little research done on factors influencing patients' acquisition and maintenance of these skills.

Research on Patients' Use of SMBG Data

Despite its central role in diabetes management, the frequency and proficiency of patients' use of SMBG data has received little research attention (8,9). Some studies have described the uses of SMBG data exhibited among specific samples of patients, whereas others have illustrated the potential benefits of patients' mastery of these skills. Delamater and colleagues (10) showed that adolescents with Type 1 diabetes used their SMBG results infrequently for insulin dose adjustments or for modifying the injection–meal interval. Rubin and Peyrot (11) reported that among adults with diabetes, insulin self-regulation based on SMBG data was associated with better diabetic control. In a 4-week prospective study of 47 families of children and adolescents with Type 1 diabetes, Wysocki et al. (12) reported that 74% of the families demonstrated at least one treatment action in response to SMBG data over that period. Among the 228 recorded treatment actions, 50% involved managing hypoglycemia, whereas the rest included adjustments to insulin (42%), diet (3%), or exercise (1%), or telephone contact with a health care provider (4%). Only 9% of the recorded actions were proactive attempts to prevent possible adverse changes in blood glucose levels. Several randomized controlled trials have shown that psychoeducational interventions targeting active use of SMBG data for diabetes problem solving improved diabetic control among children and adolescents with Type 1 diabetes (13,14). There have been no similar intervention trials conducted with adult patients.

Cox et al. (15) reported the results of a prospective study of 78 adults with Type 1 diabetes. Patients performed 50 blood glucose tests at home over a 2–3-week baseline. Episodes of severe hypoglycemia over the next 6 months were recorded in daily diaries. A higher frequency of severe hypoglycemia during the 6-month follow-up was predictable from baseline variability in blood glucose concentration and baseline frequency of low SMBG readings. In a regression analysis of these data, these two factors accounted for 44% of the variance in frequency of severe hypoglycemia during the 6-month follow-up. The risk of severe hypoglycemia could perhaps be reduced by teaching patients to attend to these factors and by sensitizing health care providers to detect patients who are at higher risk of severe hypoglycemia.

A few studies, and considerable anecdotal evidence, confirm the therapeutic value of SMBG, but there is also evidence suggesting that these potential benefits have not been fully realized. It is important, therefore, to consider behavioral, cognitive, and affective factors that may impede patients from developing and using these higher level diabetes self-management skills. A thorough understanding of the psychological prerequisites to sophisticated self-management skills could enhance the selection of patients for this approach and help marginal candidates to become more capable of these high-level responsibilities.

The Psychological Context of SMBG

Performance of a blood glucose test and reacting to its results would seem to be a relatively uncomplicated sequence of events. The SMBG enterprise, however, is in fact a very intricate system characterized by complex interactions among numerous antecedent and consequent psychological events. Several authors have offered conceptual models that illustrate this complexity. Cox et al. (16) outlined the biological, cognitive, and behavioral factors that influence the occurrence of severe hypoglycemia. They have provided an eight-step stochastic model that would account for the multiple-choice points that intercede between detection of a possible hypoglycemic episode through the actual implementation of self-treatment behaviors. Wysocki (17) presented a conceptual model of the psychological context of SMBG, which illustrated the many psychological factors that may moderate the frequency and proficiency of use of SMBG data by patients. As shown in Figure 15.1, the patient's decisions regarding when, where, and how often to test are influenced by many preexisting psychological factors, including the patient's prior knowledge and beliefs about diabetes in general and SMBG in particular; the user-friendliness of the testing equipment; the patient's aversion to obtaining blood samples; the strength of the patient's beliefs regarding accuracy of estimation of blood glucose based on subjective physical symptoms; and specific psychological characteristics including presence or absence of depression, health locus of control, self-efficacy, and availability of diabetes-specific social supports. These psychological factors can affect the quality of the patient's SMBG data by influencing the frequency of testing, accuracy of test results, logbook reliability, and the temporal regularity of testing. Without a sufficient quantity of high-quality SMBG data, no patient or health care provider can make well-reasoned treatment decisions.

Psychological appraisal of test results is a complex phenomenon that introduces another source of error into the SMBG feedback loop. This link in

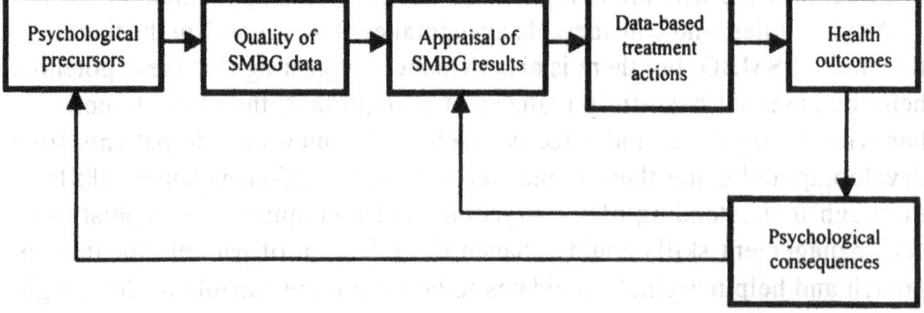

FIGURE 15.1. Conceptual model of factors influencing patients' therapeutic utilization of SMBG data.

the SMBG chain requires the patient accurately and promptly to interpret a given test result or to detect a systematic pattern within a series of results. These abilities are probably influenced by the degree of variability in the patient's SMBG data, prior experience in responding to similar situations, and accuracy of the patient's recall of those experiences. Spevack and colleagues (18) reported that even among expert diabetologists interrater reliability on judgments of diabetic control was far from perfect, with a mean of .78. If this is the case for physicians, one could speculate that the threshold for instituting a treatment action in response to SMBG data probably varies even more widely among patients. Before they can use their SMBG data effectively for therapeutic decision making, patients need explicit training in making these subtle discriminations.

Once a patient has correctly appraised the SMBG data and identified an actual or anticipated problem with blood glucose control, the patient must select and implement an appropriate treatment action. Because many diabetes problems can be solved with any of several actions alone or in combination, the patient must develop skills in recognizing the range of alternative solutions, projecting the potential consequences of each solution, and selecting the strategy that offers the best prospects for safe resolution of the identified problem. Patients must recognize the limits of their clinical judgment and know when it is appropriate to seek the guidance of a health care provider before taking definitive action.

If a selected action has been carried out, its effects on the targeted glycemic control problem will be evaluated by the patient. The effectiveness of the solution, its importance to the patient, and any adverse effects that might occur will each have psychological consequences that may influence the patient's subsequent propensity to obtain and use SMBG data for treatment adjustments and decision making. The core of this conceptual model, then, is the patient's capacity to appraise SMBG results accurately and then to carry that appraisal forward to select, implement and evaluate an appropriate and timely treatment action. As we have seen, this is an immensely complicated psychological process, with affective, cognitive, and behavioral components all playing key roles. How, then, can you evaluate your patient's capacity to assume such psychologically complex self-management responsibilities? How can you help your patients gradually to become more skilled and confident diabetes problem-solvers? I will try to give you a reasonably practical framework for helping more of your patients to achieve that level of self-management sophistication based on a well-known and widely applied taxonomy of educational objectives.

Bloom's Taxonomy and Diabetes Self-Management

Bloom's Taxonomy is a hierarchy for organizing educational objectives (19,20) according to six levels of cognitive sophistication. It could form the foundation for a systematic diabetes education program designed to assist patients to achieve self-management sophistication and independence. I have defined each cognitive level and provided examples of educational objectives at each level. Patients should master the more basic skill levels before proceeding to the more complex and sophisticated levels. Note that each successive level includes the elements of all of the lower levels. It is best to conceptualize the taxonomy as a continuum of cognitive complexity rather than as a collection of mutually exclusive categories.

Knowledge

Bloom identified *knowledge* as the lowest level of cognition, defined as the capacity to recall information accurately on demand. Instructional objectives at this level are directed at enhancing the student's ability to retrieve information from memory without any requirement for further processing of that information. Knowledge-level objectives that might be prerequisite to sophisticated diabetes self-management are:

- The student will define hypoglycemia as a metabolic state in which the blood glucose level is below 70 mg/dl.
- The student will state that the normal range for blood glucose is 70–120 mg/dl.
- The student will state the latency, duration, and peak of action of each type of insulin used by that student.

The remaining skill levels can all be thought of as higher cognitive processes because each requires some type of mental manipulation of data or facts in order to arrive at a correct answer or solution.

Comprehension

Objectives at the *comprehension* level demand more than simple retrieval of previously memorized facts and require the student to demonstrate understanding of principles or facts learned at the knowledge level. Comprehension objectives may require such operations as translation, interpretation, prediction, generalization, or explanation of examples that have not been encountered previously. Examples of diabetes educational objectives at the comprehension level are:

- When shown an actual blood glucose profile, the student will state the number or proportion of results that are above or below the normal range of 70–120 mg/dl.
- When shown a food label, the student will state the number of grams of carbohydrate contained in one serving of that food.
- The student will locate the expiration date on any vial of insulin.

Formal diabetes education all too often stops at the comprehension level.

Some patients may be able to take the next steps in becoming a sophisticated diabetes self-manager independently, but there may be many others who could benefit greatly from explicit, individualized education at the next four, higher cognitive levels.

Application

This next highest level of cognition is *application*, the ability to go beyond simple comprehension of a novel experience or event to solve a problem by selecting a tool or method that is most appropriate to the specific circumstances at hand. Here are some sample diabetes educational objectives at the application level:

- If shown a blood glucose profile with repeated episodes of hypoglycemia just after bedtime, the student will state three methods of preventing further episodes.
- When shown several foods that could be used to treat an episode of hypoglycemia, the student will be able to select the food(s) that contain 15 g of carbohydrate.
- If shown a blood glucose profile with four successive test results above 240 mg/dl, the student will state that a urine ketone test should be done.

Analysis

Analysis, the next level in Bloom's taxonomy, is the process of breaking down a complex system into its components or determining its characteristics. In the context of diabetes, this could involve recognition of the complex interactive roles that can be played by insulin dosage, caloric intake, and physical activity in yielding a specific blood glucose profile. A second critical feature of analysis-level objectives is that the student's skill mastery must be measured against some external criterion for successful performance. Here are two examples of analysis-level objectives in diabetes education:

- If shown a description of an insulin regimen consisting of three daily injections of mixed short-acting and intermediate-acting insulins and an accompanying blood glucose profile showing recurring hypoglycemia at about the same time daily, the student will correctly identify the type of insulin and time of administration that merits possible adjustment.
- If given a narrative description of a patient's usual dietary intake, physical activity, and insulin dosage, and a 14-day blood glucose profile, the student will propose and defend one or more changes in the treatment regimen that would achieve a reduction in mean blood glucose of 20 mg/dl.

Synthesis

Instructional objectives at this level are complementary to those at the analysis level. *Synthesis* is defined as the ability to combine or bring together several disparate elements to form a novel, cohesive whole. The synthesized product need only be unique to the student, not to the teacher or to those who are expert in this body of knowledge. As with analysis, the student must reach some criterion level of performance as a standard for success. Examples of diabetes educational objectives at the synthesis level are:

- The student will use food composition tables or nutritional software to develop an individualized meal plan meeting these criteria: Average daily carbohydrate intake is 90 g; calories from fat account for less than 25% of total caloric intake; and the plan includes at least three of the student's most preferred foods weekly.
- Given information on the pharmacological characteristics of several types of insulin, the student will be able to design an insulin regimen that maximizes the percentage of SMBG results within the normal range and minimizes blood glucose variability.

Evaluation

At this highest cognitive level, instructional objectives focus on teaching the student how to reach a judgment about a particular issue or problem and to provide an intellectually defensible rationale for that judgment. Examples of evaluation-level objectives for diabetes education are:

- Given a hypothetical blood glucose control problem, the student will select an appropriate adjustment to medication, diet, exercise, or some combination of these factors and provide a logical justification for the specific adjustments chosen as opposed to other alternatives.
- The student will learn to compare and contrast insulin regimens consisting of multiple daily injections versus use of an insulin pump and provide a logical rationale for which regimen best fits the student's diet and exercise habits, vocational demands, and other daily routines.
- The student will design an experiment to determine the minimum frequency of testing that enables maintenance of mean blood glucose less than 150 mg/dl and no more than one episode of moderate or severe hypoglycemia per month.

Summary and Conclusions

This chapter presented an overview of the literature on patients' utilization of SMBG data as the foundation for sophisticated diabetes self-management. A careful analysis of the SMBG enterprise revealed that this is an immensely complicated psychological system that places numerous affective, behavioral, and cognitive demands on patients. Medical management and patient education that matches this complexity with highly individualized training and psychosocial support may offer the best prospects for helping as many patients as possible to achieve greater sophistication in diabetes self-management.

References

1. American Diabetes Association. Consensus statement on self-monitoring of blood glucose. Diabetes Care 1987;10:81–87.
2. American Diabetes Association. Consensus statement on self monitoring of blood glucose. Diabetes Care 1994;17:81–86.
3. American Diabetes Association. National standards for diabetes self-management education programs and American Diabetes Association review criteria. Diabetes Care 1995;18:737–41.
4. American Diabetes Association. Clinical practice recommendations, 1996. Diabetes Care 1996;19(suppl 1):S1–118.
5. American Diabetes Association. Position statement: implications of the diabetes control and complications trial. Clinical Diabetes 1993;11:91–96.
6. Santiago JV. Perspectives in diabetes: lessons from the diabetes control and complications trial. Diabetes 1993;42:1549–54.
7. DCCT Research Group: The impact of the trial coordinator in the diabetes control and complications trial. Diabetes Ed 1993;19:509–512.
8. Wysocki T. SMBG: has the promise been fulfilled? Diabetes Spec 1988;1:83–87.
9. Wysocki T. Impact of blood glucose monitoring on diabetic control: obstacles and interventions. J Behav Med 1989;12:183–205.
10. Delamater AM, Davis S, Bubb J, Smith JA, White NH, Santiago JV. Self monitoring of blood glucose by adolescents with diabetes: technical skills and utilization of data. Diabetes Ed 1988;15:56–61.
11. Peyrot M, Rubin R. Insulin self-regulation predicts better glycemic control. Diabetes 1988;37(suppl 1):53A.
12. Wysocki T, Hough BS, Ward KM, Allen AA, Murgai N. Use of blood glucose data by families of children and adolescents with IDDM. Diabetes Care 1992;15:1041–44.
13. Delamater AM, Bubb J, Davis SG, Smith JA, Schmidt L, White NH, et al. Randomized, prospective study of self-management training with newly diagnosed diabetic children. Diabetes Care 1990;13:492–98.
14. Anderson BJ, Wolf FM, Burkhart MT, Cornell RG, Bacon GE. Effects of peer-group intervention on metabolic control of adolescents with IDDM: randomized outpatient study. Diabetes Care 1989;12:179–83.
15. Cox DJ, Kovatchev BP, Julian DM, Gonder-Frederick LA, Polonsky WH, Schlundt DG, et al. Frequency of severe hypoglycemia in insulin-dependent diabetes mellitus can be predicted from self-monitoring blood glucose data. J Clin Endocrinol Metab 79:1659–62.
16. Gonder-Frederick LA, Cox DJ, Kovatchev B, Schlundt D, Clarke WL. A biopsychobehavioral model of risk of severe hypoglycemia. Diabetes Care 1997; 20:661–69.

17. Wysocki T. The psychological context of SMBG. Diabetes Spec 1994;7: 266–70.
18. Spevack M, Johnson SB, Harkavy JM, Silverstein JH, Shuster J, Rosenbloom A, et al. Diabetetologists' judgments of diabetic control: reliability and mathematical simulation. Diabetes Care 1987;10:217–24.
19. Bloom B, (ed). Taxonomy of educational objectives, book I. Cognitive domain. White Plains, NY: Longman, 1984.
20. Vargas J. Writing worthwhile behavioral objectives. New York: Harper and Row, 1972.

16

Influence of Type 1 Diabetes on Childhood Growth and Development

JOHN I. MALONE

Insulin dependent diabetes mellitus (Type 1 diabetes) can adversely affect the growth of children. Type 1 diabetes is characterized by total insulin deficiency. Insulin is an anabolic hormone that regulates the metabolic pathways that increase the synthesis of proteins, glycogen, and fat. Insulin activates a transporter system that moves glucose into muscle cells for the production of energy and into adipocytes for both the production and storage of energy. Clinical observations indicate that insulin deficiency is associated with growth failure and that hyperinsulinemia is accompanied by weight gain and accelerated linear growth (1). Insulin promotes growth by increasing the intracellular availability of substrate (glucose) for energy production, and also exerts an indirect effect by increasing insulin-like growth factor (IGF-1), which is the primary agent that stimulates linear bone growth (2). Because Type 1 diabetes is associated with abnormal insulin production and release, it is not surprising that growth irregularities have been associated with Type 1 diabetes in growing children. Type 1 diabetes is an endocrine problem precipitated by the total absence of insulin, which contributes to the associated hormonal abnormalities seen in Table 16.1.

Tall stature at diagnosis of Type 1 diabetes was first reported in 1925 and was explained by the "hyperinsulinemia" that precedes carbohydrate intolerance (3). This hypothesis is no longer accepted because we have learned that endogenous insulin production declines during the 6–12 months prior to the clinical onset of Type 1 diabetes (4). There are studies using a comparison group of children from the same environment that show no difference in the height of newly diagnosed diabetic children (5). An evaluation of identical twins with Type 1 diabetes indicated they are shorter than their nondiabetic twins (6).

After the clinical onset of Type 1 diabetes there is little evidence of growth failure until the child has had 2 years of poor metabolic control. This is more commonly recognized after 4–7 years of diabetes (Table 16.2) (7). The growth

TABLE 16.1. Glucose homeostasis with IDDM.

- No insulin
- No amylin
- Glucagon ↑ ↓
- Growth hormone ↑
- IGF-1 ↓
- Catacholamines ↑

velocity of pubertal children has been inversely related to the degree of metabolic control during puberty (8). Growth hormone concentration is increased in association with poor metabolic control, but IGF-1 is inappropriately low (9). IGF-1 is secreted by the liver under the influence of pituitary growth hormone. It is a potent mitogen and the factor that promotes the growth of cartilage and other tissues. A significant inverse relationship has been demonstrated between hemoglobin A1c levels and IGF-1 concentrations (8). Autoimmune thyroiditis with resultant hypothyroidism is also a common problem in children who have diabetes that causes growth failure.

A group of 157 children 6–16 years of age with diabetes had their heights compared with those of an age-matched group of siblings in a cross-sectional study (10). The height percentiles of the nondiabetic children were distributed normally with 46% at or below the fiftieth percentile. The height percentiles of the children with diabetes were skewed to the left with 61% at or below the fiftieth percentile. The duration of diabetes had the greatest influence on growth failure. The heights of children became subnormal after 4 years of diabetes and significantly different after 7 years of Type 1 diabetes. In addition to the negative influence of elevated glycosylated hemoglobin, excessive loss of calcium and phosphorus in the urine of children with poorly controlled diabetes (Table 16.3) is another mechanism by which poorly controlled diabetes may result in growth failure in children (10).

Another factor influencing growth of children with diabetes is the effort to regulate blood glucose levels by calorie restriction. If one is successful in achieving near normal glucose levels by calorie restriction there will be no need to increase insulin administration which is essential for growth promotion. The social and emotional impact of nutritional limitations enforced by

TABLE 16.2. Growth failure and IDDM.

- HBA1c ↑
- Duration 4–7 years
- Calorie control
- Hypothyroidism

TABLE 16.3. Growth failure and IDDM.

• HBA1c ↓
• IGF-1 ↑
• Urine calcium ↓
• Urine phosphate ↑
• Delayed puberty

parents upon evolving adolescents frequently is counter-productive and serves as a struggle that generally results in the potentiation of overeating.

The hormonal, metabolic, and nutritional aberrations associated with type 1 diabetes results in physical growth failure is a common problem for children (10). The increased involvement of adults in the emotional and decision-making activities of maturing children has an important influence upon the development of an individuals personality (Table 16.4). The maturing child is learning by protected experience how to make successful decisions, rebound from poor decisions, improve self-confidence, and develop the capacity for independent responsibility and effective, productive living (Table 16.5).

The routine management of Type 1 diabetes fosters increased dependence of the child on an adult for day-to-day decisions on activities such as pricking ones finger to induce bleeding and making decisions about how much insulin to take as well as injecting the insulin two or more times a day. This routine self-care of a child with diabetes applies an unusual pressure and influence upon the personality and emotional development of a child. A common result of adult involvement in the complex task of managing Type 1 diabetes is the development of a overly dependent adult with a poor self-image. We who care for children who have diabetes must work to correct the metabolic defects that cause physical growth failure and other chronic complications which contribute to the morbidity of diabetes. We must not forget, however, that we are caring first of all for children who are maturing to become productive young adults.

TABLE 16.4. Personality development with IDDM.

• Physical defect
• Parents more controlling
• More failure opportunities
daily insulin administration
home glucose monitoring
• Poor self-image
• More dependence

TABLE 16.5. Personality development.

- Making choices
  - living with results
- Successful choices
  - positive self-image
- Personal responsibility
- Increasing independence
- Productive individual

References

1. Hill DJ, Milner RD. Insulin as a growth factor. Pediatr Res 1985;19:876–79.
2. Amiel SA, Sherwin RS, Hintz RL, Gertner JM, Press CM, Tamborlane WV. Effect of diabetes and its control on insulin-like growth factors in young subjects with type I diabetes. Diabetes 1984;33:1175–90.
3. Plotnick LP, Thompson RG, Beitins I, Blizzard RM. Integrated concentrations of growth hormone correlated with state of puberty and estrogen levels in girls. J Clin Endocrinol Metab 1974;38:436–39.
4. Maclaren N, Schatz D, Drash A, Grave G. Initial pathogenic events in IDDM. Diabetes 1989;38:534–38.
5. Emmerson AJ, Savage DC. Height at diagnosis in diabetes. J Pediatr 1988;147:319–20.
6. Hoskins PJ, Leslie RDG, Pyke DA: Height at diagnosis of diabetes in children: a study in identical twins. BrMed J 1985;290:278–89.
7. Vanelli M, De Fanti, Adinolfi B, Ghizzoni L. Clinical data regarding the growth of diabetic children. Horm Res 1992;37(suppl 3):65–69.
8. Rogers DG, Sherman LD, Gabbay KH. Effect of puberty on insulin-like growth factor I and HbA1 in type I diabetes. Diabetes Care 1991;14:1031–35.
9. Lanes R, Recker B, Fort P, Lipshitz F. Impaired somatomedin generation test in children with insulin dependent diabetes mellitus. Diabetes 1985;34:156–60.
10. Malone JI, Lowitt S, Duncan JA, Shah SC, Vargas A, Root AW. Hypercalciuria, hyperphosphaturia and growth retardation in children with diabetes mellitus. Pediatrics 1986;78:298–304

17

Glycosylated Hemoglobin: A Myopic View of Diabetes Care?

Suzanne Bennett Johnson

Introduction

Insulin dependent diabetes mellitus (IDDM) is characterized by complete pancreatic failure, requiring daily exogenous insulin replacement by injection for survival. It is one of the most common chronic diseases of childhood. It is far more common than pediatric AIDS, cystic fibrosis, juvenile rheumatoid arthritis, multiple sclerosis, muscular dystrophy, and childhood cancer. It affects approximately 120,000 U.S. youth (1).

Management of the disease is complex. Insulin is injected two or more times per day before meals. Short-acting and intermediate- or long-acting insulins often are mixed in an effort to manage the immediate glycemic effect of the meal and to provide a source of insulin during between-meal intervals. However, current methods of exogenous insulin replacement only crudely approximate normal pancreatic function. Both "hyperglycemia" (excessively high blood glucose levels) and "hypoglycemia" (excessively low blood glucose levels, also known as "insulin shock") consequently can and do occur. If the patient with IDDM eats too much, given the available supply of insulin, hyperglycemia will result. If the patient eats too little, given the available supply of insulin, hypoglycemia will occur. Hypoglycemia can lead to relatively rapid cognitive disorientation, convulsions, and coma. The patient is consequently told to eat small amounts frequently throughout the day. Three small meals and three snacks are recommended.

Treatment is further complicated by other factors that affect insulin action. Exercise, which is considered beneficial because it improves insulin action, may also result in hypoglycemia if insufficient calories are consumed. Illness and stress may impair insulin action, leading to hyperglycemia. Blood glucose variability is to be expected because of the interacting influences of diet, exercise, illness, emotional state, and insulin action. As a consequence, blood glucose levels must be monitored on a daily basis in order to appropriately manage hypo- or hyperglycemic episodes, should they occur. Home blood glucose (BG) monitoring is accomplished by obtaining a small sample of blood from a finger stick, which is placed on a reagent strip. The strip is then inserted into a computerized meter that "reads" the strip and reports the results. Most modern meters also hold the time, date, and result of the test in memory and can be "downloaded" by the provider at the patient's clinic appointment. The provider then uses these test results to make changes in insulin dose and timing.

The American Diabetes Association (2) recommends that a glycosylated hemoglobin (GHb) assay be performed as part of routine care for all patients with diabetes. GHb values provide an estimate of the patient's average blood glucose levels during the preceding 2–3 months and have become the "gold standard" index of a patient's glycemic control. Glycosylated hemoglobin A1C (HA1C) values of nondiabetic individuals range from 4.0 to 6.0%. The ADA recommends a HA1C goal of less than 7.0% for persons with diabetes.

Glycosylated Hemoglobin Values and Patient Health Status

Patient GHb values have been linked to a variety of biological and medical indicators of health status including other measures of glycemic control, measures of lipid metabolism, and the acute and long-term complications associated with the disease.

GHb and Other Measures of Glycemic Control

Mean blood glucose levels obtained from home BG testing meters have been shown to correlate highly with patients' GHb levels, particularly when tests are conducted before and after meals (3). GHb levels, however, show a weaker association with measures of blood glucose variability. Table 17.1 depicts the correlations between GHb levels and mean blood glucose, and between GHb and the standard deviation of blood glucose values, obtained during a 3-week period of home BG monitoring in a sample of 121 adolescent patients. GHb values correlated strongly with mean blood glucose levels, but were far less predictive of day-to-day blood glucose variability. As expected, higher levels of GHb were associated with higher mean blood glucose values and higher blood glucose variability.

GHb and Measures of Lipid Metabolism

Although disruption of glucose metabolism is the hallmark of IDDM, lipid metabolism is disturbed as well. As a consequence, patients with diabetes are at increased risk for hyperlipidemia and heart disease. GHb values ex-

TABLE 17.1. Correlations of HA1C levels with measures of glycemic control and lipid metabolism in adolescents with IDDM.

Measures of glycemic control*	r
BG mean	.60
BG standard deviation	.38
% BG tests £ 60 mg/dl	−.39
Measures of lipid metabolism	
Total cholesterol	.31
HDL cholesterol	−.06
LDL cholesterol	.30
Triglycerides	.26

*Obtained from a 3-week interval of home blood glucose (BG) monitoring; data were downloaded from One Touch Two meters, N = 120–121.

hibit a significant but weak association with measures of lipid metabolism. Table 17.1 provides these data for this same sample of 121 adolescent patients. Statistically significant but weak correlations were found between GHb and Total Cholesterol, LDL Cholesterol, and Triglyceride values, with higher GHb levels associated with poorer lipid metabolism. There was no association, however, between GHb levels and HDL Cholesterol. These data are consistent with that reported for more than 1,500 patients followed in the Diabetes Control and Complications Trial (DCCT) (4).

GHb and Measures of Acute Complications (Hypoglycemia)

Because current treatment methods only approximate normal pancreatic function, youngsters experience both hyper- and hypoglycemia. Prolonged hyperglycemia may result in fatigue, thirst, frequent urination, and, in some cases, ketoacidosis. Because of its rapid onset and debilitating consequences, however, hypoglycemia is the acute complication of primary concern to IDDM patients. Hypoglycemia occurs when blood glucose values fall below 60 mg/dl. The patient may become disoriented, and unless glucose is administered quickly, seizures, coma and even death may ensue.

Treatment regimens that attempt to maintain blood glucose levels in the near normal range unfortunately usually result in increased episodes of hypoglycemia. The DCCT successfully employed intensive therapy (consisting of three or more insulin injections a day, four or more BG tests a day, daily insulin adjustment, and frequent provider contact) to reduce GHb levels below that of conventional therapy. Adolescents in intensive therapy, however, had three times more episodes of severe hypoglycemia than did adolescents treated with conventional therapy (5).

Table 17.1 provides the correlation between GHb levels and frequency of hypoglycemia (defined as the percentage of BG tests with results of ≤ 60 mg/dl) obtained from downloaded BG testing meter data obtained from a sample of 121 adolescents treated with conventional therapy. As in the DCCT, lower levels of GHb were associated with an increased frequency of hypoglycemia.

GHb and Measures of Long-Term Complications

The DCCT was undertaken with the expressed purpose of determining whether maintaining BG levels in the near normal range would decrease the frequency and severity of the long-term complications associated with IDDM. Intensive therapy was used to reduce GHb levels to 7.0%, compared with 9% among conventionally treated patients. The trial provided strong evidence that intensive therapy could effectively delay the onset and slow the progression of diabetic retinopathy, nephropathy, and neuropathy (5,6).

Glycosylated Hemoglobin Values and Diabetes Knowledge

Although GHb levels are clearly linked to other biological indicators of patients' health status, they may be a poor indicator of patients' knowledge about diabetes and its management (7). Some studies report patients with better GHb values have greater knowledge about the disease (8); however, others report no relationship between GHb and knowledge (9,10), and still others report an inverse association (i.e., those with greater knowledge are in worse diabetes control) (11).

Knowledge is a necessary, but not sufficient, condition for diabetes regimen adherence and good glycemic control. Patients may know what to do, but not do it. Adolescents, for example, are more knowledgeable about their illness, but they are less adherent and in worse glycemic control than younger children (12). It is common for patients in poor diabetes control to be given additional education, which may explain why some studies find those with higher GHb values to be more knowledgeable.

Studies have also shown that there are different types of diabetes knowledge (e.g., general information, problem solving, and skill at insulin injection and BG testing) that are often unrelated to one another (13). Further, patient–provider communication problems are common; patients often fail to understand or recall provider recommendations (14). As a result, patient GHb values tell us little or nothing about patient knowledge about diabetes and its management (i.e., they fail to inform us as to whether a knowledge deficit exists, and they fail to detail the nature of the deficit, should one exist).

Glycosylated Hemoglobin Values and Diabetes Regimen Adherence

There is ample evidence that many patients have difficulty adhering to the diabetes treatment regimen. Although exogenous insulin replacement is necessary for good diabetes control, the literature has failed to document a consistent, strong association between other diabetes regimen behaviors and GHb values (15).

Like diabetes knowledge, diabetes daily management is complex, involving multiple behaviors (insulin injections, BG testing, exercise, dietary constraints) that are unrelated to one another. Although providers often view patients as "compliant" or "noncompliant," assuming compliance is a traitlike characteristic of the patient, the empirical evidence fails to support this view (15).

Like diabetes knowledge, diabetes regimen adherence is also a necessary, but not sufficient, condition for good glycemic control. Other factors, in addition to adherence, are known to affect blood glucose levels in IDDM patients, including endogenous insulin production, recommended insulin dose and timing, illness, stress, and hormonal changes associated with puberty. Nevertheless, providers continue to use GHb as their primary measure of patient adherence (16). Patients with high values are presumed to be nonadherent whereas those with low values are presumed to be following the provider's recommendations. Such presumptions, when incorrect, may lead to patient distrust and resentment. Patients who have been adherent and who are blamed for their poor GHb values may resent the provider's accusatory stance and may develop a sense of despair, feeling that no matter what they do, their behavior has little effect on their diabetes control. Patients who have been nonadherent and who are complimented for their good control may begin to question the provider's credibility and take provider recommendations less seriously, developing poor diabetes care habits that may have negative consequences months, or perhaps years, later.

GHb values both fail to inform the provider accurately that an adherence problem exists as well as fail to provide any information about which diabetes care behaviors are and are not occurring.

Glycosylated Hemoglobin Values and Quality of Life

Measures of quality of life, as well as physical status, are now recognized as an important health outcome. The Diabetes Quality of Life (DQOL) measure, developed for use in the DCCT, consists of four subscales: satisfaction, impact, diabetes worry, and social/vocational worry (17). Psychometric data have been reported for both adult and adolescent IDDM populations (17,18). The measure appears sensitive to type of treatment, number and severity of diabetes complications (18) but does not always correlate with GHb values (19; Perwien, Johnson, and Silverstein, unpublished manuscript).

Quality of life refers to the patient's perception of his or her ability to function physically, socially, and emotionally. Diabetes complications (e.g., blindness, kidney failure, heart disease, leg amputations) are all an obvious threat to a patient's quality of life. GHb values have been linked to diabetes complications, with those in worse glycemic control more likely to suffer. GHb values per se, however, pose no immediate threat to the patient. As a result, it is not surprising that they exhibit a poor association to measures of quality of life.

Toward a Clearer View of Diabetes Care: Placing Glycosylated Hemoglobin Values in Context

The development of the GHb assay offered an important technological advance in diabetes care because it offered the clinician and patient a reliable measure of the patient's average glycemic control over a time interval of 2–3 months. Prior to the availability of this assay, clinicians were forced to rely on a single momentary BG test conducted during a clinic visit that often failed to provide a reliable estimate of the patient's "usual" glycemic control. In their enthusiastic acceptance of the GHb assay, however, clinicians often presume it measures far more than average glycemic control, including patient knowledge, adherence, and quality of life. This had led to the myopic view of diabetes care depicted in Figure 17.1: an exaggerated emphasis on GHb results with inaccurate presumptions about links between GHb results and patient knowledge, adaptation, and behavior.

To place a patient's GHb value in an appropriate context is to understand what kinds of information it can, and cannot, provide. A patient's GHb value *is* an excellent estimate of average blood glucose over the preceding 2–3 months. It is *not* an excellent measure of blood glucose variability, frequency of hypoglycemia, lipid metabolism, or diabetic complications. A patient with a high GHb value, however, compared with a patient with a low GHb value, is *more likely* to have higher blood glucose variability, less frequent hypoglycemia, higher cholesterol, LDL and triglyceride values, and earlier onset of diabetes complications.

A patient's GHb value is *not* a measure of patient's knowledge about diabetes, adherence with the treatment regimen, or perceived quality of life, although all may be *indirectly* related to a patient's GHb value. Accurate knowledge about diabetes, skill at diabetes management tasks, and adherence to the treatment regimen are necessary, but not sufficient, conditions for good glycemic control to occur. As depicted in Figure 17.2, GHb values

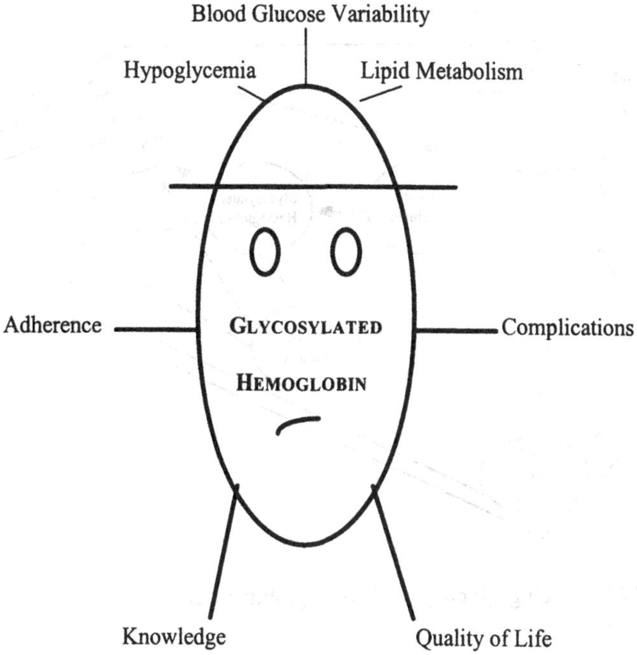

FIGURE 17.1. Glycosylated hemoglobin: A myopic view of patient care.

are the product of a complex system of variables that include provider behavior, biologic factors, as well as patient behavior. A high GHb value tells the provider that something is wrong, but not what is wrong. Perhaps the insulin dose and timing recommended by the provider is wrong. Perhaps the patient failed to understand the provider's recommendation. Perhaps the patient is measuring and delivering the insulin incorrectly. Perhaps the patient has just entered puberty, and so on. To successfully impact the patient's GHb levels, the provider must understand and assess the components of this complex system.

The patient's quality of life is a function of the impact of daily disease management demands, acute and long-term diabetic complications, as well as the patient's personal, family and social resources. Because GHb values have been related to diabetic complications, they are indirectly related to patients' quality of life. Quality of life, however, is the product of a complex system (see Fig. 17.2); GHb is only one of many parameters involved.

To place the GHb assay in an appropriate context, the provider must understand what information the GHb assay *does* and does *not* provide, and be willing to collect the information it does not provide. The myopic view of diabetes care, with the GHb assay as its core element, has appeal because of its simplicity. Diabetes, however, is a complex disease to manage and to live with. We do our patients a disservice when we behave otherwise.

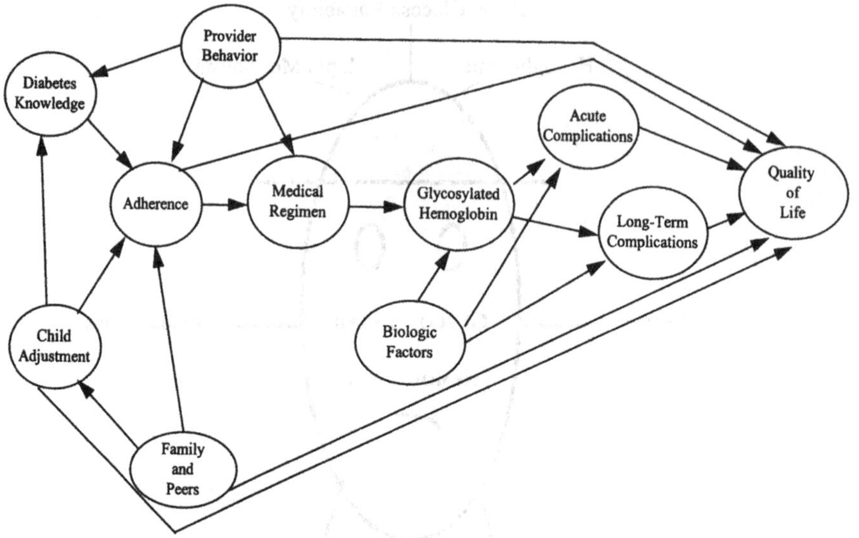

FIGURE 17.2. Placing glycosylated hemoglobin in context: A complex of diabetes management.

Acknowledgment. Supported by Grant No. R01HD 13820 from the National Institute of Child Health and Human Development.

References

1. LaPorte R, Matsuchima M, Chang Y. Prevalence and incidence of insulin-dependent diabetes. In: Harris M, ed. Diabetes in America, second edition. NIH Publication No. 95-1468, 1995:37–46.
2. American Diabetes Association. Position statement: standards of medical care for patients with diabetes. Diabetes Care 1997;20(suppl 1):5–13.
3. Nathan D, Singer D, Hurxthal K, Goodson J. The clinical information value of the glycosylated hemoglobin assay. N Engl J Med 1984;310:341–46.
4. DCCT Research Group. Lipid and lipoprotein levels in patients with IDDM: diabetes control and complications trial experience. Diabetes Care 1992;15:886–94.
5. DCCT Research Group. Effect of intensive diabetes treatment on the development and progression of long-term complications in adolescents with insulin-dependent diabetes mellitus: diabetes control and complications trial. J Pediatr 1994;125: 177–88.
6. DCCT Research Group. The effect of intensive treatment of diabetes on the development and progression of long-term complications in insulin-dependent diabetes mellitus. N Engl J Med 1993;329:977–86.
7. Glasgow R, Osteen V. Evaluating diabetes education: are we measuring the most important outcomes? Diabetes Care 1992;15:1423–32.
8. McCulloch D, Young R, Steel J, Wilson E, Prescott R, Duncan L. Effect of dietary compliance on metabolic control in insulin dependent diabetics. Hum Nutr Appl Nutr 1983;37:157–61.

9. Beggan M, Cregan D, Drury, M. Assessment of the outcome of an educational programme of diabetes self-care. Diabetologia 1982;23:246–51.
10. Wysocki R, Hough B, Ward K, Green L. Diabetes mellitus in the transition to adulthood: adjustment, self-care, and health status. J Dev Behav Pediatr 1992;13:194–201.
11. Weist M, Finney J, Barnard M, Davis C, Ollendick T. Empirical selection of psychosocial treatment targets for children and adolescents with diabetes. J Pediatr Psychol 1993;18:11–28.
12. Johnson SB. Managing insulin-dependent diabetes mellitus in adolescence: A developmental perspective. In: Wallander J, Siegel L, ed. Adolescent health problems: behavioral perspectives. New York: Guilford Press, 1995:265–88.
13. Johnson SB. Knowledge, attitudes, and behavior: correlates of health in childhood diabetes. Clin Psychol Rev 1984;4:503–24.
14. Page P, Verstraete D, Robb J, Etzwiler D. Patient recall of self-care recommendations in diabetes. Diabetes Care 1981;4:96–98.
15. Johnson SB. Insulin-dependent diabetes mellitus in childhood. In: Roberts M, ed. Handbook of pediatric psychology, second ed. New York: Guilford Press, 1995: 263–85.
16. Clarke W, Snyder A, Nowacek G. Out-patient pediatric diabetes: I. Current practices. J Chron Dis 1985;38:85–90.
17. DCCT Research Group. Reliability and validity of a diabetes quality-of-life measure for the diabetes control and complications trial. Diabetes Care 1988;11: 725–32.
18. Jacobson A, De Groot M, Samson J. The evaluation of two measures of quality of life in patients with type I and type II diabetes. Diabetes Care 1994;17:267–74.
19. Ingersoll G, Marrero D. A modified quality-of-life measure for youths: psychometric properties. Diabetes Ed 1991;17:114–18.

Part V

Treatment of Congenital Adrenal Hyperplasia: Efficacy, Innovation and Quality of Life

18

Congenital Adrenal Hyperplasia Due to 21-Hydroxylase Deficiency (Salt-Losing Form and Simple Virilizing Form): Long-Term Results of Treatment

CLAUDE J. MIGEON

Congenital adrenal hyperplasia (CAH) is a group of disorders, each one having a defect of one of the specific enzymes involved in adrenal steroidogenesis, which leads to the biosynthesis of cortisol (1).

Physiology of Steroid Secretion by Adrenal Cortex

All steroids are derived from cholesterol. Its stepwise conversion to hormones requires the sequential secretion of a series of enzymes (2). The genes encoding these enzymes are now known. The first step is the conversion of cholesterol to pregnenolone by a specific cytochrome P450—the *cholesterol side-chain cleavage enzyme*—encoded by the CYP IIA gene. Next, pregnenolone is transformed into progesterone by *3b-hydroxysteroid dehydrogenase*, the only enzyme in steroidogenesis that is not a cytochrome P450. Three more enzymes will be necessary for the formation of cortisol: *17-hydroxylase* (CYP 17 gene), *21-hydroxylase* (CYP 21) and *11-hydroxylase* (CYP 11 B1). The intermediate products are 17-hydoxyprogesterone, 11-deoxycortisol, and, finally, cortisol.

In adrenal cells with absent 17-hydroxylase, the same series of enzymes will permit the formation of the salt-retaining hormones, corticosterone and aldosterone. The CYP17 enzyme can also carry out the removal of the side chain of the steroid molecule that results in the formation of adrenal androgens (androstenedione and dehydroepiandrosterone). The secretion of cortisol is under the control of pituitary ACTH, which in turn is under the control of hypothalamic corticotropin releasing hormone (CRH). These three hormones are under homeostatic regulation, with cortisol having a negative feedback on CRH and ACTH. The secretion of aldosterone is mainly under the control of the renin–angiotensin system.

The secretion of adrenal androgens is under an unknown temporal system. During fetal life there is a large androgen production that is prolonged in early neonatal life. This secretion then ceases and will not resume until adolescence. It is known as *adrenarche* at that time. Maximal adrenal androgen secretion occurs in the teens and twenties. By 30 years of age it decreases and becomes almost nil in 45–50-year-old subjects.

The Various Forms of Congenital Adrenal Hyperplasia and the Pathophysiology of 21-Hydoxylase Deficiency

As defined earlier, CAH is a disorder of the secretion of cortisol by the adrenal cortex. There are several different forms of CAH, each related to one of the enzymes necessary to transform cholesterol to cortisol. Among these various forms, the 21-hydroxylase deficiency is by far the most frequent, representing more than 90% of CAH cases (2,3).

A 21-hydroxylase deficiency results in decreased or completely absent secretion of cortisol. This, in turn, reduces the negative feedback at the hypothalamic/pituitary level, which is then translated into increased secretions of CRH and ACTH. The increased ACTH secretion is responsible for the hyperplasia of the adrenal cortex and for the increased secretion of the precursors of cortisol, particularly 17-hydroxyprogesterone and the adrenal androgens.

The most important adrenal androgen secreted in large amounts in CAH is androstenedione. This steroid is not androgenic by itself, as it does not bind to the androgen receptor. Ten percent of it, however, is metabolized peripherally to testosterone. Testosterone will in turn be metabolized into dihydrotestosterone in the target cells and it will masculinize the external genitalia of the female fetus. The large amounts of androstenedione secreted in patients with CAH can be measured as such in peripheral blood or as its metabolites in urine (urinary 17-ketosteroids).

The increased secretion of 17-hydroxyprogesterone and, to a lesser extent, progesterone produces a salt-losing tendency in all patients with CAH. The salt loss will bring about an increased secretion of renin and angiotensin II. If the 21-hydroxylase deficiency is only partial, then the adrenal cortex will be able to produce compensatory amounts of aldosterone, and the patient will be considered as presenting the *simple virilizing form* (4). In contrast, if the 21-hydroxylase deficiency is very marked or complete, then the adrenal cortex is unable to produce any amount of aldosterone and the

CAH patient will present the *salt-losing form* (4) of the syndrome. It follows that when 21-hydroxylase deficiency is partial (in simple virilizing CAH), the increased ACTH secretion permits a normal or close to normal secretion of cortisol. When the 21-hydroxylase deficiency is complete (in salt-losing CAH), however, the increased ACTH secretion will be unable to return the cortisol secretion to normal.

In summary, in the simple virilizing form, the partial 21-hydroxylase deficiency, permits an almost normal secretion of cortisol and increased secretion of aldosterone that compensates for the salt-losing tendency. As a consequence, the major symptoms in this form are related to increased androgen secretion. During fetal life, female genitalia are masculinized. Virilism will be noted postnatally and the metabolic effects of androgens will result in rapid growth and increases in muscle mass.

In the salt-losing form, the signs of hypersecretion of androgens will also be present. In addition, the lack of salt-retaining hormone results in acute adrenal crisis shortly after birth. The situation is further complicated by the absence of cortisol secretion, which results in hypoglycemia.

Treatment of Congenital Adrenal Hyperplasia

In the late 1940s, cortisone was synthesized and made available for therapeutic purposes. It was first tried in rheumatoid arthritis with what was reported as miraculous results. It was used in 1950 for CAH with no less striking results: (1) cortisone could supress urinary 17-ketosteroids of patients with the virilizing form, and (2) in combination with deoxycorticosterone acetate, it could also keep alive the patient with the salt-losing form (5–7). Multiple additional studies confirmed these findings.

The basic modality of treatment involves glucocorticoid replacement therapy and, when necessary, mineralocorticoid replacement. Studies of cortisol secretion rate at various ages in normal infants and children (8) found that this secretion was fairly constant at various ages when corrected for body surface area. The mean ± SD was 12.1 ± 1.5 mg/pM^2 of body surface area per 24 hours.

In the past, mineralocorticoid replacement was obtained by using deoxycorticosterone acetate i.m., usually 1 mg daily. At presently, 9-alpha - fluorocortisol is universally used at a dose of 0.1–0.15 mg daily. Salt supplement is often added to the diet, at least in early life.

Monitoring of Treatment

It is most important, because of large individual variation in cortisol secretion and therefore dose replacement, to monitor treatment very carefully (2). The means for determining the appropriate dose of glucocorticoid include the determination of plasma 17-hydroxyprogesterone and androstenedione concentrations, and the measurement of the urinary excretion of pregnanetiol and 17-ketosteroids. It is also important to follow somatic growth (bone age and height age).

The goal of treatment in children is to suppress plasma androstenedione and urinary 17-ketosteroids. A complete suppression of plasma 17-hydroxyprogesterone and urinary pregnanetiol, however, are indicative of overtreatment.

After about 1 month of glucocorticoid therapy, the CRH-ACTH system is fully suppressed and cortisol secretion is almost nil. Under such conditions, the patient is unable to respond to stress by a physiologic increase in secretion of cortisol. Hence, additional glucocorticoids must be provided. Minor infection and/or low-grade fever (i.e., sore throat, runny nose, temperature up to 38°C) may not require a change in dosage. During conditions of moderate stress (i.e., upper respiratory infections, with lung congestion and temperatures above 38°C), the dose should be double, whereas in major stress, the cortisol requirement is three times the normal replacement.

When infants or children are unable to retain oral therapy, the parents are advised to administer an intramuscular injection of approximately 50mg/m^2 of cortisol sodium succinate (SoluCortef). This measure will give the parents 6 hours to get in touch with a physician or to go to a hospital emergency room.

In female patients, treatment also includes surgical correction of the external genitalia. Masculinization is usually greater in salt losers than it is in simple virilizers.

At 6–12 weeks of age, efforts will be made to feminize the appearance of the genitalia. This is done by size reduction of the phallus to make it look as a clitoris. This often involves the removal of the posterior part of the corpora and the recession of the glans, keeping appropriate vascular and nerve connections.

Some urologists feel that correction of the vaginal opening can be performed at the same time. In our observation, early correction often results in a ring of scar tissue that interferes with sexual intercourse. Postsurgical use of dilators may prevent this condition, but the pain related to this maneuver and the psychological trauma to the patient and parents have made us recommend correction at adolescence when the patient is ready to begin her sex life.

Life-Saving Treatment for Salt Losers

It must be remembered that prior to 1950 all infants with the salt-losing form of CAH would die, usually in early infancy. Indeed, Iversen (9) reported on the age at the time of death of more than 70 infants, most of them in the first year of life. In 1951, Dr. Lawson Wilkins, with Drs. Lytt Gardner, John Crigler, and myself, celebrated the first birthday of the first treated salt-losing child and who is still alive today (7).

It is appropriate to state, however, that the treatment of salt losers can still be very troublesome in infancy and early childhood. Later, in adulthood, the patients are much less prone to salt-losing crisis, although they continue to require their mineralocorticoid replacement therapy.

In the first 15 years of treatment of 50 salt losers, 7 young patients died—five of adrenal crisis, one of hyperatremia, and one of encephalitis. Although better understanding of the disorder has resulted in improved results, incidents can still occur. Indeed, most of these patients have visited the hospital emergency room on a number of occasions. Further complications can arise from additional disorders such as protein allergy or asthma.

Status of Adult Female Patients

Almost 50 years after treatment became available, it is important to evaluate the long-range results of therapy (10,11). We have specifically reviewed the status of patients of our clinic who have reached adulthood. Good results have generally been obtained, although there are some specific problem areas.

Adult Height

The mean ± adult height of the salt loser was 156.8 ± 6.6 cm. This was significantly greater than the mean height of patients with virilizing form (153.3 ± 5.4 cm). This small difference in outcome is probably related to the fact that the salt losers were generally treated earlier in life than were the simple virilizing patient. Height in both groups was significantly lower than that of normal adult American females and of the mean parental height. Among a group of 80 women, 31.25% were below the third percentile, 42.5% were between –1 and –2 SDs, 17.5% were between –1 SD and the mean, whereas only 8.75% were above the mean.

Causes of loss of stature can be overtreatment as well as undertreatment. Administration of glucocorticoids in amounts greater than normal replacement can result in poor statural growth. Suboptimal therapy may result in abnormal secretion of androgens with early bone maturation. The means for monitoring proper therapy are unfortunately not very sensitive.

Puberty

Pubarche, in almost one third of the patients, was somewhat premature (i.e., before 8 years of age). This probably reflected the fact that some of the patients were poorly controlled in childhood, resulting in an early appearance of body hair.

In contrast, thelarche was somewhat delayed when compared with normal girls. In most patients, breast development followed pubarche, which is contrary to the normal timing of pubertal events in girls. Menarche occurred at

13.77 years, compared with 12.9 years in the normal U.S. population. We believe that it was related to a poor suppression of adrenal androgens rather than a slow rate of growth because most of the patients tended to be taller and heavier than average at that age.

Menses

In a few patients, amenorrhea was a difficult problem, various types of therapy being unsuccessful. Indeed, one third of the women had no or irregular periods (11). This has been observed by others as well (12,13).

Adequacy of Vaginal Reconstruction

A satisfactory introitus to the vagina was present in 66% of the patients with the simple virilizing form and 47.5% of those with the salt-losing form. This difference is statistically significant. We believe that it is a reflection of the greater masculinization observed in the salt losers and therefore of the greater difficulty in correcting the external genitalia. Among the women with adequate vaginal reconstruction, 25% of them reported having no sexual experience. In the rest of the 28 women with inadequate vaginal reconstruction, 65% reported having no sex life. In addition, three patients volunteered the information that they were homosexual.

The lack of sexual experience in a rather large percentage of women, whether their genitalia were appropriately corrected (25% with no experience) or not (65% with no experience) has not been adequately explained (11,14,15). Poor surgical repair in itself was probably a major factor. One could also hypothesize that surgery on the external genitalia had been a psychological trauma to the libido of some women. One could also consider the effects of androgens on the fetal brain.

Marital Status and Fertility

Instances of marriage were low in both the simple virilizing form and the salt-losing form. Only 50% of the women were married in the first group and 20% in the second.

Fertility was considered only among patients who reported having heterosexual activity and who had a normal introitus. In the simple virilizing form (24 women), the fertility rate was 60%, whereas the fertility rate was about 30% among the salt-losing subjects (12 women).

Treatment Compliance

Although not always stated, our study strongly suggested that compliance was far from perfect in many subjects. Some patients reported erratic clinical follow-up, whereas others complained of virilization. It was occasionally stated that little difference in health was noted with or without treatment.

Some of the unsatisfactory results are clearly related to poor compliance. Disorders that require life-time treatment are often subject to poor compliance.

Status of Adult Male Patients

Among a group of 52 male patients with CAH only 30 had reached adulthood at the time of this study. Five of them could not be located, so the study group was therefore 25 patients ranging from 18.2 to 37.2 years of age (16).

Adult Height

The mean ± adult height was 164 ± 7.6 cm, with an average of 150–178.6 cm. This was significantly lower than was that of normal adult American men and of the mean parental height.

The most probable explanation for the short stature was early sexual maturation, which was itself related to lack of compliance with treatment or undertreatment.

Puberty

It is somewhat difficult to appreciate sexual maturation in boys. It requires a precise evaluation of testicular enlargement because the appearance of pubic hair can be related to abnormal secretion of adrenal androgens or to testicular androgens. Whatever the cause, the appearance of pubic hair was generally earlier than normal.

Fertility

Among the younger male patients, many were not married and not eager to have children. For this reason, fertility was judged either by paternity or by sperm count. Twenty patients were studied, and 18 of them were considered fertile. Two had low sperm counts: One was due to his drug addiction, and the other was for no apparent reason.

Steroid Hormones

The plasma concentration of testosterone was normal in all patients, whereas androstenedione values were elevated in half this group. Plasma 17-hydroxyprogesterone and urinary pregnanetriol were elevated in almost all subjects. Serum FSH and LH were within the normal range; however, LH values were below the mean.

The elevated concentration of androstenedione and 17-hydroxyprogesterone demonstrate that most of the patients were not entirely controlled by therapy. It is probable that the testosterone production of these men was the summation of testicular secretion and of peripheral metabolism of androstenedione to testosterone.

Therapeutic Compliance

The lack of therapeutic compliance was readily admitted by many patients. Although they received treatment regularly as children while under control of their parents, they became lax in later life. For unknown reasons, two were never treated and four others stopped therapy between 7 and 15 years prior to our evaluation. In contrast, two patients complied very strictly because missing as few as one or two doses resulted in headaches or malaise.

Summary

Our study of the long-range results of CAH treatment in 80 female patients showed a number of problems. These included the inability to reach their height potential because 33% of the subjects were below the third percentile of normal American women. Another problem was virilization as expressed by early pubarche and adult hirsutism. Surgery for vaginal reconstruction was widespread in 35% of the subjects. Amenorrhea or irregular menses was reported by one third of the patients. This partially accounts for the low fertility rate. Finally, there appeared to be psychosexual problems because a high percentage of women reported a lack of sexual activity. In male patients, the main problems were related to short stature.

Alternative therapies including adrenalectomy and blockage of adrenal action with testolactone have been proposed, but their efficacy remains to be demonstrated (17).

References

1. Donohoue PA, Parker K, Migeon CJ. Congenital adrenal hyperplasia. In: Scriver CR, Beaudet AL, Sly WS, Valle D, eds. The metabolic and molecular bases of inherited disease, seventh ed. McGraw Hill: New York, 1995:2929.
2. Migeon CJ, Donohoue PA. Adrenal disorders. In: Kappy MS, Blizzard RM, Migeon CJ, ed. Wilkins the diagnosis and treatment of endocrine disorders in childhood and adolescence. Springfield, IL: Charles C Thomas, 1994:782.
3. New MI. Steroid 21-hydroxylase deficiency (congenital adrenal hyperplasia). Am J Med 1995;98:2S–8S.
4. Kowarski A, Finkelstein JW, Spaulding JS, Holman GS, Migeon CJ. Aldosterone secretion rate in congenital adrenal hyperplasia. A discussion of the theories of pathogenesis of the salt-losing form of the syndrome. J Clin Invest 1965;44:1505.
5 Wilkins L, Lewis RA, Klein R, Rosemberg E. The suppression of androgen secre-

tion by cortisone in a case of congenital adrenal hyperplasia. Bull Johns Hopkins Hosp 1950;86:249.
6. Bartter FC, Albright F, Forbes AP, Leaf AP, Dempsey E, Carroll E. The effects of adrenocorticotrtophic hormone and cortisone in adrenogenital syndrome associated with congenital adrenal hyperplasia: an attempt to explain and correct its disordered hormonal pattern. J Clin Invest 1951;30:237.
7. Wilkins L, Lewsi RA, Klein R, Gardner LI, Crigler JF, Rosemberg E, et al. Treatment of congenital adrenal hyperplasia with cortisone. J Clin Endocrinol Metab 1951;11:1.
8. Kenny FM, Preeyasombat C, Migeon CJ. Cortisol production rate. II. Normal infants, children, and adults. Pediatrics 1966;37:34.
9. Iversen T. Congenital adrenocortical hyperplasia with disturbed electrolyte regulation. Pediatrics 1955;16:875.
10. Klingensmith GJ, Garcia SC, Jones HW Jr, Migeon CJ, Blizzard RM. Glucocorticoid treatment of girls with congenital adrenal hyperplasia: effects on height, sexual maturation and fertility. J Pediatr 1977;90:996–1004.
11. Mulaikel RM, Migeon CJ, Rock JA. Fertility rates in female patients with congenital adrenal hyperplasia due to 21-hydroxylase deficiency. N Engl J Med 1987;316:178–82.
12. Helleday J, Siwers B, Ritzen EM, Carlstrom K. Subnormal androgen and elevated progesterone levels in women treated for congenital virilizing 21-hydroxylase deficiency. J Clin Endocrinol Metab 1993;76:933.
13. Holmes Walker DJ, Conway GS, Honour JW, Rumsby G, Jacobs HS. Menstrual disturbance and hypersecretion of progesterone in women with congenital adrenal hyperplasia due to 21-hydroxylase deficiency. Clin Endocrinol 1995;43:291.
14. Federman DD. Psychosexual adjustment in congenital adrenal hyperplasia. N Engl J Med 1987;316:209.
15. Kuhnle U, Bullinger M, Schwarz HP, Knorr D. Partnership and sexuality in adult female patients with congenital adrenal hyperplasia. First results of a cross-sectional quality-of-life evaluation. J Steroid Biochem Mol Biol 1993;45:123.
16. Urban MD, Lee PA, Migeon CJ. Adult height and fertility in men with congenital virilizing adrenal hyperplasia. N Engl J Med 1978;299:1392.
17. Van Wyk JJ, Gunther DF, Ritzen EM, Wedell A, Cutler GB, Migeon CJ, et al. Therapeutic controversies. The use of adrenalectomy as a treatment for congenital adrenal hyperplasia. J Clin Endocrinol Metab 1996;81:3180.

19

Psychological Outcome in Congenital Adrenal Hyperplasia

SHERI A. BERENBAUM

Studies of psychological outcome in congenital adrenal hyperplasia due to 21-hydroxylase deficiency (CAH) are important for three reasons.* First, this information helps in the medical management of the patients, as well as in educating patients and their families about the likely course and consequences of the disease. This is a particular concern in CAH because changes in physical appearance and growth (including virilization in girls and short stature in both boys and girls) may affect psychological development. Second, CAH provides a unique opportunity to examine the effects of prenatal and neonatal hormones on the development of the brain and behavior because individuals with CAH are exposed to high levels of androgen beginning early in gestation and continuing throughout important periods for brain development. Thus, studies of CAH allow us to confirm studies in nonhuman mammalian species, which indicate that gonadal hormones play a major role in the development of sex differences in behavior and in the brain (1,2). Third, resolutions of controversies in the treatment of girls with CAH depend on adequate data. This includes the benefits versus the costs of prenatal treatment and the best age for surgical reconstruction of virilized genitalia. These issues have become increasingly important with the addition of CAH to many state and national newborn screening programs and the increased number of cases detected (3,4).

John Money and Anke Ehrhardt were the first to demonstrate the importance of systematic study of girls and women with CAH (5,6). Their findings had pronounced effects on both science and clinical practice. Subsequent studies with systematic behavioral methods have confirmed many of their findings, but not all. This chapter will summarize the findings on behavior

*The focus of this chapter is congenital adrenal hyperplasia due to 21-hydroxylase deficiency, which results in an increase in adrenal androgens beginning early in gestation and continuing until the diagnosis is made and corticosteroid replacement initiated, usually in the early neonatal period. For further discussion of the disease and treatment, see References 51 and 52.

in children and adults with CAH, consider whether these changes reflect the effects of prenatal androgens or other factors that are unique to CAH, indicate the clinical significance of the findings; and point out where additional evidence is needed about psychological outcome in CAH.

Behavioral Changes Associated with CAH

Behavioral studies of individuals with CAH vary in many ways, the most important of which are the objectivity, reliability, and validity of the measures used, the comparison groups, and statistical power for detecting differences. These methodological issues will not be discussed in detail, but they have been considered in the summaries that follow.

Some of the following results reported come from my own studies of individuals with CAH and their unaffected relatives recruited through university-affiliated pediatric endocrine clinics in the midwestern United States. One study was conducted in collaboration with Dr. Susan Resnick and involved assessment of cognitive abilities and aggression in adolescents and adults (see Ref. 7 for details). The other, more extensive study, involves repeated, longitudinal assessment of children and adolescents on a variety of sex-typed behaviors. The initial testing included observations of toy preferences and rough play in children between the ages of 3 and 8, and was conducted in collaboration with Dr. Melissa Hines (8,9). Many of these children were then seen on several subsequent occasions and new subjects were added, so that, over the 12 years of this study, data are available on 182 children between the ages of 3 and 18 for multiple measures of sex-typed behaviors (as described shortly) (10–12).

The sample involved in this systematic long-term follow-up includes 52 girls with CAH, 39 boys with CAH, 37 unaffected sisters or female first cousins, and 54 unaffected brothers or male first cousins.[†] Most patients with CAH had the salt-wasting form of the disorder, and were diagnosed in the early newborn period. All girls had had some degree of genital virilization, but no girl had ever been reared as a boy.

Childhood and Adolescent Activities and Interests

One of the striking characteristics of CAH girls noted by Money and Ehrhardt was their interest in outdoor sports and boys' toys. In one study (6), 59% of girls with CAH—but no sisters—were considered to be tomboys. Other studies based on interviews confirm these findings (13). More compelling evidence comes from observational studies with unaffected

---

[†]Unaffected relatives serve as the best comparison for general genetic and environmental background. Because not all patients had a same-sex control, relatives of male and female patients were combined to form control groups.

relatives serving as controls. In a structured playroom where children are presented with a set of sex-typed toys and allowed to play for 10 minutes, girls with CAH play more with boys' toys and less with girls' toys than do female relatives (8,10). When presented with a set of sex-typed toys and allowed to choose one to keep, girls with CAH make very different choices than do their controls (10). Across two test sessions, 41% of girls with CAH picked a toy vehicle at least once, compared with none of the control girls (who generally picked a doll or markers) and 65% of boys (CAH and unaffected relatives). Children's self-reports and parent's reports of children's toy and activity choices confirm these observational findings (10). It is important to emphasize that these sex-atypical preferences characterize both the group of CAH girls as well as most individuals within the group. For example, as shown in Figure 19.1, there is very little overlap between girls with CAH and unaffected girls on a composite measure of sex-typed activities (derived from observations, child self-report, and parent-report); the few girls with CAH whose scores are in the range of control girls have a mild form of the disease (data from Ref. 10). Boys with CAH do not differ from their unaffected male relatives in sex-typed play or activities (8,10).

Observations from our follow-up study suggest that this interest in boy-typical activities extends into adolescence, and that the differences between girls with CAH and unaffected female relatives remain quite large (see Ref. 53). Activities were not directly observed; rather, they were measured by questionnaires. Girls with CAH differed from unaffected female relatives by more than a standard deviation, which was higher on boy-typical interests and lower on girl-typical interests. Boys with CAH did not differ from unaffected male relatives. Future investigations will involve direct measures of adolescents' activities.

It is interesting that despite this clear interest in boy-typical activities, most girls with CAH appear to prefer girls as playmates (9,10). This may reflect their female-typical gender identity (see later) and their lack of interest in rough play (9). Results on playmate preferences are based only on self-report, however, and it would be interesting to observe the peer interactions of girls with CAH. In particular, it is important to know how reported preference interacts with responses from peers to affect actual behavior. For example, it would be interesting to see whether girls with CAH spend more time alone because their sex-atypical interests are not appealing to other girls, and their identity as girls and low interest in rough play also make them unattractive playmates to boys.

Gender Identity

The overwhelming majority of females with CAH develop normal (female) gender identity, and they do not wish to be male, but the picture may be more complicated than was originally suggested (5). A small minority of

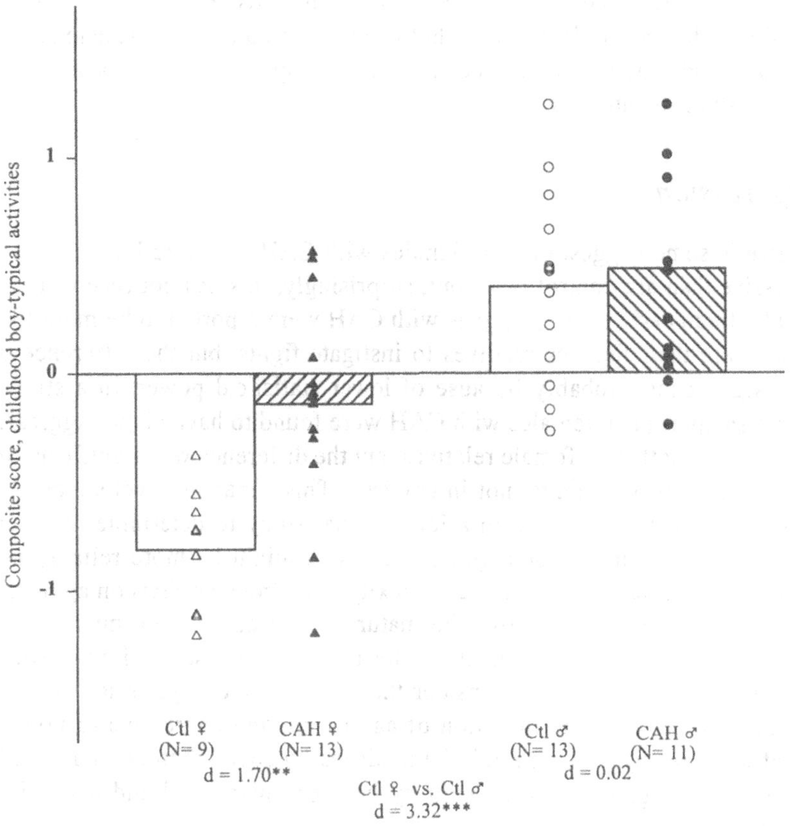

FIGURE 19.1. Scores on composite measure of boy-typical play activities of female and male patients with CAH and unaffected relatives. Bars represent group means. CAH = congenital adrenal hyperplasia; Ctl = control (unaffected same-sex relatives); *d* = difference between group means/average standard deviation. Group differences were evaluated by *t* test; $^{**}p < .01$; $^{***}p < .001$, one-tailed. Data from Berenbaum and Snyder (10).

females with CAH develop male gender identity (14) and it is not clear how they differ from the majority who develop female identity. Further, CAH girls' responses to questions about gender identity reveal the complexity of gender identity and the difficulty in assessing it. This is illustrated by some of our results obtained in collaboration with Dr. J.M. Bailey. Many girls with CAH expressed some dissatisfaction with aspects of the female role (e.g., a dislike of dresses). Girls with CAH were also more likely to consider being a boy temporarily, but, importantly, none was interested in becoming a boy permanently. On a continuous measure of gender identity (obtained by adding scores on 10 interview items), girls with CAH were significantly more masculine than were control girls. Future studies of gender identity need to consider separate aspects of gender identity (e.g., the affect associated with being a girl), the way that gender is used to make decisions about oneself and others, and whether masculine responses reflect basic identity or boy-typical interests.

Aggression

There is some suggestion that females with CAH are more likely to be aggressive than are control girls, but, surprisingly, this has not received much study. In an early study (6), girls with CAH were reported to be more likely than were their females relatives to instigate fights, but the difference was not significant, probably because of lower statistical power. In a study of three samples (11), females with CAH were found to have higher aggression than were unaffected female relatives, but the difference was significant only in adolescents and adults, not in children. This apparent developmental effect needs to be replicated in a longitudinal study to determine whether it reflects measurement issues (e.g., aggression might be more reliably measured in older subjects), or the complexity of androgen effects on aggression (e.g., androgen might control the maturation of aggression, much as hormones control the development of physical characteristics). Future studies of aggression also need to consider the complexity of aggression (e.g., the distinction between the initiation of aggression and aggressive response to conflict), how aggression might be modified by social factors, and the likelihood that aggression is affected by both organizational and activational hormones (15).

Maternal Interest

There have been more studies of androgen effects on male-typical behavior (behaviors that are higher or more common in males than in females) than on female-typical behavior (behaviors that are higher or more common in females than in males), and it is typical to conceptualize the effects of androgens to be masculinizing (i.e., to facilitate male-typical behavior). This probably stems from analogy with physical development of the external genitalia, but, because sex-typed behavior is not a single continuum with masculine at one end and feminine at the other (e.g., Ref. 16), it is reasonable to consider how androgens may differentially affect male-typical and female-typical behavior. In fact, studies in rodents clearly show that hormones can differentially affect masculine and feminine behaviors as well as the different components of these behaviors (for review and discussion, see Ref. 17).

One of the most important female-typical behaviors relates to readiness to care for infants and young children. Several studies suggest that girls and women with CAH have reduced interest in activities related to maternal behavior. Compared with controls, CAH females play less with dolls (e.g.,

Ref. 6,10), and, on single interview items, are reported by themselves and their mothers to be less interested in infants and in motherhood, and more interested in pursuing a career (6,13). They have also been found to score lower than controls on personality measures on which females typically score higher than males and which may relate to maternal behavior. This includes scales measuring empathy, intimacy, the need for social relations, and maternal/nurturant behavior (18), as well as response to another's need for help or comfort (7).

In our sample of children with CAH and their unaffected relatives, we studied interest in infants using a parent-report questionnaire. As hypothesized, girls with CAH were reported by their parents to be less interested in infants compared with control girls, with the difference of substantial size (approximately two-thirds of a standard deviation). Boys with CAH were similar to their unaffected male relatives. These findings are consistent with studies in other species and suggest that high levels of androgens in the prenatal and/or early postnatal period acts to inhibit the development of maternal behavior (see Ref. 12 for details of the study and review of the literature).

Cognitive Abilities

There have been a number of studies of intelligence and specific cognitive abilities in patients with CAH. Early studies (19) reported that patients with CAH had higher overall intelligence (IQ) than would be expected (compared with population norms), but further study (19–21) revealed that relatives of patients with CAH also had higher than average IQ, which suggests sampling selection in the families seen at pediatric endocrine clinics. Nass and Baker (22) summarized data (including their own) suggesting that patients with salt-wasting (SW) CAH have IQ scores below that of patients with simple-virilizing (SV) CAH, which they proposed resulted from brain damage in SW patients. Nevertheless, most studies reveal that patients with CAH do not differ from their siblings in overall intelligence. This is not surprising because there are no sex differences in overall intelligence and thus no theoretical reason to expect patients with CAH to differ from controls.

On the other hand, it is reasonable to expect the *pattern* of cognitive abilities to be affected by early androgens because there are sex differences in specific cognitive abilities, with males outperforming females on measures of spatial and mathematical abilities, and females outperforming males on measures of verbal fluency, verbal memory, and perceptual speed (23,24). Consistent with the hypothesis that early androgens affect neural substrates of cognitive abilities, females with CAH appear to have higher spatial abilities than do control females in childhood, adolescence, and adulthood (25,26). Although differences have not always been observed between females with CAH and controls, it is important to note that the studies failing to find differences have generally used measures that do not show sex differences, small samples (and thus low statistical power to see differences), and/or subjects varying in age (see Ref. 27 for review). Female-typical abilities have not been well studied with respect to effects of early androgens.

It is interesting to note that males with CAH appear to have lower spatial ability than do their unaffected male relatives (25). This finding is consistent with studies of spatial ability in relation to circulating hormones in normal samples suggesting that spatial ability is enhanced by androgens in the mid-range: high spatial ability associated with relatively high testosterone in females but relatively low testosterone in males (28). On the other hand this reduced spatial ability in males with CAH may reflect consequences of the disease because boys are generally diagnosed later than girls and as a result of salt-wasting episodes. This issue clearly requires further study.

Sexuality

It is common for families of girls with CAH to wonder about later sexual behavior, especially sexual orientation, given the genital anomalies and possible androgen effects on the brain (29,30). Early studies on sexual orientation in women with CAH were inconsistent, with some suggesting increased rates of bi- or homosexuality compared with controls, and others failing to find differences between women with and without CAH (for review, see Ref. 31). Sexual orientation has been difficult to study for several reasons: Rates of homosexuality or bisexuality are low and it takes fairly large samples to detect increased rates in women with CAH; subjects need to be old enough to have established sexual orientation, and many lesbians do not acknowledge their orientation until their thirties; women with CAH need to have the disease in good control, to ensure that changes in sexual behavior result from effects of early hormones rather than circulating hormones; it is difficult to assess sexuality because of its very personal nature and, given the social constraints against homosexual behavior, it is necessary to assess arousal and fantasy as well as actual behavior.

In a study of women with CAH and their sisters, Zucker and colleagues (31) addressed most of these problems. Compared with their sisters, women with CAH had less sexual experience with men, but they did not have more experience with women. It is interesting to note, compared with their sisters, women with CAH reported both less sexual arousal to men and more sexual arousal to women. These results emphasize the importance of assessing arousal and fantasy, and not just behavior. It is important to note that, although women with CAH were more likely than their sisters to express sexual interest in women, the majority of women with CAH had heterosexual interests, whereas the others had bisexual—not exclusively homosexual—interests. For example, on a lifetime global rating of sexual orientation in fantasy, 66% of women with CAH were classified as exclusively heterosexual, 27% as bisexual, and 7% had no sexual fantasies; 100% of controls were classified as exclusively heterosexual (31, Table 8).

Although there is good reason to think that the reduced heterosexuality of women with CAH is directly related to their prenatal exposure to high levels of androgens, other factors may also affect sexual responses in CAH women, particularly psychological responses to the repeated examination of the genitalia, body image problems resulting from the abnormal genitalia, and the quality of the surgical repair of the genitalia (32,33). Most studies included women who had less than optimal surgery, so it has not been possible to separate the effects of genital virilization and surgery from androgen effects on the brain. The data from Zucker et al. (31) are important in this regard because it seems unlikely that women would become sexually aroused to women as a psychological response to genital anomalies. Nevertheless, this issue requires further study in a sample of females who received reconstructive surgery aimed at preserving clitoral sensitivity and vaginal introitus and maximizing sexual potential (34).

What Causes These Behavioral Changes?

Overall, behavioral studies of females with CAH suggest that early androgens contribute to the development of some aspects of human sex-typed behavior. Androgens appear to facilitate male-typical behaviors, such as interest in boys' toys and activities, aggression, spatial ability, and sexual arousal to women. Androgens also appear to inhibit female-typical behaviors, such as interest in girls' toys and activities, and maternal behavior. On the other hand, androgens appear to have only small effects on aspects of gender identity and playmate preference.

There are several reasons to think that the behavioral changes found in females with CAH specifically reflect exposure to moderately high levels of androgens in the prenatal and neonatal periods, rather than other factors that differ between individuals with CAH and controls (35). First, the findings are consistent with theoretical expectations and with studies in other populations. Differences between CAH and control females are consistent with those in other species where hormones have been directly manipulated (1,2), and are found only on measures that show sex differences and thus would be reasonably expected to be sensitive to effects of early hormones. Further, data from other samples (both clinical samples and normal individuals with typical variations in prenatal hormones) confirm some of the behavioral effects found in CAH females (36–38).

Second, behavioral changes cannot be attributed to the disease itself. The other hormones that are abnormal in CAH, such as progesterone and corticosteroids, have smaller and less consistent behavioral effects than androgen, and they may actually prevent masculinization (39). Behavioral similarities between CAH and control males make it unlikely that behavioral changes in CAH females reflect general disease characteristics or other hormonal abnormalities.

Third, it is unlikely that behavioral changes in CAH females result from social responses to their virilized genitalia. Degree of genital virilization has not always been found to relate to behavior in CAH girls (8,12,13,40) or in androgenized female rhesus macaques (41). Parents do not report that they treated CAH girls in a masculine fashion (6–8) and may actually encourage feminine behavior (42), which is consistent with data showing maternal behavior to be unrelated to offspring behavior in androgenized female macaques (41). It would be valuable, however, to observe parents' behavior directly.

Fourth, behavioral changes are unlikely to result from excess androgens later in postnatal life because CAH females may actually have subnormal androgen levels (43), and behavior has not been found to relate to aspects of disease control or treatment (13; Berenbaum, Duck, and Korman, unpublished observations). Nevertheless, we are continuing to investigate this question.

Fifth, some behavioral changes in CAH females relate to the severity of the disease. For example, females with SW-CAH appear to be more behaviorally masculinized than females with SV-CAH (31,40,44). Because SW-CAH is associated with lower enzyme activity than SV-CAH, and consequently with a more severe disease (45), it is likely that behavioral differences between SW-CAH and SV-CAH reflect differences in levels of androgens present early in life.

Nevertheless, there are several issues that require further study regarding relative influences on psychological outcome in individuals with CAH. First, it would be valuable to have direct evidence that behavioral changes in CAH result from the action of early androgens on the brain. Data suggest that neuroendocrine function in CAH women results in part from elevated androgens early in life (46), and it is likely that there will soon be direct studies of brain structure in individuals with CAH. Second, it is essential to study directly how parents treat their daughters with CAH. This would include information about parent knowledge, expectations, and attitudes, and direct observations of interactions between parents and children. Third, it is important to examine the generality of the results to date that have been obtained from patients recruited through academic medical centers. Toward that goal, we are involved in behavioral follow-up studies of children who have been identified through newborn screening.

Psychological Adjustment

Clinical reports suggest that females with CAH have problems in psychological adjustment as a result of genital virilization, genital surgery, and repeated inspections of the genitalia. In fact, prenatal treatment for CAH is justified in part for its benefit for adjustment (47). On the other hand, the Intersex Society of North America (48) has suggested that emotional problems are the consequences of early surgery to correct the anomalies. Psychological adjustment has not been extensively studied, but data from several countries do not support the supposition that females with CAH have poor overall adjustment (49,50), although they may have problems in specific areas, including body image and psychosexual adjustment (33,50). Previous studies should have detected problems if they exist because participants were older women with suboptimal medical and surgical treatment. Nevertheless, methodological limitations, especially insensitive measures, small samples, and lack of sibling controls, may have made it difficult to detect problems. Psychological adjustment is one of the most important topics for further study, and it should be examined in relation to age as well as quality of genital surgery and follow-up medical care.

Summary and Conclusions

Overall, the evidence strongly suggests that prenatal or neonatal androgens affect the development of various aspects of sex-typed behavior. The interesting questions now become ones of mechanism (i.e., how hormones affect behavior). This means finding the neural substrates that mediate androgen effects, the basic behavioral processes that mediate androgen effects on complex behaviors (e.g., what basic processes underlie preference for toy trucks vs. dolls?), and the ways in which hormonally influenced predispositions guide individuals' selections of and responses to the environment (see Ref. 38 for a discussion of these issues).

The greatest controversies about the nature and causes of behavioral changes in CAH females concern sexual behavior, psychosexual adjustment, and general psychological adjustment. It is important to conduct systematic studies of psychological and psychosexual adjustment in females with CAH, and to determine whether adjustment is related to the age and quality of corrective genital surgery. The answers to these questions will affect medical treatment.

In sum, psychological outcome in CAH is generally good. Individuals with CAH show some behavioral changes that appear to be associated with the effects of early androgens on the development of the brain. Most salient is the interest in boy-typical play and activities that characterizes most girls with CAH. It is important to remember that gender identity and psychological adjustment are typical in the majority of cases.

Acknowledgments. Preparation of this chapter and my own research reported here were supported by National Institutes of Health Grant HD19644. I thank the following people for their contributions to my research: Kristina Korman provided outstanding research assistance, including coordination of the project, and data collection, processing, and management; Drs. Stephen Duck, Deborah Edidin, Orville Green, David Klein, Ora Pescovitz, Gail Richards, Julio Santiago, Bernard Silverman, and David Wyatt generously provided access to their patients and answered medical questions; Elizabeth Snyder, Kathleen Bechtold, Jackie Ewing, Kim Ketterling, Robyn Reed, Cindy Tubbs, and George Vineyard assisted in data collection and/or processing; Dr. Stephen Duck examined medical records and provided ratings on androgen excess and disease characteristics; Dr. Brad Therrell and Kristina Korman provided thoughtful and helpful comments on an earlier version of this chapter. I am particularly grateful to the children and their parents for their continuing cooperation and enthusiastic participation in the study.

References

1. Arnold AP, Gorski RA. Gonadal steroid induction of structural sex differences in the central nervous system. Ann Rev Neurosci 1984;7:413–42.
2. Goy RW, McEwen BS. Sexual differentiation of the brain. London: Oxford University Press, 1980.
3. Pang S, Clark A, et al. Congenital adrenal hyperplasia due to 21-hydroxylase deficiency: newborn screening and its relationship to the diagnosis and treatment of the disorder. Screening 1993;2:105–39.
4. Therrell BL Jr., Berenbaum SA, Manter-Kapanke V, Simmank J, Korman K, Prentice L, et al. Results of screening 1.9 million Texas newborns for 21-hydroxylase-deficient congenital adrenal hyperplasia. Pediatrics 1998;101:583–90.
5. Money J, Ehrhardt AA. Man and woman, boy and girl. Baltimore: Johns Hopkins University Press, 1972.
6. Ehrhardt AA, Baker SW. Fetal androgens, human central nervous system differentiation, and behavior sex differences. In: Friedman RC, Richart RR, Vande Weile RL, ed. Sex differences in behavior. New York: Wiley, 1974:33–51.
7. Resnick, S. M. Psychological functioning in individuals with congenital adrenal hyperplasia: Early hormonal influences on cognition and personality. Unpublished doctoral dissertation, University of Minnesota, Minneapolis, 1982.
8. Berenbaum SA, Hines M. Early androgens are related to childhood sex-typed toy preferences. Psych Sci 1992;3:203–6.
9. Hines M, Kaufman, F. Androgen and the development of human sex-typical behavior: rough-and-tumble play and sex of preferred playmates in children with congenital adrenal hyperplasia (CAH). Child Dev 1994;65:1042–53.
10. Berenbaum SA, Snyder E. Early hormonal influences on childhood sex-typed activity and playmate preference: implications for the development of sexual orientation. Dev Psych 1995;31:31–42.
11. Berenbaum SA, Resnick SM. Early androgen effects on aggression in children and adults with congenital adrenal hyperplasia. Psychoneuroendocrinology 1997; 22:505–15.
12. Leveroni C, Berenbaum SA. Early androgen effects on interest in infants: evidence from children with congenital adrenal hyperplasia. Dev Neuropsych 1998;14: 321–40.
13. Dittmann RW, Kappes MH, Kappes ME, Borger D, Stegner H, Willig RH, et al.

Congenital adrenal hyperplasia I: gender-related behaviors and attitudes in female patients and their sisters. Psychoneuroendocrinology 1990;15:401–20.

14. Meyer-Bahlburg HFL, Gruen RS, New MI, Bell JJ, Morishima A, Shimshi M, et al. Gender change from female to male in classical congenital adrenal hyperplasia. Horm Behav 1996;30:319–32.
15. Monaghan EP, Glickman SE. Hormones and aggressive behavior. In: Becker JB, Breedlove SM, Crews D, eds. Behavioral endocrinology. Cambridge: MIT Press, 1992:261–85.
16. Huston AC. Sex-typing. In: Mussen PH, ed. Handbook of child psychology: Vol. 4. Socialization, personality, and social development. New York: Wiley, 1983: 387–467.
17. Fitch RH, Denenberg VH. A role for ovarian hormones in sexual differentiation of the brain. Behav Brain Sci 1998;21:311–52.
18. Helleday J, Edman G, Ritzen EM, Siwers B. Personality characteristics and platelet MAO activity in women with congenital adrenal hyperplasia (CAH). Psychoneuroendocrinology 1993;18:343–54.
19. Money J, Lewis V. IQ, genetics, and accelerated growth: adrenogenital syndrome. Bull Johns Hopkins Hosp 1966;118:365–73.
20. Baker SW, Ehrhardt AA. Prenatal androgen, intelligence, and cognitive sex differences. In: Friedman RC, Richart RR, Vande Weile RL, eds. Sex differences in behavior. New York: Wiley, 1974:53–76.
21. McGuire LS, Omenn GS. Congenital adrenal hyperplasia. I. Family studies of IQ. Behav Genet 1975;5:165–73.
22. Nass R, Baker SW. Androgen effects on cognition: congenital adrenal hyperplasia. Psychoneuroendocrinology 1991;16:189–201.
23. Halpern DF. Sex differences in cognitive abilities, second ed. Hillsdale, NJ: Erlbaum Associates.
24. Kramer JH, Delis DC, Daniel M. Sex differences in verbal learning. J Clin Psychol 1988;44:907–15.
25. Hampson E, Rovet JF, Altmann, D. Spatial reasoning in children with congenital adrenal hyperplasia due to 21-hydroxylase deficiency. Dev Neuropsych 1998; 14:299–320.
26. Resnick SM, Berenbaum SA, Gottesman II, Bouchard TJ. Early hormonal influences on cognitive functioning in congenital adrenal hyperplasia. Dev Psych 1986;22:191–98.
27. Berenbaum SA, Korman K, Leveroni C. Early hormones and sex differences in cognitive abilities. Learning Indiv Diffs 1995;7:303–21.
28. Kimura D, Hampson E. Cognitive pattern in men and women is influenced by fluctuations in sex hormones. Curr Dir Psychol Sci 1994;3:57–61.
29. LeVay S. The sexual brain. Cambridge: MIT Press, 1993.
30. Money J. Sin, sickness, or status? Homosexual gender identity and psychoneuroendocrinology. Am Psych 1987;42:384–99.
31. Zucker KJ, Bradley SJ, Oliver G, Blake J, Fleming S, Hood J. Psychosexual development of women with congenital adrenal hyperplasia. Horm Behav 1996;30: 300–18.
32. Mulaikal RM, Migeon CJ, Rock JA. Fertility rates in female patients with congenital adrenal hyperplasia due to 21-hydroxylase deficiency. N Engl J Med 1987;316:178–82.
33. Slijper FME, van der Kamp HJ, Brandenburg H, de Muinck Keizer-Schrama SMPF,

Drop SLS, Molenaar JC. Evaluation of psychosexual development of young women with congenital adrenal hyperplasia: a pilot study. J Sex EdTher 1992;18:200–7.
34. Donahoe PK, Schnitzer JJ. Evaluation of the infant who has ambiguous genitalia, and principles of operative management. Semin Ped Surg 1996;5:30-40.
35. Quadagno DM, Briscoe R, Quadagno JS. Effects of perinatal gonadal hormones on selected nonsexual behavior patterns: a critical assessment of the nonhuman and human literature. Psychol Bull 1977;84:62–80.
36. Collaer ML, Hines M. Human behavioral sex differences: a role for gonadal hormones during early development? Psych Bull 1995;118:55–107.
37. Reinisch JM, Ziemba-Davis M, Sanders SA. Hormonal contributions to sexually dimorphic behavioral development in humans. Psychoneuroendocrinology 1991;16: 213–78.
38. Berenbaum SA. How hormones affect behavioral and neural development: introduction to the special issue on "gonadal hormones and sex differences in behavior." Dev Neuropsychol 1998;14:175–96.
39. Hull EM, Franz JR, Snyder AM, Nishita JK. Perinatal progesterone and learning, social and reproductive behavior in rats. Physiol Behav 1980;24:251–56.
40. Slijper FME. Androgens and gender role behavior in girls with congenital adrenal hyperplasia (CAH). In: DeVries JG, DeBruin JPC, Uylings HBM, Corner MA, eds. Progress in brain research, vol 61. Amsterdam: Elsevier, 1984:417–22.
41. Goy RW, Bercovitch FB, McBrair MC. Behavioral masculinization is independent of genital masculinization in prenatally androgenized female rhesus macaques. Horm Behav 1988;22:552–71.
42. Ehrhardt AA, Meyer-Bahlburg HFL. Effects of prenatal sex hormones on gender-related behavior. Science 1981;211:1312–18.
43. Helleday J, Siwers B, Ritzen EM, Carlstrom K. Subnormal androgen and elevated progesterone levels in women treated for congenital virilizing 21-hydroxylase deficiency. J Clin Endocrinol Metab 1993;76:933–36.
44. Dittmann RW, Kappes MH, Kappes ME, Borger D, Meyer-Bahlburg HFL, Stegner H, et al. Congenital adrenal hyperplasia II: gender-related behaviors and attitudes in female salt-wasting and simple-virilizing patients. Psychoneuroendocrinology 1990;15:421–34.
45. Wedell A, Thilen A, Ritzen EM, Stengler B, Luthman H. Mutational spectrum of the steroid 21-hydroxylase gene in Sweden: implications for genetic diagnosis and association with disease manifestation. J Clin Endocrinol Metab 1994;78:1145–52.
46. Barnes RB, Rosenfield RL, Ehrmann DA, Cara JF, Cuttler L, Levitsky L, et al. Ovarian hyperandrogenism as a result of congenital adrenal virilizing disorders: evidence for perinatal masculinization of neuroendocrine function in women. J Clin Endocrinol Metab 1994;79:1328–33.
47. Mercado AB, Wilson RC, Cheng KC, Wei J, New, MI. Prenatal treatment and diagnosis of congenital adrenal hyperplasia owing to steroid 21-hydroxylase deficiency. J Clin Endocrinol Metab 1995;80:2014–20.
48. Intersex Society of North America. Web page. www.isna.org 1997.
49. Berenbaum SA. Congenital adrenal hyperplasia: intellectual and psychosexual functioning. In: Holmes C, ed. Psychoneuroendocrinology: brain, behavior, and hormonal interactions. New York: Springer-Verlag, 1990:227–60.
50. Kuhnle U, Bullinger M, Schwarz HP. The quality of life in adult female patients with

congenital adrenal hyperplasia: a comprehensive study of the impact of genital malformations and chronic disease on female patients life. Eur J Ped 1995;154:708–16.

51. Miller WL. The adrenal cortex. In: Rudolph AM, Hoffman JIE, Rudolph CD, Sagan P, eds. Rudolph's pediatrics, twentieth ed. Stamford, CT: Appleton and Lange, 1996: 1711–42.
52. White PC, New MI, Dupont B. Congenital adrenal hyperplasia. N Engl J Med 1987;316:1519–24.
53. Berenbaum SA. Effects of early androgens on sex-typed activities and interests in adolescents with congenital adrenal hyperplasia. Horm Behav 1999;35:102–10.

20

Psychosexual Quality of Life in Adult Intersexuality: The Example of Congenital Adrenal Hyperplasia (CAH)

An Invited Contribution

Heino F.L. Meyer-Bahlburg, Sonia Gidwani, Ralf W. Dittmann, Curtis Dolezal, Susan W. Baker, Akira Morishima, Jennifer J. Bell, and Maria I. New

Introduction

A fundamental aspect of the quality of life in adolescence and adulthood is psychosexuality. It comprises three interrelated aspects: (1) gender role behavior and gender identity; (2) sexual life, with its four components of sexual orientation, courtship, partner bonding, and genital sexuality; (3) reproduction and parenting. Intersexuality tends to affect all three aspects of psychosexuality. In this chapter, we will use data on the syndrome of classical congenital adrenal hyperplasia (CAH) in 46,XX individuals with 21-hydroxylase deficiency as an illustrative example.

Concerning gender-role behavior of CAH females, a number of studies have demonstrated significant shifts in the direction of masculinization, most markedly so in childhood (1,2). The shift is much more pronounced in the salt-wasting (SW) than the simple virilizing (SV) form (3). The extreme degree is patient-initiated gender change in midadulthood (4). In the latter paper, we combined two cases of SW-CAH (including one of the 13 patients of the current report) with one SV case and one case of 11-beta-hydroxylase deficiency. Four features distinguished these four patients with gender change from the remaining 12 SW patients: (1). All four experienced very delayed genital surgery or, in one case, none at all (i.e., their apparent genital ambiguity persisted well into childhood or adolescence). (2)

All underwent glucocorticoid replacement therapy only intermittently or not at all; therefore, they were all postnatally exposed to markedly elevated androgen levels for prolonged periods. (3) In childhood gender-role behavior, these four gender-change patients tended to be even less feminine (and slightly more masculine) than the SW-CAH group, which already differed markedly from normal controls by itself. (4) All four gender-change patients were sexually attracted exclusively to women (i.e., were homosexual relative to their chromosomal sex). Nevertheless, it was not before adulthood that these 4 CAH females fully faced up to the issue of gender change. The quality of life as a female was obviously so inadequate for these patients that they intended to switch to the male role. This finding underlines the need for long-term follow-up studies well into midlife, if one wants to obtain a comprehensive database for optimal patient management.

Reproductive outcome in women with classical CAH was studied by means of a postal questionnaire survey by Mulaikal, Migeon, and Rock (5). It was found to be particularly low for women with the SW form. The authors offered insufficient hormonal regulation by glucocorticoid replacement and the status of the vagina as the most plausible explanation, and Federman (6) emphasized the potential additional contribution of effects of prenatal sex-hormone abnormalities on brain and behavior to this outcome.

The sexual life of women with classical CAH and especially their genital sexual functioning are the focus of this chapter because of the fact that a large percentage of CAH females undergo genital surgery of their genitalia at some time between infancy and young adulthood, often more than once. Two aspects of the genital status are of particular interest here: the status of the vagina and the status of the clitoris. The status of the vagina—specifically its length and the width of the introitus—has obvious implications for coital capacity. The continued presence of an enlarged clitoris or its regrowth after resection is associated with increased rates of "gender transposition" (7; see also Ref. 4) (i.e., gender change and/or bi-/homosexuality). Moreover, we have learned from our clinical work that clitoral surgery, especially total clitorectomy, may be associated with impaired erotic sensitivity with negative implications for sexual enjoyment and the overall sex life.

The data for this report come from a pilot project on adult CAH females. In contrast to the postal survey of Mulaikal et al. (5), we set up a comprehensive psychologic/psychiatric protocol for a face-to-face evaluation along with a detailed review of the medical chart complemented by additional medical examinations where indicated and feasible. To maximize the potential effect sizes, we planned to contrast women with SW as the most severe form of classical CAH to women with nonclassical (NC) late-onset CAH, and to compare both with a sample of normal women from our research data bank.

Method: Sample Selection

Thirteen females with SW CAH and six women with NC CAH were recruited from two pediatric endocrine clinics in New York City. All adult women with CAH under 52 years of age were eligible, although recruitment for the pilot study was started with the relatively older and geographically more easily accessible women. A SW CAH woman with psychosis was excluded. A group of 30 normal control (CO) women was selected from a data bank of a project on the long-term psychological sequels of prenatal diethylstilbestrol exposure (see Ref. 8) that had used a similar protocol. These CO women had been selected from the records of women who visited a gynecologist's private practice for routine gynecological care and who had no history of prenatal hormone abnormalities or prenatal DES exposure, nor did they have any gynecological disorders such as infertility or a positive PAP smear. The CO women had to be 18 years of age or older, of white race, and capable of speaking English; women with mental retardation, severe congenital anomalies, and debilitating chronic diseases were excluded (for recruitment details, see Ref. 9).

Method: Assessment

All women underwent a full-day protocol of systematic interviews (both structured and qualitative), standard self-report questionnaires, and psychometric tests. For the clinical patients, the medical data were excerpted from the hospital charts and complemented in most cases by a physical examination that focused on somatic androgen effects as part of the study protocol. In the case of the control women, data from their medical charts were supplemented by a structured medical history. The psychologic data of the current report come primarily from the Sexual Behavior Assessment Schedule (SEBAS-A) (10), a semi-structured interview covering psychosexual milestones, sexual orientation, sexual activity level, and sexual dysfunctions, as well as a qualitative interview concerned with the patient's experience of her endocrine condition, including surgery and hormone treatment and the effects on several aspects of her life.

Method: Data Analysis

Standard parametric and nonparametric three-group and two-group statistical comparison tests were used for exploratory analysis.

Results

All participating women were white except for one African-American and two Latina women in the SW group and one Latina woman in the NC group. Most women were in their twenties and thirties, but the NC women were significantly older (mean, 37 years) than the other two groups (SW: 30 years; CO: 27 years). Socioeconomic status was mostly middle-class.

All of the SW women had been born with some degree of ambiguous genitalia, and all had undergone some type of surgical correction. Table 20.1 shows that almost all SW women had undergone surgery of the clitoris, but none of the NC women and none of the controls had done so. Many of the SW women underwent multiple surgeries of the clitoris that, for most, extended into the developmental period of initial gender identity formation and later, for some, even into the teenage years. Three SW women, as compared with none of the NC women, rated the erotic sensitivity of their clitoris as low.

As Table 20.2 shows, 10 of the SW women had undergone vaginal surgery, most during the adolescent years (i.e., at an age when a young woman is likely to be at least somewhat aware that such surgery may have implications for her sex life and reproductive outcome). Only two of the SW women (17% of those with data) considered the width of the introitus as fully adequate for intercourse, as compared with four (67%) of the NC women.

The quality of hormonal control in these females was highly variable (not shown). The majority of our CAH women, both SW and NC, had various indications of at least intermittent (and, in NC cases, treatment-preceding) deficiencies in the androgen control, as indicated by signs of virilization such as hirsutism, acne, menstrual irregularities, receding hairline, and short stature.

TABLE 20.1. Clitoral surgery and status.

Variable	SW (N = 13)	NC (N = 6)
Has had operation		
Ever	11	
Never	2	6
Type of operation		
Clitorectomy	5	
Clitoral resection	3	
Unclear which	3	
Age at most recent operation		
< 1 yr	2	
1–2 yrs	2	
2–5 yrs	3	
> 10 yrs	3	
No information	1	
Erotic sensitivity at present		
Low	3	
Don't know	2	
Average	6	
Not asked	2	

TABLE 20.2. Vaginal surgery and status.

Variable	SW (N = 13)	NC (N = 6)
Has had operation		
Ever	10	
Never	2	6
No information	1	
Age at most recent operation		
≤ 1 yr	1	
1–3 yrs	1	
> 10 yrs	8	
No information	1	
Vaginal width, current		
Adequate	2	4
Dubious	5	2
Tight	5	
(Too tight for coitus)	2	
No information	1	

The overall heterosexual romantic involvement of SW women appears to be lower than it is in the other two groups (Table 20.3). Fewer SW women reported having had a heterosexual crush, ever. Those who did, experienced it later. Similar differences hold for the experience of love. Fewer of the SW women than those of the other groups had ever been heterosexually active. Among women who had ever been heterosexually active, the SW women had fewer sex occasions in their lifetime (LT). Differences in age at first intercourse and in the number of LT partners went in the same direction, but did not reach statistical significance.

Sexual orientation was assessed by the Kinsey scale, which ranges from 0, exclusively heterosexual, to 6, exclusively homosexual. The rating is based on erotic imagery, attractions, and actual partners. Four of the SW women, but none of the others, had Kinsey scores above K2 (one K3, one K4,and two K6), and the difference in means (SW: 1.7; NC: 0.8; CO: 0.5) is statistically significant (not shown).

Table 20.4 contains the findings on sexual functioning. Current functioning refers to the past 12 months. In comparison to the other two groups, the SW women rated their sex drive—assessed regardless of sexual orientation—on average as lower, although there was also one NC woman who rated her sex drive as "none." The self-rating of sexual interest in terms of the frequency of sexual thoughts replicates the findings on the sex drive rating. The SW group does not seem to suffer from increased problems with vaginal lubrication (the NC women report a longer lubrication latency), nor from dyspareunia, but note that the data on these variables are limited to women who are hetero-

TABLE 20.3. Heterosexual romance and activity.

	SW	NC	CO	Three groups	SW v. CO	NC v. CO	SW v. NC
Crush:							
Had ever (N)[1]	10/13	6/6	29/30	(*)	(*)		
(%)	77%	100%	97%				
Age at first, mean[2]	12.4	8.5	11.0	(*)		(*)	*
Love:							
Had ever (N)[1]	5/13	6/6	28/30	***	**		*
(%)	38%	100%	93%				
Age at first, mean[2]	20.5	16.2	17.4		(*)		
Intercourse:							
Had ever (N)[1]	8/13	5/6	27/30	(*)	*		
(%)	62%	83%	90%				
Age at first, mean[2]	19.7	18.9	18.1				
#LT partners, mean[2]	1.5	2.7	2.4				
#LT occasions, mean[2]	3.3	5.0	5.3	*	**		

[1]Statistical test: Chi-square or Fisher's Exact Test.
[2]Statistical test: ANOVA.
(*) $p < 0.10$; *$p < 0.05$; **$p < 0.01$; ***$p < 0.001$.

TABLE 20.4. Sexual dysfunctions.

					p (ANOVA)		
	SW	NC	CO	Three groups	SW v. CO	NC v. CO	SW v. NC
Current[1]							
Sex drive	2.8	4.2	4.4	**	*		
Sex interest	4.0	6.0	5.7	**	*		*
Vaginal response: degree	4.8	4.0	4.7				
Vaginal response: speed	4.0	3.0	4.1	(*)		*	(*)
Orgasmic frequency	2.7	4.2	3.9		(*)		
Dyspareunia[2]	4.5	4.0	4.8				
Lifetime[3]							
Lack of sex interest	3.5	3.5	4.4			(*)	
Lack of vaginal response	4.2	4.8	4.7				
Lack of orgasm	3.5	5.0	4.1				(*)
Vaginismus	4.5	4.2	4.8				
Dyspareunia	4.4	3.4	4.7	*			

[1]Categorized variables.
[2]High score = absent.
[3]Five-point response scale: e.g., 1 = Always; 3 = Two such phases (of at least four weeks duration); 5 = No such phase.
(*) $p < 0.10$; *$p < 0.05$; **$p < 0.01$.

sexually active. There is a statistical tendency for SW women to have an overall lower orgasmic frequency than the other two groups. The LT data show similar trends. There is some suggestion in the data that the genital procedures and the genital status are related to the sexual functioning, but the database is yet too small for appropriate statistical analysis within the SW CAH sample.

In regard to reproduction and parenthood (not shown), only one of the 13 SW women versus 4 of the 6 NC women had ever been pregnant ($p < .05$); the CO women had not been asked. None of the SW women versus 50% of the NC women and 34% of the controls had at least one child ($p < .05$).

Discussion

Our findings show that psychosexuality is broadly affected in the SW CAH condition. Apart from changes in gender-role behavior (which were not the focus of this report), heterosexual initiation was delayed, current heterosexual activity was lower than in controls, and sexual orientation shifted toward increased rates of bi- and homosexuality. Sex drive was diminished and overall orgasmic frequency was reduced. Finally, childbearing was decreased. The prenatal and postnatal hormonal milieu, genital surgeries, and resulting genital status, all are likely contributors to this outcome. In our qualitative interviews, several women reported that frequent genital examinations, especially those performed by male physicians, and often by unfamiliar ones, also contributed by making them shy and avoidant of all sexual contacts.

Concerning the reproductive outcome, one has to note the variability in age of the participants. For most women in the study, the reproductive years are not yet over, and some women are too young really to have tried to become pregnant. Nevertheless, the SW women seem to be markedly lower in childbearing, especially when one considers that they are older than the normal controls and have, therefore, theoretically more years of opportunity for childbearing. (In another, slightly older, normal control group from the same databank—with a mean age of 31 years—the rate of women having their own children was even higher, 54%.)

Our data are compatible with the suggestion by Mulaikal et al. (5) that, apart from the endocrine situation, the vaginal status may contribute to the low reproductive outcome in SW CAH women. Our data suggest that clitoral status also has to be considered. It seems plausible that all three biological factors influence psychosexual development in adolescence. Other data from our study, as yet unpublished, indicate an additional factor; an unusually low interest in having children and related variables dating back to childhood on the part of the SW CAH women. This supports Federman's (6) comments regarding contributing behavioral effects.

Although preliminary and in need of replication with a larger sample, our data from this study carry significant implications. Early gender-confirming genital surgery and consistent hormonal regulation remain important in preventing gender identity problems. Emphasis in the evaluation of genital surgical procedures has to move away from evaluating mostly cosmetic results and to include courtship and sexual functioning in adulthood. Frequency of genital examinations, especially by multiple examiners, needs to be rigorously curtailed. Reduced fertility is only in part secondary to problems of the sex-hormone regulation after puberty and may have at least as much to do with behavioral factors in SW CAH women. Global quality of life measures as used by Kuhnle, Bullinger, and Schwarz (11) appear to be unsuited to capture all of these details and should be complemented by syndrome-specific measures. Finally, there is an urgent need for cross-center and interdisciplinary collaboration to obtain *long-term* follow-up data on sufficient sample sizes that might firm up these conclusions.

Acknowledgments. This research was supported in part by USPHS NIMH CRC Grant MH-30906, NYSPI BRSG Grant 10/89, NIH Grant HD00072, and NIH CRC Grant 06020. Rhoda S. Gruen served as interviewer, Robin Faigeles and Sherri Cohen as research assistants, and Patricia Connolly provided word processing.

References

1. Money J, Ehrhardt AA. Man and woman, boy and girl: Differentiation and dimorphism of gender identity from conception to maturity. Baltimore (MD): Johns Hopkins University Press, 1972.
2. Berenbaum S. Psychological outcome in congenital adrenal hyperplasia. In: Stabler B, Bercu BB, editors. Therapeutic outcome of endocrine disorders: efficacy, innovation and quality of life. New York: Springer-Verlag, 2000:186–99.
3. Dittmann RW, Kappes MH, Kappes ME, Börger D, Meyer-Bahlburg HFL, Stegner H, et al. Congenital adrenal hyperplasia II: gender-related behavior and attitudes in female salt-wasting and simple-virilizing patients. Psychoneuroendocrinology 1990;15:421-34.
4. Meyer-Bahlburg HFL, Gruen RS, New MI, Bell JJ, Morishima A, Shimshi M, et al. Gender change from female to male in classical CAH. Horm Behav 1996;30:319–32.
5. Mulaikal RM, Migeon CJ, Rock JA. Fertility rates in female patients with congenital adrenal hyperplasia due to 21-hydroxylase deficiency. New Engl JMed 1987;316:178–82.
6. Federman DD. Psychosexual adjustment in congenital adrenal hyperplasia [editorial]. New Engl JMed 1987;316:209–11.
7. Money J, Devore H, Norman BF. Gender identity and gender transposition: longitudinal outcome study of 32 male hermaphrodites assigned as girls. J Sex Marital Ther 1986;12:165–81.

8. Meyer-Bahlburg HFL, Ehrhardt AA, Rosen LR, Gruen RS, Veridiano NP, Vann FH, et al. Prenatal estrogens and the development of homosexual orientation. Dev Psychol 1995;31:12–21.
9. Lish JD, Ehrhardt AA, Meyer-Bahlburg HFL, Rosen LR, Gruen RS, Veridiano NP. Gender-related behavior development in females exposed to diethylstilbestrol (DES) in utero: an attempted replication. J Am Acad Child Adol Psychiatr 1991;30:29–37.
10. Meyer-Bahlburg HFL, Ehrhardt AA. Sexual behavior assessment schedule–adult (SEBAS-A). New York: Authors 1983. Available through the Columbia University College of Physicians and Surgeons.
11. Kuhnle U, Bullinger M, Schwarz HP. The quality of life in adult female patients with congenital adrenal hyperplasia: a comprehensive study of the impact of genital malformations and chronic disease on female patients life. Eur J Pediatr 1995;154:708–16.

21

Male Fertility in Congenital Adrenal Hyperplasia

An Invited Contribution

César Bergadá, Ana Claudia Keselman, Stella Maris Campo, María Gabriela Ropelato, and Héctor Edgardo Chemes

It has been shown that the majority of noncentral precocious sexual developments in boys are due to overproduction of adrenal androgens in patients with late onset congenital adrenal hyperplasia (CAH) with 21-hydroxylase deficiency. In these cases the diagnosis is easily suspected because the testes size remains prepubertal. This characteristic has diagnostic value, especially in patients with bone ages of 13 or more years (1). This can be physiologically explained by the inhibitory effect that high levels of circulating adrenal androgens exert on the secretion of gonadotropins.

In 1954 Wilkins and Cara (2), demonstrated that the pituitary inhibition produced by androgens was responsible for the lack of testicular development. This was ascertained because of the rapid testicular growth that took place after treatment with cortisone acetate in boys under 9 years of age with bone age over 13 years. Gonadotropin suppression was also reported by Penny et al. in 1973 (3) in a 6-year-old boy with bone age of 13, who increased his gonadotropin levels and testicular volume after 6 months of cortisone therapy. This situation is now very well understood and treated with gonadotropin releasing hormone (GnRH) analogs as in other cases of central precocious puberty.

Patients who have never been treated reach adulthood with underdeveloped testes and are infertile. Adequate corticoid treatment, however, can reverse that situation and promote fertility (4–11). When the diagnosis is made early in infancy or soon after the appearance of pubic hair, and adequate treatment is instituted throughout late adolescence, these patients undergo normal puberty and become fertile (1). On the other hand, it has also been reported that some men who discontinue corticoid therapy in adult-

TABLE 21.1. Clinical evolution of Cases 1 to 5 from childhood to adulthood: onset of pubic hair, period of treatment, final height, and fertility.

	Childhood		Adolescence		Adult	
	Onset of pubic hair (years)	Onset of therapy (years)	Early	Late	Height (cm)	Fertility
Case 1	4	6	Treated	?	162	Complete spermat. in childhood
Case 2	6	None	Nontreated	Nontreated	163	Infertile
Case 3	8	8.8	Treated	Withdrawal	158	Fertile
Case 4	6	6	Treated	Withdrawal	157	Fertile
Case 5	4	4.6	Treated	Treated	167	Fertile

hood for several years may remain fertile (4,5,12,13). This chapter will report and comment on some situations that may clarify the effect of androgens on spermatogenic function in patients with CAH.

Case Reports

Five male patients with late onset CAH—one prepubertal child and four adults—were studied at the division of endocrinology of the Hospital de Niños Ricardo Gutierrez of Buenos Aires. Three of the latter were being followed since their diagnosis in early childhood (Table 21.1).

Case 1

A 5-year-old boy consulted for sexual precocity and acceleration of growth in 1962. Pubic hair development was first noticed at age 4. He had a height of 123 cm and bone age of 11 years, pubic hair Tanner 3, marked androgenic stimulation of external genitalia with a penis 12 cm in length and testicular volume of 3 ml. At 6 years of age he had a height of 140 cm, growth velocity of 15 cm/year a bone age of 13 years. His external genitalia and pubic hair were Tanner stage 4, with testicular volume of 5 ml. Urinary 17-ketosteroids (17 KS) were 21 mg/24 hours. Prednisone therapy at a dose of 7.5 mg/day was started. One year later, growth rate fell to 3 cm/year and 17-KS decreased to 3.2 mg/24 hours. At 8 years he showed catch-up growth of 14 cm/year, height of 154 cm, bone age of 15 years, and the testes increased to a volume of 15 ml with a rise of 17-KS to 25 mg/24 hours. Prednisone was augmented to 10.0 mg/day. Testes became even larger (20 ml) and hard, and a testicular biopsy was obtained that showed mature testes, with normal Leydig cells and seminiferous tubules of normal adult diameter containing complete spermatogenesis (Fig. 21.1). The boy remained on corticoid therapy,

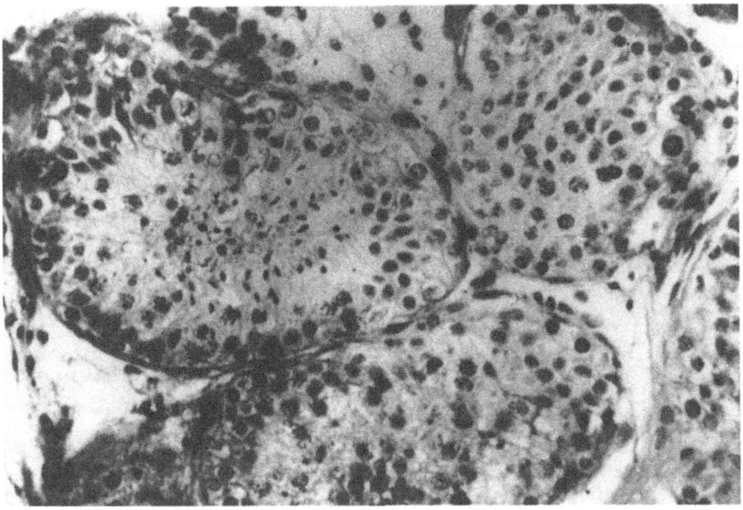

FIGURE 21.1. Testicular biopsy from Case 1. See text for description of this and all subsequent figures.

and at 10.4 years he was seen for the last time with a height of 162 cm and bone age of 16 years.

Case 2

A 23-year-old man was examined at the endocrine division in 1997 because of the diagnosis of CAH made on his 6-year-old brother. The patient was married, and the couple was under study for infertility. Past history revealed that he started to develop pubic hair at age 6 and completed his sexual development and growth at 10 years of age. At 23 he measured 163 cm and weighed 61 kg. He had genitalia and pubic hair Tanner stage 5, and testicular volume of 5-6 ml each. Plasma testosterone: 1830 ng/dl; 17-OHProgesterone: 170 ng/ml; DHEAS: 7830 ng/ml; androstenedione: 400 ng/dl; cortisol: 8.1 ug/dl; GnRH test: LH; basal, 1.1, at 30 minutes: 2.0, and at 60 minutes: 2.5 mIU/ml and FSH-basal: < 1.0, at 30 minutes: 1.3, and at 60 minutes: 1.4 mIU/ml. Urinary 17-KS: > 20 mg/24 hours; pregnanetriol: 13.3 mg/24 hours. Various semen analysis revealed azoospermia. A bilateral testicular biopsy showed little hormonal stimulation (Fig. 21.2). The seminiferous tubule diameter was between 100 and 150 um (adult range: 170–250; prepubertal: 50–70) with slight thickening and hyalinization of the tubular wall. The Sertoli cells were mature, and spermatogenesis had developed until the meiotic prophase in 90% of the tubules with small numbers of spermatocytes and some spermatids. There were very few differentiated Leydig cells and many precursor cells in

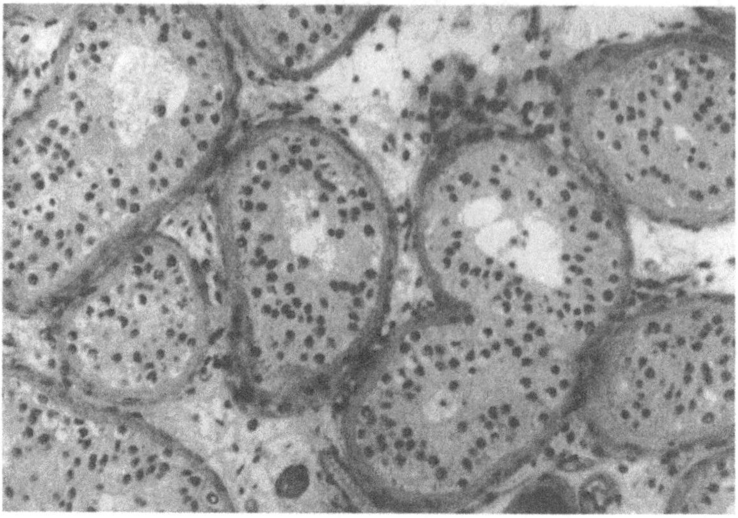

FIGURE 21.2. Testicular biopsy from Case 2.

the interstitium. The conclusion was that the testes showed marked hypospermatogenesis with a poorly stimulated interstitial tissue. Treatment with 30 mg of hydrocortisone (t.i.d.) was started and 3 months later the testes reached a volume of 15 ml and semen analysis showed the presence of sperms for the first time.

Cases 3 and 4 were brothers who came to the hospital in 1961 at ages 8 years, 8 months and 4 years, 10 months, respectively, after the birth of a sister with ambiguous external genitalia due to non–salt-losing or simple virilizing CAH.

Case 3

He was seen at age 8 years, 8 months. He started the development of pubic hair 1 year previously before. He had a height of 148.3 cm, bone age of 12.5 years, pubic hair Tanner 4, a penis 12 cm long, and testicular volume of 10 ml. Urinary 17-KS were 9.4 mg/24 hours. Treatment with 10 mg of prednisone daily was started which was then taken sporadically until age 17 when he decided to stop therapy, when his height was 158 cm and testicular volume 20 ml. He was re-evaluated at age 21 after 4 years off therapy. His testes remained the same size; Plasma testosterone was 1620 ng/dl, and he had low basal levels of gonadotropins with poor response to GnRH: LH (LER 907) basal, 48, at 30 minutes 68, and at 120 minutes: 25 ng/ml and FSH-basal, 42, at 30 minutes 82, and at 120 minutes: 70 ng/ml. Testicular biopsy showed seminiferous tubules of normal diameter with complete spermatogenesis (Fig. 21.3). The interstitial tissue contained mainly precursor Leydig cells and very few mature cells. The patient got married and fathered a normal child.

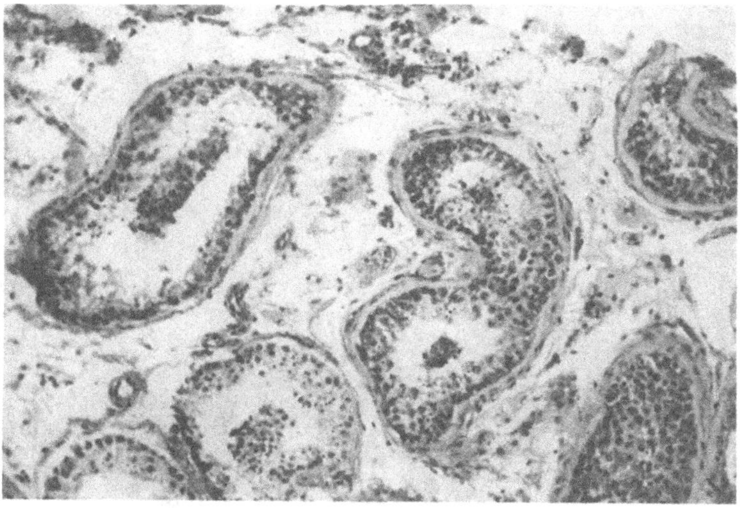

FIGURE 21.3. Testicular biopsy from Case 3.

Case 4

Brother of Case 3, was first seen at age 4 years, 10 months, with a height of 112 cm, bone age of 6 years, genitalia Tanner 1, testicular volume of 2 ml, and 17-KS of 6.9 mg/24 hours. He was followed for 1 year, during which he grew 9.7 cm and bone age advanced 2 years, but there was not any change in the external genitalia, nor any pubic hair. Treatment with 10 mg of prednisone was given. At age 11 years 3 months he had a height of 147.5 cm and a bone age of 12.6, started to develop pubic hair, and had a testicular volume of 6 ml. At 14 years of age he stopped treatment, and at 18 years he was 159 cm tall and had complete sexual development with adult testicular volume. Urinary 17-KS were 10.1 mg/24 hours, preganetriol: 19.9 mg/24 hours, plasma testosterone: 1430 ng/dl; GnRH test showed lack of response of gonadotropins: LH (LER 907) basal, 42, at 20 minutes: 40, at 120 minutes: 48 ng/ml; FSH-basal, 48, at 30 minutes: 55, at 60 minutes, 80, and at 120 minutes: 58 ng/ml. A testicular biopsy revealed normal size seminiferous tubules with full spermatogenesis and almost absence of mature Leydig cells (Fig. 21.4). The patient got married 4 years later, and fathered a child without corticoid treatment.

Case 5

The diagnosis of non–salt-losing CAH was made at the age of 4 years because of premature pubarche, advanced bone age, and elevated urinary 17-KS and pregnanetriol. He started prednisone therapy, which was administered throughout childhood and adolescence and continued during adulthood. He

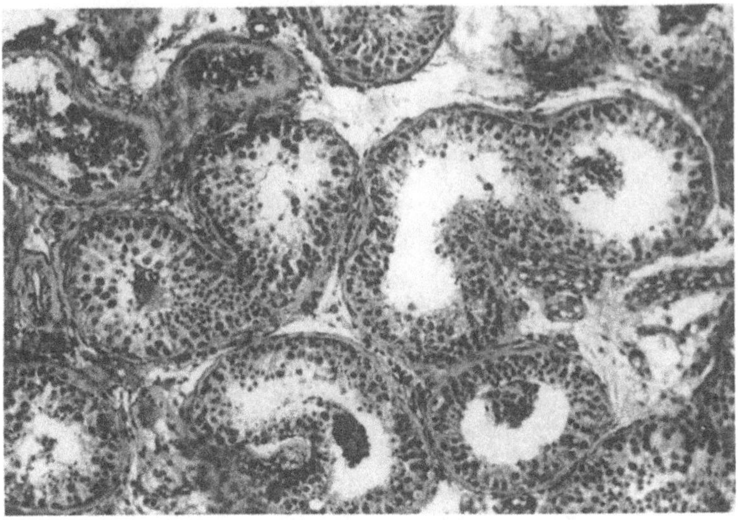

FIGURE 21.4. Testicular biopsy from Case 4.

was studied again at 23 years of age. GnRH test showed normal LH and FSH responses. Sperm count was normal, and a testicular biopsy demonstrated normal seminiferous tubules with full development of spermatogenesis and normal amount of mature Leydig cells.

Discussion

The negative feedback mechanism between sex steroids and gonadotropins is well known and explains the inhibition of LH and FSH by the high levels of circulating adrenal androgens in patients with CAH. These androgens are secreted in high concentrations of androstenedione which is peripherally converted to testosterone (14), and in turn suppresses gonadotropin production. This is the hormonal profile of the adult patient with 21-hydroxylase deficiency never treated with corticoids.

The diagnosis of simple virilizing or late-onset CAH should be made when prepubertal patients develop pubic hair, have acceleration of their growth velocity, and advanced bone age, although their testes remain small. The diagnosis is easily confirmed with the detection of elevated values of plasma 17-hydroxyprogesterone and urinary 17KS and pregnanetriol. This was the case with Patient 1, who after starting treatment with prednisone at age 6 had a marked increase in testicular volume several months later. Full spermatogenesis and normal Leydig cells development were observed in the testicular biopsy, revealing pubertal activation of the pituitary-gonadal function with the clinical, hormonal, and histological picture of central precocious puberty. This situation is now succesfully treated with GnRH analogs. A similar case had been described by Wilkins and Cara in 1954 (2), but at that time there was no treatment available for this precocious sexual development in patients with CAH.

Case 2 started at a similar age with the same clinical picture, but because no diagnosis was made, corticoid therapy was never instituted. Due to his advanced bone age, he stopped growing at age 10 with complete pubertal virilization. At age 23 he was 163 cm tall, was azoospermic, and had a testicular volume of 6 ml. He had high levels of plasma testosterone, androstenedione and 17-hydroxyprogesterone with low values of LH and FSH that did not respond to acute administrationof GnRH. Testicular hystology, however, showed development of spermatogenesis until meiotic prophase. After starting corticoid therapy all hormones became normal, the testes increased their size, and spermatozoa appeared in his semen. The same reversible infertility with corticoid treatment has been reported in other patients whose diagnosis was made late in adolescence or adulthood (4–11). The biopsy findings in this patient showing small seminiferous tubules with normal amounts of spermatogonia and arrest of spermatogenesis can be explained by the hormonal condition of depressed gonadrotropin secretion. It is possible that some of the high circulating testosterone levels enter the testes directly and contribute to the initiation of the first steps of spermatogenesis that cannot develop further in the absence of adequate amounts of LH and especially FSH. It has been experimentally demonstrated that testosterone and its 5 alpha reduced compounds are needed to stimulate spermatogenesis to the end of the meiotic division throughout all reproductive life (15–24). FSH is necessary for spermatogonial renewal and to complete spermiogenesis (17,18,20,23), although it seems not to be needed to maintain spermatogenesis in the adult (24–26). This would explain why untreated CAH patients with pubertal or adult bone age, and spermatogenesis arrested at the meiotic stage, complete it soon after begining corticoid therapy because of reactivation of gonadotropin function.

The evaluation of Cases 3 and 4 is more interesting because they were fertile, even though they had not had corticoid treatment for several years. Similar cases have also been published in the literature (4,5,12). The major difference compared with Case 2 is that these two patients started treatment during childhood and they were adequately treated until late adolescence, thus allowing for a normal testicular development induced during puberty by endogenous gonadotropins. They stopped corticoid therapy after their testes had reached complete development of spermatogenesis.

Experimental studies have demonstrated that hypophysectomy performed in adult rats impairs normal meiotic and spermiogenic development. This can be restored with LH and FSH administration, as well as with testosterone propionate alone in high doses (21–24). These observations indicate that testosterone administration can maintain adult spermatogenesis with supressed levels of LH and FSH.

Tapanainen et al. (25) have published studies performed in 13 families with an inactivating point mutation in the FSH receptor gene. Homozygous females were infertile, whereas males were oligospermic but not necessarily infertile. The five men studied had low testicular volume. Two had fathered two children each. All had elevated serum FSH concentrations, moderately elevated LH, and normal testosterone. Kumar et al. (25) obtained transgenic mice deficient in FSH using embryonic stem cells technology. FSH-deficient females were infertile due to a block in folliculogenesis prior to antral follicular formation, whereas male mice were fertile with normal Sertoli and Leydig cells and spermatogenesis, despite having small testes. These authors concluded that spermatogenesis can start without significant action by FSH. The reduced testicular size, however, indicates that Sertoli cell proliferation is affected and therefore partially dependent on FSH. Chemes et al. (17,20) and Almiron et al. (18) have demonstrated that even though the first spermatogenic wave can start in the absence of FSH, Sertoli and spermatogonial proliferation and spermiogenesis are severely affected. It seems, therefore, that in the absence of FSH, spermatogenesis can start, but its quantitative yield is significantly compromised.

Adult patients with CAH who remain fertile after withdrawal of corticoid treatment have gonadotropins suppressed by high levels of circulating testosterone. They represent the human counterpart of hypophysectomized experimental animals maintained on high testosterone administration. Although we do not know how much intratesticular testosterone is present in these patients, it could be assumed that some testosterone may reach the seminiferous tubules, and, with the low levels of circulating FSH, contribute to maintain spermatogenesis. The two fertile patients described by Urban et al. (5) who had never been treated do not fit this hypothesis, and they are the only cases reported in the literature who have normal testicular size and are fertile. A possible explanation for this could be that they developed a pubertal or postpubertal "late-onset" CAH after complete testicular maturation.

In conclusion, overproduction of adrenal androgens has two effects in men with CAH, depending on the age of the onset of the disease and treatment: (1) LH and FSH inhibition with testicular immaturity and sterility in patients who have been never treated, remaining infertile and (2) maintenance of spermatogenesis and fertility after withdrawal of corticoid therapy in adult patients, despite gonadotropin deficiency. As a result, patients who have received adequate treatment throughout infancy and adolescence may discontinue therapy in adult life without affecting their fertility, although the possible development of adrenal or testicular adenomas (adrenal rest tumors) should be periodically evaluated (13,27,28).

References

1. Wilkins L. The diagnosis and treatment of endocrine disorders in childhood and adolescence. Springfield, Ill Thomas, 1965;401–5.
2. Wilkins L, Cara J. Further studies on the treatment of congenital adrenal hyperplasia with cortisone. V. effects of cortisone-therapy on testicular development. J Clin Endocrinol Metab 1954;14:287–96.
3. Penny R, Olambiwonnu NO, Frasier SD. Precocious puberty following treatment in a six year old male with congenital adrenal hyperplasia: studies of serum luteinizing hormone (LH) and follicle stimulating hormone (FSH) and plasma testosterone. J Clin Endocrinol Metab 1973;36:920–24.
4. Molitor JT, Chertow BS, Fariss BL. Long-term follow up of a patient with congenital adrenal hyperplasia and failure of testicular development. Fertil Steril 1973;24:319–23.
5. Urban MD, Lee PA, Migeon CJ. Adult height and fertility in men with congenital adrenal hyperplasia. N Engl J Med 1978;199:1392–96.
6. Glenthoj A, Damkjaer M, Neilsen M, Starup J. Congenital adrenal hyperplasia due to 11β hydroxylase deficiency: final diagnosis in adult age in three patients. Acta Endocrinol 1980;93:94–99.
7. Wischusen J, Baker HWG, Hudson B. Reversible male infertility due to congenital adrenal hyperplasia. Clin Endocrinol (Oxf) 1981;14:571–77.
8. Mirsky HA, Hines JH. Infertility in a man with 21-hydroxylase deficient congenital adrenal hyperplasia. J Urol 1989;142(1):111–13.
9. Augarten A, Weissenserg R, Pariente C, Sack J. Reversible male infertility in late onset congenital adrenal hyperplasia. J Endocrinol Invest 1991;14:237–40.
10. Iwamoto T, Yajima M, Tanaka H, Minagawa N, Osada R. A case report: reversible male infertility due to congenital adrenal hyperplasia. Nippon-Hinyokika-Gakkai-Zasshi 1993;84:2031–34.
11. Bonacorsi AC, Adler I, Figueiredo JC. Male infertility due to congenital adrenal hyperplasia: testicular biopsy findings, hormonal evaluation and therapeutic results in three patients. Fertil Steril 1987;47:664–70.
12. Prader A, Zachmann M, Illig R. Normal spermatogenesis in adult males with congenital adrenal hyperplasia after discontinuation of therapy. In: Congenital adrenal hyperplasia. Lee PA, Plotnick LP, Kowarski, et al., eds. Baltimore: Baltimore University Park Press, 1977:397–401.
13. Willi V, Atares M, Prader A, Zachmann M. Testicular adrenal-like tissue (TALT) in congenital adrenal hyperplasia detection by ultrasonography. Pediatr Radiol 1991;21(4):284–87.
14. Rivarola MA, Saez JM, Migeon CJ. Studies of androgens in patients with congenital adrenal hyperplasia. J Clin Endocrinol Metab 1967;27:624–30.
15. Chowdhury AK, Steinberger E. Effect of 5 alpha reduced androgens on sex accesory organs, initiation and maintenance of spermatogenesis in the rat. Biol Reprod 1975;12:609–17.
16. Chemes HE, Podestá E, Rivarola MA. Action of testosterone, dihydrotestosterone in 5 alpha androstane, 3 alpha, 17 beta diol on the spermatogenesis of immature rats. Biol Reprod 1976;14:322–38.
17. Chemes HE, Dym M, Raj HGM. The role of gonadotropins and testosterone on initiation of spermatogenesis in the immature rats. Biol Reprod 1979;21:241–69.

18. Almiron I, Domené H, Chemes HE. The hormonal regulation of premeiotic steps of spermatogenesis in the newborn rat. J Androl 1984;5:235–42.
19. Ahmad N, Haltmeyer GC, Eiknes KB. Maintenance of spermatogenesis in rats with intratesticular implants containing testosterone or dihydrotestosterone. Biol Reprod 1973;8:111–19.
20. Chemes HE. Cambios testiculares asociados al comienzo y desarrollo de la pubertad humana. In: Fisiopatología de la Pubertad. Bergadá C, Rivarola M, eds. Buenos Aires: Ergón, 1986;49–67.
21. Clermont Y, Harvery SC. Duration of the cycle of the seminiferous epithelium of normal hypophysectomized and hypophysectomized hormone treated albino rats. Endocrinology 1965;76:80–89.
22. Boccabella AV. Reinitiation and retardation of spermatogenesis with testosterone propionate and other hormones after long term post hypophysectomy regression period. Endocrinology 1963;72:787–98.
23. Steinberger E, Duckett GE. Hormonal control of spermatogenesis. J Reprod Fert 1967;(suppl 2):75–87.
24. Dym M, Raj HGM, Lin YC, Chemes HE, Kotite NJ, Hayfeh SM, et al. Is FSH required for maintenance of spermatogenesis in adult rat? J Reprod Fert 1979;(suppl 26):175–81.
25. Tapanaimen JS, Aittomãki K, Vaskivmo T, Huhtaniemi I. Men homozygous for an inactivating mutation of the follicle-stimulationg hormone (FSH) receptor gene present variable suppression of spermatogenesis and fertility. Nature Genet 1997; 15:205–6.
26. Rajendra Kumar T, Wang Y, Lu N, Matzuk MM. Follicle stimulating hormone is required for ovarian follicle maturation but not male fertility. Nature Genet 1997;15:201–4.
27. Radfar N, Bartter FC, Easley R, et al. Evidence for androgens LH suppression in a man with bilateral testicular tumors and congenital adrenal hyperplasia. J Clin Endocrin Metab 1977;45:1194–204.
28. Cutfield RG, Bateman JM, Odell WE. Infertility caused by bilateral testicular masses secondary to congenital adrenal hyperplasia. Fertil Steril 1983;40:809–14.

Part VI

Treatment of Congenital Hypothyroidism: Efficacy, Innovation and Quality of Life

22

Growth and Development of Hypothyroid Infants

Delbert A. Fisher

Introduction

Congenital hypothyroidism (CH) is classified as permanent and transient, and as sporadic and endemic (Table 22.1). The most common cause worldwide is iodine deficiency. It is estimated that there are 5.7 million cases of endemic cretinism worldwide (1,2). The prevalence of sporadic CH approximates 1 in 4,000 newborn infants in developed countries conducting newborn screening (3–5), and assuming a worldwide population of 6 billion persons, there are about 1.5 million sporadic hypothyroid individuals worldwide and probably 150,000–200,000 CH infants born yearly. The most common cause of sporadic CH is thyroid dysgenesis, accounting for 85–90% of cases; thyroid dyshormonogenesis accounts for about 10%, and other disorders for a variable 1–5% (4–6). Thyroid hormone resistance syndromes are uncommon; In 1993, Refetoff and colleagues reported 296 patients from 98 families (7).

Screening for CH was introduced in the early 1970s (4–6). Prior to that time, the diagnosis usually was delayed, often many months, and clinical manifestations of thyroid hormone deficiency in affected infants increased progressively in the absence of treatment (Table 22.2) (5–20). The most profound effects were growth failure and dwarfism, mental retardation, and neurological dysfunction. With the advent of newborn screening, early diagnosis, and early treatment with thyroxine, these effects have largely been ameliorated. This chapter will review information about treatment efficacy to date.

Growth Effects

Studies in the rat model have characterized a profound effect of thyroid hormones on growth hormone (GH) secretion and action (12,21). Hypothyroidism decreases pituitary GH content, impairs the pituitary GH response to

TABLE 22.1. Causes of congenital hypothyroidism.

A. Permanent hypothyroidism
Thyroid dysgenesis
Ectopia
Hypoplasia
Aplasia
Thyroid dyshormonogenesis
TSH deficiency
TSH receptor mutation
Iodide symporter defect
Organification defect
Thyroglobulin abnormality
Iodotyrosine deiodinase defect
Thyroid hormone resistance
B. Transient hypothyroidism
Maternal TSH receptor blocking antibody
Drug induced
Hypothyroidism with prematurity
Iodine deficiency
C. Endemic cretinism
Iodine deficiency
Iodine deficiency plus (endemic) goitrogen(s)

GHRH, reduces basal and pulsatile GH secretion, and decreases circulating GH levels (12). Similar effects have been observed in hypothyroid human subjects. Hypothyroid patients show limited GH responses to insulin hypoglycemia, arginine, and GHRH, reduced nocturnal GH secretion, and reduced circulating levels of IGF-I, IGF-II, IGF-binding protein-3, GH binding protein, and bioactive IGF (22,23). Table 22.3 shows the effect of thyroid hormone treatment on nocturnal GH secretion and IGF-I concentrations in hypothyroid children (24). There is also evidence that thyroid hormones stimulate production of other growth factors, including epidermal growth factor, nerve growth factor, and erythropoietin, and have direct actions on bone, potentiating the cartilage response to IGF-I, and stimulating osteoblastic bone resorption and remodeling (14,22,25,26).

These hormonal and growth factor deficiencies contribute importantly to the disordered growth of hypothyroid infants and children, including the decreased long-bone growth, delayed bone maturation, decreased carcass growth, delayed tooth eruption, and anemia. The actions of thyroid hormones and GH are synergistic. Growth hormone administered to neonatal hypophysectomized rats increases body weight, but it has a limited effect on skeletal growth; in contrast, thyroxine accelerates skeletal growth and potentiates the GH effects. Combined treatment optimizes growth and development (27). The vast majority of infants with CH are born with normal or increased length and weight, and early adequate thyroid hormone treatment prevents development of growth retardation. There may be a transient period of growth deceleration during the early weeks of treatment (28), but even in infants with

TABLE 22.2. Manifestation of congenital hypothyroidism in infancy and early childhood.

A. Metabolic effects
Lethargy
Constipation
Feeding problems
Myxedema (with respiratory distress)
Prolonged hyperbilirubinemia
Hypothermia
Bradycardia
Decreased sweating
Carotinemia
Anemia
Decreased metabolic rate
Dry, thickened skin
Muscular dystrophy (hypertrophy, weakness)
B. Growth/skeletal effects
Decreased long bone growth
Delayed bone maturation
Epiphyseal dysgenesis
Increased head circumference
Increased bone density
Delayed tooth eruption
C. Hormone dysfunction
Decreased growth hormone secretion
Decreased somatomedin production
Other growth factor deficiencies (EGF, NGF, erythropoietin, etc.)
Hyperprolactinemia
Increased LH/FSH secretion
Precocious puberty
Insensitive TSH negative feedback control system
D. Central nervous system maturation
Decreased IQ
Deafness
Neurological dysfunction (spasticity, incoordination, hyperreflexia, tremor)
Strabismus, nystagmus
Attention Deficit Disorder

severe CH, manifested by very low serum T4 concentrations and delayed bone maturation at birth, early, adequate treatment results in mean height and body mass index equal to or greater than values in normal children (29–32). Bone age values also are normalized by 2–3 years (33). Bone mineral density and metabolism also are normal in treated children given adequate nutrition (34).

The effects of thyroid hormones on growth and physical development extend through most of the second decade, and delayed or inadequate replacement therapy during childhood or adolescence can reduce adult height (35,36). Thyroxine treatment in children with growth retardation due to a prolonged period of untreated hypothyroidism induces usually

TABLE 22.3. Effects of thyroxine treatment on GH secretion and IGF levels in hypothyroid children.*

	Hypothyroid	Thyroxine treated
Noctural GH secretion (μg/L)	1.48 (± 0.38)	3.54 (± 0.71)
Plasma IGF-I levels (U/ml)	0.46 (± 0.20)	1.5 (± 0.34)

*Data from Chernausek and Turner (24).

marked catchup growth, but in some instances this is inadequate to normalize adult height (3,36). Adult height is generally inversely correlated with the duration of untreated hypothyroidism prior to the advent of puberty (36). This is thought to be due to the onset of puberty, limiting the chance to achieve full growth catchup before epiphyseal fusion. Suppression of pubertal development by administration of gonadotropin releasing hormone plus GH was shown to improve height gain in a juvenile hypothyroid patient (36).

Metabolic Effects

Thyroid hormones are required for normal homeothermy in mammalian species including humans and for maintaining body temperature via two major mechanisms: effects on brown adipose tissue (BAT) thermogenesis and effects on basal metabolism mediated via mitochondrial energy production (37). Thyroid hormones increase mitochondrial size, number, and surface area in association with increased substrate utilization and oxygen consumption (37). BAT thermogenesis is directly stimulated by norepinephrine, and expression of the key molecule in the BAT thermogenic response, the uncoupling protein (or thermogenin), is dependent on triiodothyronine produced locally via thyroxine monodeiodination (10). Both systems are active in the newborn with CH, and hypothermia in these infants, if observed, is minimal in degree. Hypothermia accrues progressively in the absence of treatment. Other metabolic effects of thyroid hormone deficiency (Table 22.2) in the newborn period, like the defects in thermogenesis, usually are mild or absent and rapidly corrected by thyroxine replacement therapy. The tendency to minimal clinical signs and symptoms of hypothyroidism in the athyroid newborn is due, in part, to the limited, but significant, placental transfer of maternal thyroxine to the fetus; serum total T4 concentrations in the cord blood of athyroid infants approximate 30% of normal newborn levels (38). In addition, thyroid hormone effects on various metabolic systems become manifest during critical ontogenic windows of development during the third trimester and neonatal period (25). In any event, early treatment is essential to prevent or correct the progressive manifestations of the hypothyroid state.

Hormone Dysfunction

A variety of functional changes in hormone metabolism are observed in hypothyroid patients. These include decreased growth hormone and somatomedin production as already discussed. Hyperprolactinemia, with or without galactorrhea, may occur, usually in prolonged, severe hypothyroidism associated with sellar enlargement and thyrotroph hyperplasia (22). On rare occasions, severe juvenile hypothyroidism with marked TSH hypersecretion and hyperprolactinemia may be associated with precocious puberty (13). The mechanism remains unclear, but it has been postulated that the high levels of TSH, perhaps with alterations of glycosylation, may cross-stimulate gonadal gonadotropin receptors (39). On the other hand, marked TRH hypersecretion may evoke second messenger paracrine stimulation of pituitary gonadotrophic cells, since serum gonadotrophic hormone levels may be elevated in association with the precocious puberty (13).

In adults, hypothyroidism reduces the hepatic clearance of cortisol which, in the presence of a normal level of cortisol binding globulin, results in mild hypercortisolemia; however, diurnal rhythmicity and endogenous cortisol production rate are normal (40). The mild hypercortisolemia with a normal cortisol production rate suggests a decreased negative feedback effect of cortisol on corticotropin-releasing hormone-ACTH secretion (40). Cortisol metabolism is normalized within weeks or months by thyroxine therapy. Feedback regulation of ACTH secretion in infants with CH has not been studied.

Elevated TSH levels at birth are the hallmark of primary CH, which indicates an operative negative feedback control system for TSH secretion. In many infants, however, although the system is operative, the setpoint for feedback regulation of TSH is altered. The first report was by Sato and colleagues in 1976, and this has been followed by several subsequent studies that indicates that serum TSH concentrations tend to be elevated in infants and children with treated CH despite serum total thyroxine (T4) concentrations in the normal range (41–45). Figure 22.1 shows serum TSH plotted versus total T4 concentrations measured during the first 4 years of thyroxine treatment of 979 CH children in England studied by Grant et al. (45). These data were plotted relative to the TSH-T4 line plot for normal children in California and show a significant displacement to the right (e.g., decreased T4 sensitivity of the negative feedback control mechanism in the CH infants and children). In their study, Grant and co-workers observed that 1280 (43%) of 2960 TSH results measured in their 979 children were greater than 7mU/L; levels were relatively higher during the first year (45). The patients were divided into severe and less severe cases on the basis of pretreatment plasma T4 concentrations (<30 nmol/L vs. >30 nmol/L, respectively), and there was a tendency for the proportion of TSH concentrations above 7 mU/L to be greater in the children with severe hypothyroidism (45).

The significance of the elevated serum TSH levels in treated CH infants remains controversial because it is difficult to distinguish an elevation in

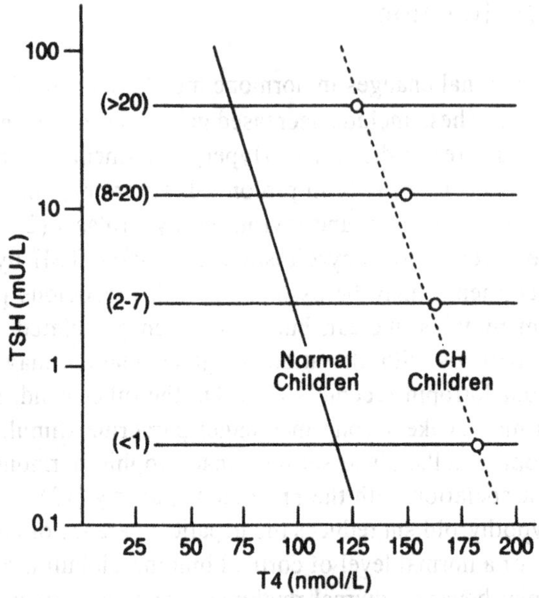

FIGURE 22.1. Serum TSH concentrations plotted versus serum total T4 levels in children with a normal hypothalamic-pituitary thyroid axis and acquired hypothyroidism or hyperthyroidism versus serum TSH and total T4 values in children with CH treated with Na-l-thyroxine. The plot in the CH infants is displaced to the right, which suggests decreased sensitivity of the hypothalamic-pituitary T4 negative feedback TSH regulatory system. The CH data were derived from Grant and co-workers (45). The data for non-CH (normal axis) children were developed by The Nichols Institute Clinical Correlations Department, San Juan Capistrano, California.

serum TSH in the individual patient due to altered feedback control from elevation associated with inadequate therapy. Grant and colleagues reflect this dilemma in their discussion (45). It is clear that all infants with CH do not have an altered TSH control system, and to identify those infants who do it is necessary to plot their T4 (and preferably free T4) versus TSH relative to a normal population. The normal range (for that child) of serum TSH relative to the normal or desirable T4 or free T4 level can then be determined and considered in therapy management. The additional problem is that the feedback axis matures so that TSH levels for a given serum T4 decrease with age. McCrossin and co-workers, however, have demonstrated persistence of the altered feedback control set-point through the second decade (42).

Nervous System Maturation

Thyroid hormones are essential for normal development of the nervous system, including the brain and peripheral nervous system. Hypothyroidism during the critical period of CNS maturation is associated with a variety of developmental abnormalities (18–20). These include disrupted and delayed patterns of cell migration, reductions in cell densities, decreased axonal/dentritic arborizations and synaptic densities, delayed myelinogenesis and impaired neurotransmitter development (18–20). Resulting neurologic dysfunction includes delayed motor development, behavioral disturbances, speech disorders, deafness, hypotonia or spasticity, tremors and convulsions, and variable mental deficiency (18–20). The critical (thyroid dependent) period of brain maturation in the human extends from fetal life to age 2–3 years (46).

Prior to the advent of newborn thyroid screening the average IQ in CH infants due to delayed treatment approximated 75, and the rate of IQ loss in the early months of life approximated five points per month (6). Intrauterine hypothyroidism in infants with CH (manifested as delayed bone maturation at birth), if inadequately treated in the neonatal period, can add an additional 5–10 points of IQ deficit (47). The mothers of these infants, however, have normal thyroid function in the vast majority of cases; the full extent of thyroid hormone deficiency on brain maturation and final IQ in circumstances of combined maternal and fetal thyroid hormone deficiency remains to be quantified. The most important interval in therapy for infants with sporadic CH is the first year of life. This is the period of most rapid brain growth and maturation. The second and third years are important, but not as critical, and the impact of hypothyroidism or brain maturation after 3 years is minimal (46).

There are numerous reports of intellectual and behavioral outcomes of infants with CH detected early (by neonatal screening) and treated with exogenous Na-l-thyroxine. Seven reports were evaluated by Derkson-Lubsen and Verkerk; these included 675 CH patients and 570 controls (48). Meta-analysis showed a lower IQ and poorer motor skills in the CH children, with a mean IQ deficit of 6.3 points (95% confidence interval 4.7–7.8 points). Table 22.4 summarizes factors that have been considered to impact IQ in treated infants. The most important risk factor for IQ outcome in the meta-analysis was severity of CH, defined as serum T4 level and skeletal maturation at the time of diagnosis; behavioral differences were not detected, but they have been reported in other studies (17,20,21).

All of the factors in Table 22.4 are involved in CH infants. The impact of social class and parental IQ are not unique to hypothyroid infants, and they account for much of the spectrum of IQ in the normal population. Thyroid agenesis, low initial T4 value, and neonatal bone age focus on the issue and significance of intrauterine hypothyroidism. Thyroid dependency of brain maturation extends to fetal life, but as already mentioned the exact timing and total significance, relative to the first 2–3 years of extrauterine life are not clear. Dubuis and co-workers have shown that treatment of infants with severe CH using a median initial dose of 12.1 μg/kg/day of Na-l-thyroxine improves IQ relative to a mean treatment dose of 6 μg/kg/day; the mean IQ values in infants with moderate and severe CH for treatment doses of 12.1

TABLE 22.4. Factors impacting IQ in infants treated for congenital hypothyroidism.*

• Initial serum T4 concentration
• Skeletal maturation at birth
• Thyroid agenesis (vs. dyshormonogenesis, hypoplasia/ ectopia)
• Age at onset of treatment
• Thyroxine dose
• Mean serum T4 during treatment
• Social class
• Parental IQ

*Data from Derksen-Lubsen and Verkerk (48).

versus 6.0 μg/kg/day Na-l-thyroxine were 110 and 107 in the moderate group versus 98 and 111 for the infants with more severe disease (49).

Thus, the higher treatment dose reduced the impact of severe hypothyroidism from 13 IQ points to three points. This would suggest that the impact of intrauterine hypothyroidism in infants with CH approximates 10 points of IQ and that this can be retrieved in such infants with early intensive therapy. The goal of therapy is to maintain the serum T4 level (and free T4 level) in the upper half of the normal range (10–16 μg/dL; 128–206 nmol/L during the first year). Heyerdahl and co-workers have shown that infants with CH and mean serum T4 levels approximating 10 μg/dL during the 6 month to 24 month age interval have lower mean IQ than CH infants with mean serum T4 approximating 13 μg/dL (verbal IQ < 80 vs. IQ > 94) (50). The neurological and behavioral sequellae in CH infants are more difficult to assess and tend to correlate with the degree of initial hypothyroidism and with attained IQ (17). These features will be reviewed in more detail in Chapter 23.

Hypothalamic-Pituitary Hypothyroidism

Hypothalamic-pituitary hypothyroidism (HPH) includes hypothalamic thyrotropin releasing hormone (TRH) deficiency and pituitary thyroid stimulating hormone (TSH) deficiency. Severe TSH deficiency with early onset hypothyroidism occurs with a prevalence approximately 1 in 30,000 births (51). Less severe disease, usually associated with TRH deficiency, seems to be nearly as common as isolated GH deficiency, occurring 1 in 5000–10,000 newborns (52). In the less severe patients, mild reductions in T4 and free T4 serum concentrations are associated with normal range TSH levels and diagnosis is often difficult. The only clinical manifestation may be retarded growth. The most reliable diagnostic test is the absence of the nocturnal TSH surge that occurs between 10 P.M. and midnite (52). Using this test, children with apparent idiopathic short stature with free T4 values in the lowest third of the normal range have a 32% incidence of HPH and manifest significant improvement in growth velocity with thyroxine treatment (52). Infants with severe HGH and neonatal hypothyroidism may develop brain damage without treatment; the children with milder HGH usually do not (52).

Thyroid Hormone Resistance

Resistance to thyroid hormone (RTH) is a genetic disorder due to mutations in the beta form of the nuclear thyroid hormone receptor gene (8,16,53). The clinical manifestations are variable and have been reviewed in detail by Refetoff and colleagues and by Usala (8,53). Variable tissue resistance is reflected in differing phenotypes, including generalized resistance and more selective pituitary resistance. Both groups of patients manifest elevated serum free thyroid hormone concentrations in association with inappropriately normal serum TSH levels (8). In most cases, the elevated serum thyroid hormone levels fully compensate the RTH and the patients appear euthyroid with normal growth and mental development. In some patients, compensation may be incomplete and variable among different tissues in a particular patient and given tissues in different patients (8,53). High levels of thyroid hormones can more rarely produce toxic effects in some or most tissues and a clinical state resembling hyperthyroidism. Symptoms attributed to hypothyroidism include congenital deafness, congenital nystagmus, infantile hypotonia, delayed bone maturation, growth retardation, learning disabilities, delayed speech, and mental retardation; manifestations suggesting hyperthyroidism include failure to thrive, diarrhea, agitation, hyperactivity, nervousness and tremulousness, goiter, and tachycardia (8).

Treatment has included high levels of replacement with thyroxine or triiodothyonine (T3) in patients with predominance of hypothyroid features and administration of antithyroid drugs, T3, thyroid hormone analogs, dopamine agonists or antagonists, somatostatin, glucocorticoids, iodide, or thyroidectomy in patients with prominent hyperthyroid signs and symptoms. Management of these patients can clearly be difficult and outcome will reflect early diagnosis, careful assessment and prolonged, detailed follow-up, and reevaluation. In patients with generalized RTH, treatment aimed at reduction of thyroid hormone levels should be avoided. Routine thyroid hormone treatment is controversial, but treatment of infants with growth retardation and delayed bone maturation using pharmacological doses of thyroxine may be beneficial, and improved behavior of children with attention deficit hyperactivity disorder (ADHD) has been reported with such treatment (8). Patients with predominant pituitary resistance and prominent hyperthyroid manifestations usually require treatment, so none of the approaches mentioned earlier is ideal.

Transient Hypothyroidism

The causes of transient hypothyroidism in term or preterm infants are summarized in Table 22.5 (4,54,55). Transient primary hypothyroidism is characterized by elevated serum levels of TSH and low values of total and free T4 persisting for several weeks. Goiter and clinical manifestations of hypothyroidism are observed only occasionally. Thyroid function returns to normal either spontaneously or after a short period of therapy with iodide or thyroxine (4). In term infants, in the absence of iodine deficiency, the growth, developmental and neurological effects of short term or treated transient hypothyroidism are minimal. The most common cause of transient hypothyroidism in term infants, worldwide, is iodine deficiency in geographic areas of low iodine intake/availability (4). When the iodine deficiency is severe, the neonatal hypothyroid state may be severe and prolonged and result in loss of intellectual capacity (4). The particular sensitivity of the newborn to transient hypothyroidism is due to the low thyroid iodine content and rapid turnover of thyroidal thyroglobulin and organic iodine stores and immaturity of the autoregulatory mechanisms (4).

Hypothyroidism in premature infants is of particular concern. For premature infants the stresses of extrauterine transition are superimposed on an immature thyroid axis (56). Hypothalamic TRH production/secretion is relatively reduced, the thyroid gland response to TSH is not yet mature, the capacity of the thyroid follicular cell to iodinate the tyrosyl residues of thyroglobulin (organify iodine) remains inefficient, and the capacity to convert thyroxine (T4) to active triiodothyronine (T3) is low. Thyroxine-binding globulin levels also are low and the premature infant in the extrauterine environment is relatively hypothyroxinemic with low levels of serum TSH and T3 (56). This has been referred to as the *hypothyroxinemia of prematurity* (56). Serum free T4 levels also are low and thyroglobulin values increased, reflecting the low iodine and iodothyronine stores and rapid iodothyronine turn-

Table 22.5. Causes of transient hypothyroidism.

- A. Term infants
  - Iodine deficiency
  - Drug exposure
    - Antithyroid drugs
    - Iodine overload
    - Radiographic contrast agents (iodinated)
    - Amiodarone
    - TSH Receptor antibodies
- B. Preterm infants
  - Primary hypothyroidism
    - Iodine deficiency
    - Iodine excess
  - Secondary/tertiary hypothyroidism

over. The increased thyroid hormone requirement associated with extrauterine exposure stresses an already compromised system (56). Thus, the premature infant is particularly susceptible to development of transient primary hypothyroidism. This tendency is augmented by a relatively low iodine intake or exposure to excess iodine.

Transient primary hypothyroidism in premature infants increases in prevalence with decreasing gestation age (GA), from 0.12% in low birthweight (LBW; 1501–2499 gm) to 0.41% in very low birthweight (VLBW; < 1500 gm) infants (57). These prevalence rates are derived from New England, which is an area of iodine sufficiency. The prevalence in iodine deficient areas can be much higher. VLBW infants also tend to develop low serum levels of free T4 in the absence of hyperthyrotropinemia, and this presumably reflects transient secondary/tertiary hypothyroidism due to hypothalamic-pituitary axis immaturity. Approximately 5–10% of premature infants of less than 29 weeks gestation age manifest free T4 concentrations (by immunoassay) less than 5 pmol/L in association with normal range TSH concentrations (56,58).

The significance/impact of transient hypothyroidism in the premature infant remains unclear. Treatment of transient primary hypothyroidism persisting beyond 2 weeks is recommended, but there are no long-term followup studies of such infants. A prospective study of Van Wasseaer and colleagues was conducted to assess the effect of thyroxine treatment on the physiological hypothyroxinemia of prematurity (56,59). One group of premature infants was treated with thyroxine and a control group with placebo. Results showed that thyroxine treatment of infants of more than 27 weeks gestation age has no beneficial effect on mental development assessed at 24 months (59). However, a subgroup of 13 treated infants of 25–26 weeks gestational age, and at risk for transient secondary/tertiary hypothyroidism, showed a 24 month IQ score 18 points higher than that of 18 control infants (59). This suggests a possible beneficial effect of thyroxine treatment of small premature infants, but further studies are necessary to determine whether and which infants require treatment.

References

1. Delange FM. Endemic cretinism. In: Braverman LE, Utiger RD, eds. The thyroid, seventh ed. Philadelphia: Lippincott-Raven, 1995:756–67.
2. Hetzel BS, Pandov CS. S.O.S. for a billion: the conquest of iodine deficiency disorders. New York: Oxford University Press, 1994.
3. Toublanc JE. Comparison of epidemiological data on congenital hypothyroidism in Europe with two other parts of the world. Horm Res 1992;38:230–35.
4. Delange F. Neonatal screening for congenital hypothyroidism: results and perspectives. Horm Res 1997;48:51–61.
5. Fisher DA. Management of congenital hypothyroidism. J Clin Endocrinol Metab 1991;72:523–29.
6. Delange F, Fisher DA, The thyroid gland, In: Brook CD, ed. Clinical pediatric endocrinology, third ed. Oxford: Blackwell Science, 1995:397–433.

7. Fisher DA. The hypothyroxinemia of prematurity. J Clin Endocrinol Metab 1997;82:1701–3.
8. Refetoff S, Weiss RE, Usala SJ. The syndrome of resistance to thyroid hormones. Endocr Rev 1993;14:348–99.
9. Fisher DA, Pickering DE. Infantile hypothyroidism: diagnosis and treatment. Pediatr Clin N Am 1957;November: 863–72.
10. Bianco AC, Silva JE. Intracellular conversion of thyroxine to triiodothyronine is required for the optimal thermogenic function of brown adipose tissue. J Clin Invest 1987;79:295–300.
11. Najjar SS. Muscular hypertrophy in hypothyroid children; the Kocher-Debre-Semelaigne syndrome. J Pediatr 1974;85:236–39.
12. Giustina A, Wehrenberg WB. Influence of thyroid hormones on the regulation of growth hormone secretion. Eur J Endocrinol 1995;133:646–53.
13. Winters SJ, Berga SL. Gonadal dysfunction in patients with thyroid disorders. Endocrinologist 1997;7:167–73.
14. Huang SM, Chan SH, Wu TJ, Chow NH. Effect of thyroid hormone on urinary excretion of epidermal growth factor. Eur Surg Res 1997;29:222–28.
15. Fisher DA. Thyroid hormone effects on growth and development, In: Delange F, Fisher DA, Malvaux P, ed. Pediatric thyroidology. Switzerland: Karger 1985: 75–89.
16. Kopp P, Kitajima K, Jameson JL. Syndrome of resistance to thyroid hormone: insights into thyroid hormone action. Proc Soc Exp Biol Med 1996;211:49–61.
17. Kooistra L, Van der Meere JJ, Vulsma T, Kalverboer AF. Sustained attention problems in children with early treated congenital hypothyroidism. Acta Paediatr 1996;85:425–29.
18. Bernal J, Nunez J. Thyroid hormones and brain development. Eur J Endocrinol 1995;133:390–98.
19. Timiras PS, Nzekwe EU. Thyroid hormones and nervous system development. Biol Neonate 1989;55:376–85.
20. Porterfield SP, Hendrich CE. The role of thyroid hormones in prenatal and neonatal neurological development, current perspectives. Endocr Rev 1993;14:94–106.
21. Weiss RE, Refetoff S. Effect of thyroid hormone on growth: lessons from the syndrome of resistance to thyroid hormone. Endocr Metab Clin N Am 1996;25: 719–29.
22. Snyder PJ. The pituitary in hypothyroidism. In: Braverman LE, Utiger RD, eds. The thyroid. Philadelphia: Lippincott-Raven, 1995:836–40.
23. Meill J, Taylor A, Zini M, Maheshwari HG, Ross RJM, Valcavi R. Effects of hypothyroidism and hyperthyroidism on insulin-like growth factors (IGFs) and growth hormone and IGF binding proteins. J Clin Endocrinol Metab 1993;76:950–55.
24. Chernausek SD, Turner R. Attenuation of spontaneous nocturnal growth hormone secretion in children with hypothyroidism and its correlation with plasma insulin-like growth factor-I concentrations. J Pediatr 1989;114:968–72.
25. Fisher DA. Thyroid hormone effects on growth and development. In: Grave GD, Cassorla FG, eds. Disorders of human growth. Springfield: Charles Thomas, 1988:266–80.
26. Britto J, Fenton A, Holloway W, Nicholson GC. Osteoblasts mediate thyroid hormone stimulation of osteoclastic bone resorption. Endocrinology 1994;134: 169–76.

27. Glasscock GF, Nicoll CS. Hormonal control of growth in the neonatal rat. Endocrinology 1981;109:176–84.
28. Leger J, Czernichow P. Congenital hypothyroidism: decreased growth velocity in the first weeks of life. Biol Neonate 1989;55:218–23.
29. Bucher H, Prader A, Illig R. Head circumference, height, bone age, and weight in 103 children with congenital hypothyrodism before and during thyroid hormone replacement. Helv Paediatr Acta 1985;40:305–16.
30. Aronson R, Erhlich RM, Bailey JD, Rovet JF. Growth in children with congenital hypothyroidism detected by neonatal screening. J Pediatr 1990;116:33–37.
31. Grant DB. Growth in early treated congenital hypothyroidism. Arch Dis Child 1994;70:464–68.
32. Chiesa A, de Papendieck LG, Keselman A, Heinrich JJ, Bergada C. Growth followup in 100 children with congenital hypothyroidism before and during treatment. J Pediatr Endocrinol 1994;7:211–17.
33. Heyerdahl S, Kase BF, Stake G. Skeletal maturation during thyroxine treatment in children with congenital hypothyroidism. Acta Paediatr 1994;83:618–22.
34. Leger J, Ruiz JC, Guibourdenche J, Kindermans C, Garabedian M, Czernichow P. Bone mineral density and metabolism in children with congenital hypothyroidism after prolonged L-thyroxine therapy. Acta Paediatr, 1997;86:704–10.
35. Rivkees SA, Bode HH, Crawford JD. Long term growth in juvenile acquired hypothyroidism: the failure to achieve normal adult stature. N Engl J Med 1988;318:599–602.
36. Boersma B, Otten BJ, Stoelinga GBA, Wit JM. Catchup growth after prolonged hypothyroidism. Eur J Pediatr 1996;155:362–67.
37. Loeb JN. Metabolic changes in thyrotoxicosis. In: Braverman LE, Utiger RD, eds. The thyroid. Philadelphia: Lippincott-Raven, 1995:687–93.
38. Vulsma T, Gons MH, deVijlder JJM. Maternal transfer of thyroxine in congenital hypothyroidism due to a total organification defect or thyroid agenesis. N Engl J Med 1989;321:1–6.
39. Grossman M, Weintraub BD, Szkudlinski MW. Novel insights into the molecular mechanisms of human thyrotropin action: structural, physiological, and therapeutic implications for the glycoprotein hormone family. Endocr Rev 1997;18: 476–501.
40. Iranmanesh A, Lizarralde G, Johnson L, Veldhuis JD. Dynamics of 24 hour endogenous cortisol secretion and clearance in primary hypothyroidism assessed before and after partial thyroid hormone replacement. J Clin Endocrinol Metab, 1990;70:155–61.
41. Sato T, Suzuki Y, Taketani T, Ishiguro K, Nakajima H. Age related change in pituitary threshold for TSH release during thyroxine replacement for cretinism. J Clin Endocrinol Metab 1977;44:553–59.
42. McCrossin RB, Sheffield LJ, Robertson EF. Persisting abnormality in the pituitary-thyroid axis in congenital hypothyroidism. In: Nogataki S, Stockijt JHR, eds. Thyroid research VIII. Canberrt: Australian Academy of Science, Canberra 1980:37–40.
43. Shultz RM, Glassman MS, MacGillivray MH. Elevated threshold for thyrotropin suppression in congenital hypothyroidism. Am J Dis Child 1980;134:19–24.
44. Walker P, Dussault JH. Long term effects of neonatal thyroid dysfunction in the rat: implication for neonatal screening. In: Dussault JH, Walker P, eds. Congenital hypothyroidism. New York: Marcel Dekker, 1983:397–410.

45. Grant DB, Fuggle DW, Smith I. Increased plasma thyroid stimulating hormone in treated congenital hypothyroidism: relation to severity of hypothyroidism, plasma thyroid hormone status and daily dose of thyroxine. Arch Dis Child 1993;69: 555–58.
46. Dobbing J, Sands J. Quantitative growth and development of human brain. Arch Dis Child 1973;48:757–67.
47. Dubuis JM, Glorieux J, Richer D, Deal CL, Dussault JH, VanVliet G. Outcome of severe congenital hypothyroidism: closing the developmental gap with early high levothyroxine treatment. J Clin Endocrinol Metab 1996;81:222–27.
48. Derksen-Lubsen G, Verkerk PH. Neuropsychological development in early treated congenital hypothyroidism: analysis of literature data. Pediatr Res 1996;39: 561–66.
49. Dubuis JM, Glorieux J, Richer F, Deal CL, Dussault JH, VanVliet G. Outcome of severe congenital hypothyroidism: closing the developmental gap with early high dose levothyroxine treatment. J Clin Endocrinol Metab 1996;81:222–27.
50. Heyerdahl S, Kase BF, Lie SO. Intellectual development in children with congenital hypothyroidism in relation to recommended thyroxine treatment. J Pediatr 1991;118:850–57.
51. Hanna CE, Krainz PL, Skeets MR, Miyahara RS, Sesser DE, LaFranchi SH. Detection of congenital hypopituitary hypothyroidism: ten years experience in the Northwest Regional Screening Program. J Pediatr 1986;109:959–64.
52. Pitukcheewanont P, Rose SR. Nocturnal TSH surge: a sensitive diagnostic test for central hypothyroidism in children. Endocrinologist 1997;7:226–32.
53. Usala SJ. Thyroid hormone resistance. In: Weintraub BD, ed. Molecular endocrinology. New York: Raven Press, 1995:393–409.
54. De Catte L, De Wolf D, Smitz J, Bougatif A, De Schepper J, Foulon W. Fetal hypothyroidism as a complication of amiodarone treatment for persistent fetal supraventricular tachycardia. Prenatal Diagnosis 1994;14:762–65.
55. Daniels GH. Thyroid disease and pregnancy: a clinical overview. Endocr Prac 1995;1:287–301.
56. Fisher DA. The hypothyroxinemia of prematurity. J Clin Endocrinol Metab 1997;82:1701–3.
57. Frank JE, Faix JE, Hermos RJ, Mullaney DM, Rojan DA, Mitchell ML, et al. Thyroid function in very low birthweight infants: effects of neonatal hypothyroid screening. J Pediatr 1996;128:548–54.
58. Rooman RP, DuCaju MVL, Op De Beeck L, Docx M, Van Reempts P, Van Acker RT. Low thyroxinemia occurs in the majority of very preterm newborns. Eur J Pediatr 1996;155:211–15.
59. Van Wassenaer AG, Kok JH, De Vijlder JJM, Briet JM, Smit BJ, Tamminga P, et al. Effects of thyroxine supplementation on neurologic development in infants born at less than 30 weeks gestation. N Engl J Med 1997;336:21–26.

23

Neurobehavioral Consequences of Congenital Hypothyroidism Identified by Newborn Screening

JOANNE F. ROVET

Thyroid hormone is an essential hormone for growth, metabolism, and brain development. Children who lack thyroid hormone in utero or early life have poorer physical and neurological development. Some of the more common conditions leading to low pre- and postnatal thyroid hormone levels are congenital hypothyroidism, maternal thyroid disease during pregnancy, prematurity, and intrauterine exposure to substances such as maternal thyroid autoantibodies and environmental toxins (e.g., PCBs) (1). These groups are at varying risk of inadequate growth and neurodevelopment (2–4).

In congenital hypothyroidism (CH), thyroid hormone is lacking during the perinatal period and early infancy, as well as in late gestation in some cases. CH affects 1 in 3000–4000 newborns in North America, with a marked female preponderance. It is caused by a defect in the thyroid gland, which can be missing (athyrosis), ectopic, or dysfunctional, or, less commonly, a defect in the hypothalamus or pituitary that regulate the thyroid. Because of its characteristically late presentation of outward signs and symptoms, the diagnosis of CH was typically delayed until quite late in infancy, past the time to prevent extensive and permanent brain damage. As a result, CH (also known as cretinism) was a leading cause of children's mental retardation (5).

The developed world, however, has witnessed a remarkable advance in the care and outcome of children with CH. With the implementation of regional or statewide newborn thyroid screening programs, most children with CH are now diagnosed and treated before ever manifesting any disease signs. As a result, the devastating effects of cretinism have been almost totally eliminated, and these children now develop normally, both physically and mentally. Nevertheless, as they still undergo a transitory period when thyroid hormone is unavailable, which can begin in late pregnancy and extend for up to several months postnatally until thyroid hormone levels have normalized, there is still the potential for deficits in later cognitive, academic, and behavioral functioning.

Since the advent of neonatal CH screening in the late 1970s and early 1980s, a number of research teams have been the studying the children so identified. In 1980, Robert Ehrlich and I began a follow-up study of a large cohort of children living in the greater Toronto area diagnosed with CH at birth. The oldest children were identified through an experimental program conducted at several Toronto hospitals (6) and the remainder by a provincewide screening program, which was also one of the earliest regional programs. More than 100 children were recruited and followed throughout childhood and into early adolescence. Until age 9, they were evaluated on an annual basis with age-appropriate standardized psychometric tests. When they were in grades 3 and 6 at school, they were also tested with a large battery of psychoeducational tasks, and, as adolescents, they received a thorough neuropsychological evaluation. Siblings initially served as controls, whereas classmates participated in the psychoeducational phase, and unaffected teenagers matched for age, gender, and SES, were places in the adolescent neuropsychological phase. Because of the detail in which our children with CH were studied, our research represents one of the most (if not the most) comprehensive of its kind worldwide. Our results, however, are both highly descriptive and have also served to generate a number of further questions on the role of thyroid hormone on brain development and later cognitive functioning. They have spawned several new research ventures in our lab on more recent cohorts. The latter include detailed studies of thyroid hormone and attention in school-age children and in infants.

Our findings have conclusively demonstrated that newborn screening has nearly eliminated mental retardation totally. Nevertheless, present-day CH children do demonstrate a variety of *subtle* selective neuromotor and cognitive impairments, the nature of which reflect the type and severity of their thyroid disorder as well as the timing of thyroid hormone insufficiency. Our studies have also revealed specific relationships between aspects of therapy and subsequent outcome, including different (and sometimes opposite) effects of initial versus maintenance dosages.

This chapter will serve to integrate findings from our previous and current studies with those reported in the literature by other research teams. The chapter begins with a review of the major findings on thyroid hormone effects on brain development and the mechanisms by which these are achieved. This is followed by an examination of disease and treatment parameters that impact on outcome. The findings (both our own and others) on children with CH diagnosed by newborn screening are presented next. In this section, a number of domains of function are examined including growth and development, general intelligence and specific cognitive abilities, hearing, school achievement, and behavior. Wherever possible, this section aims to relate specific deficits to different disease- and treatment-related factors.

Finally, the chapter concludes with a discussion of critical and outstanding issues related to the general care, management, and study of children with CH.

Thyroid Hormone and Brain Development

An abundant literature on thyroid hormone and the brain currently exists. This literature relies almost exclusively on animal models, mainly the rat. The studies show that thyroid hormone plays a major role in neurodevelopmental processes and subsequent brain functioning (7,8), including cell division and neurogenesis (9), axon and dendrite formation (10), neuronal migration (11), synaptogenesis (12), myelination (13), and neurotransmission (14). Moreover, both animal and human autopsy studies show that cerebellum, striatum, hippocampus, corpus callosum, thalamus, and cortex are brain structures that are directly affected by a lack of thyroid hormone in early life (15,16).

Thyroid hormone regulates the timely expression of genes that produce essential neurodevelopmental proteins (17). Thyroid hormone binds to nuclear receptors of the steroid-retinoic acid-thyroid hormone superfamily (18). Some of the genes under thyroid control include those for myelin-associated glycoprotein and myelin-basic protein (19–21), tau, which is important for cytoskeleton development (22), microtubule-associated proteins involved in neuronal migration (23), and the protein kinase C substrate, RC3/neurogranin, which is important for synaptogenesis (24). Of the four nuclear receptors for thyroid hormone that have now been isolated, three are localized in critical brain regions for mental and motor functioning, including the caudate, hippocampus, cortex, corpus callosum, and cerebellum (25–31). Thyroid hormone receptors have also been localized in different structures of the ear (32,33) and in brain structures that comprise the auditory pathways (34), which suggests a role for thyroid hormone in auditory processing. Similar findings have also been observed in the retina (35), which suggests a role of thyroid hormone in vision. In addition, as different thyroid hormone receptors have unique ontogenies (36) in different cerebral areas (31), unique and discrete critical periods appear to exist when thyroid hormone is essential both pre- (31) and postnatally (30).

Thyroid hormone is also involved in the development and regulation of different neurotransmitter systems (14,37–39). Perinatal thyroid hormone deficiency disrupts dopaminergic systems in the striatum and cholinergic systems in basal forebrain (40). Findings that thyroid hormone receptor density is largest in the locus coeruleus (the major noradrenergic nucleus in the brain) and in noradrenergic projections (41), signify that thyroid hormone possibly shares a co-transmitter relationship with norepinephrine (42). It has been proposed that the neurotransmitter pathways may themselves be vehicles for thyroid hormone distribution and action in the brain (43).

Screening, Diagnosis, and Treatment

Screening for CH involves assaying for either low levels of thyroxine (T4) or for elevations of pituitary thyrotropin (TSH). For either approach, the alternate hormone is assayed when a value exceeds an established cutoff value or falls within the lowest (or highest for TSH) percentiles. In North America, T4 screening is used mostly, whereas TSH is evaluated in Europe. Our program in Ontario is based on TSH screening.

There are advantages and disadvantages to each mode of screening. Screening T4 allows for the detection of hypothalamic and pituitary forms of hypothyroidism and thyroid hormone binding deficiencies. By contrast TSH screening detects children with compensated or subclinical hypothyroidism who produce low normal levels of T4 at birth due to overstimulation by the pituitary and are missed by programs screening for T4. Some investigators propose that TSH screening may be superior to T4 because TSH screening identifies a greater number of hypothyroid children. These are children with ectopic and hypoplastic thyroids that produce enough hormone to pass the initial screening test, but progressively lose functional capacity and become hypothyroid by about 3–4 months (44). Some T4 screening programs counteract this by providing a second test at 3–4 months of age at the time of a well-baby visit (45). Because different screening programs include different groups of children, this may account for different findings in outcome observed among the various follow-up studies.

The identification of a child with CH requires immediate attention. The screening lab or a delegated representative usually notifies the primary physician, who in turn notifies the family. In some cases, families may be notified directly. Confirmatory diagnosis requires further thyroid function tests and determination of etiology using technetium scans or ultrasonography (46). Serum thyroglobulin (TBG) measurement is useful in confirming athyrosis because TBG is absent in these children. About 60% of children with CH have significantly delayed ossification, which suggests intrauterine hypothyroidism; in fact, bone age is a useful marker of timing of disease onset and period of prenatal hypothyroidism (see later). Although most newborns with CH appear to be perfectly normal at the time of diagnosis, some do show mild symptoms and signs of hypothyroidism (e.g., jaundice, umbilical hernias, and constipation), but the pattern is neither specific nor diagnostic.

It is important to commence treatment as quickly as possible. The exact duration reflects disease severity, age when treatment was initiated, and dosage of replacement hormone. CH is treated with levothyroxine (L-T4) using one of two commercial preparations, synthroid (Knoll Pharmaceuticals) or Levoxine (Daniels Pharmaceuticals), which are interchangeable and do not differentially affect TH levels or thyrotropin concentrations (47). When treatment is optimal, it takes about 3–6 weeks from birth (or 1–2 weeks from the start of therapy) to achieve euthyroidism (48). In some children with confirmed CH, TSH levels may remain elevated for a considerable period of time. In our experience, there is a small subset with elevated TSH levels and normal-to-high T4 levels at birth who are at increased risk of lower intelligence and behavior problems; the etiology of this resistance-like profile is not known.

American Pediatric Association guidelines recommend a relatively high starting dosage (10–16 mg/kg or 50 mg) so that serum T4 can reach target levels very quickly (49). Although this high dose usually achieves euthyroidism within 2 weeks versus 4 weeks for a moderate dose (50), the issue of proper dose levels is still controversial (50–54) because of the potential for hyperthyroxinemia and its associated adverse events. Because the initial dose of L-T4 determines the period of hypothyroidism, different sequelae are expected to reflect different dose levels. In addition, because mother's milk contains small amounts of thyroxine (55,56), breast feeding is thought to provide an alternate source of thyroid hormone and has been shown to offset the effects of thyroid hormone insufficiency to a slight degree (57).

Subsequent maintenance requires gradually raising dose levels of L-T4 until adult levels of 88–125 mg are achieved when body proportions reach adult size. As these levels are not based on empirical evidence and may be too high for certain aspects of cognitive functioning (see later), however, it important that patients be continuously monitored. It is especially important to monitor patients closely during adolescence when problems with compliance may arise in as many as 50% of affected teenagers (58).

Because some children identified by newborn thyroid screening programs may have transient hypothyroxinemia at birth, it is necessary to identify these children by taking them off medication at a safe age (59). In our program, children are routinely given a 1-month trial off-therapy with subsequent reevaluation at age 3 (60).

Growth and Development

Overall, growth and development are normal in children with early treated CH (61,62); however, there may be a lag of several months in the onset of the childhood growth phase that normally occurs between 8 and 9 months of age (63). This delay is associated with age at start of treatment and initial dose (63). In our cohort, growth assessed to age 9 was within normal limits and children's projected adult heights matched their parents' (64). Nevertheless, height was inversely correlated with factors reflecting timing, duration, and severity of early hypothyroidism. Adequately treated CH was associated with slightly increased head circumference in childhood (64).

There are no formal reports of pubertal and sexual development in this population; however, the children in our study, who were evaluated physically at time of psychological testing during adolescence, demonstrated appropriate-for-age growth and development and no indication of delays or abnormalities. Several mothers of female patients also reported heightened premenstrual syndrome symptoms, but it is not clear whether this observation exceeds normality and therefore requires further clarification.

Neurobehavioral Outcome

General Intelligence

Most studies of children with CH identified by newborn screening have used global IQ as the primary, and often only, endpoint (see Ref. 65 for a review). Because IQ is a composite score based on many underlying abilities that reflect the involvement of multiple heterogeneous brain regions, this is a relatively crude parameter for assessing time-limited effects of an inadequate TH supply. In the computed IQ, subtle but significant effects of TH deficiency on selective neurocognitive domains could be masked by nonsignificant effects in the other domains.

Prospective studies of children with CH clearly confirm that the mental retardation formerly associated with cretinism has been prevented by newborn screening and early treatment (65–68). Across studies, IQ falls in the normal range but it is about 5–10 points lower. Degree of lowering appears to depend on a number of factors, including initial CH severity (69,70), etiology (71), fetal hypothyroid duration (72), starting dose levels (52), and compliance (73). Based on a summary of 675 cases with CH from seven studies in the literature (including our own), Derksen-Lubsen and Verkerk (74) have reported that IQ was 6.3 points lower in children with CH diagnosed by screening than in controls' and that disease-related factors were more potent risk factors (for global IQ) than were treatment-related variables.

Specific Abilities

A number of studies have examined selective neurocognitive functions in children with CH. The findings have concurred that despite screening and normal intelligence, the children still are at risk for delays or persisting deficits in neuromotor (75), visuomotor and visuospatial (71), speech and language (79), and attention and memory areas (80–82). Studies using multivariate techniques demonstrated correlations between (1) poor motor performance and more severe prenatal hypothyroidism, (2) weak visuomotor abilities and severity of hypothyroidism in the first few weeks of life, and (3) poor auditory processing and language skills and the period of postnatal hypothyroidism (71). Problems in attention are associated with (high) thyroid hormone levels at time of testing, whereas memory deficiencies reflect both early and later thyroid factors (52).

In the motor domain, problems reflect weaker or less-adequate lower-limb control (75–77), although difficulty with upper-limb coordination and guided motion has also been observed (78). In our program, which assessed motor ability annually from 1 to 6 years of age, children with CH performed significantly below controls at almost every age (except 2 years). When tested with a sensitive measure of specific neuromotor skills at age 6, they performed worse on indexes of gross than they did on fine motor function, which reflected their decreased agility, balance, bilateral coordination, and strength. Children with athyrosis represented the most-affected CH etiology in terms of motor performance (77). As fine motor coordination was less impaired than gross, this suggested to us that CH impacted on *selective* aspects of the motor system, at least within the time frame when these children were hypothyroid.

Our studies have also revealed problems in the visuomotor domain (71) that were especially evident during the middle childhood years and seemed to wane in adolescence. Between 6 and 9 years of age, we noted that children with CH were significantly less competent than controls in copying complex visual designs; however, they seemed to catch up by adolescence. Despite this catch-up, their poorer performance during the elementary school years can have implications for school achievement, given the high demands for blackboard copying during these years.

In the language domain, we observed that children with CH showed delayed development relative to controls beginning at age 2 (71). Their speech development was most delayed relative to controls at age 3, which is anecdotally when many parents have sought consultation and neuropsychological evaluation. An examination of children by the severity of their language impairment, however, has revealed that fewer than 5% actually had what is considered to be a severe language impediment even though 22% had impairments of moderate severity (and 74% were normal). Regarding receptive language, approximately 50% showed mild-to-moderate deficits at age three (unpublished findings), which suggests of an auditory processing deficit (see later).

On spatial tasks, our findings have revealed the existence of problems throughout childhood, which have persisted into adolescence. Tasks with high demands on visual working memory (e.g., mental rotation) that are particularly difficult for children with CH are spatial. Children with CH also demonstrated difficulty with certain aspects of memory. Both their parents and their teachers have reported a concern for memory problems on questionnaires they completed. At 4 and 6 years of age children with CH performed significantly below controls on standardized memory tests (71). Preliminary (unpublished) analyses of specific memory task results show that visual and verbal rote repetition skills (short-term memory) may be more problematic than visual or verbal long-term memory skills based on various recall paradigms.

Attention is additionally an area of concern in children with CH. As early as first grade both parents and teachers acknowledged poorer attention. Not all children are equally affected, however, and of those who are affected, most have mild to moderate impairments. A preliminary analysis of the questionnaire data from our current study comparing 7–12 year olds with CH or ADHD showed that in the CH group, 30–40% suggested an attention disorder compared with 2–8% of controls. By our criteria, 98% of children in the ADHD group had a bona fide disorder. Using parent rating scales, we found a significantly increased risk of ADHD among children with CH, although this was much less than in a group of children determined to have ADHD and be taking ritalin. Figure 23.1, which presents the results from the Conners Parent and Conners Teacher Rating Scales, shows that children with CH had significantly elevated scores compared with controls on scales of cognitive problems, hyperactivity, and attention disorders. The effects were much smaller, however, than were those for children with ADHD, who also had behavior and social problems. Teachers, on the other hand, rated children with CH and ADHD similarly. These findings suggest moderately increased risk of an attention disorder in children with CH, with about one third of cases suggesting concern.

We previously showed that a (high) concurrent T4 level was the strongest predictor of poorer attention (83) and that children with a high T4/high TSH hormone profile (as in resistance to thyroid hormone) obtained lowest psychometric attention scores, despite better test results in other domains (80,81). On computerized attention tests, children and adolescents with CH showed greater difficulty focusing and sustaining attention than controls, but they were not impulsive, as was the ADHD group (84). Children with CH demonstrated most difficulty with stimulus processing aspects of attention (e.g., focus, select), whereas children with ADHD had difficulties inhibiting motor responses. In addition, the groups also displayed different relations between attention and thyroid hormone, with poorer performance being associated with higher T4 levels in CH and with lower levels in ADHD (84).

Hearing

Because of the association between thyroid and auditory function in several abnormal thyroid conditions and laboratory findings on animals that show that TH plays a significant role in the maturation of inner ear structures (85,86), several groups have studied hearing in children with CH identified by screening. Residual hearing impairments are observed in 20% of these children (87,88), with a sensorineural hearing loss for high frequencies the commonest problem. We previously reported that even though these hearing problems were not associated with speech delays nor poorer language facility, hearing problems did contribute to poorer auditory discrimination, word recognition, and phonemic awareness skills (88). This suggests the possiblity of distorted auditory signals in the brains of these children.

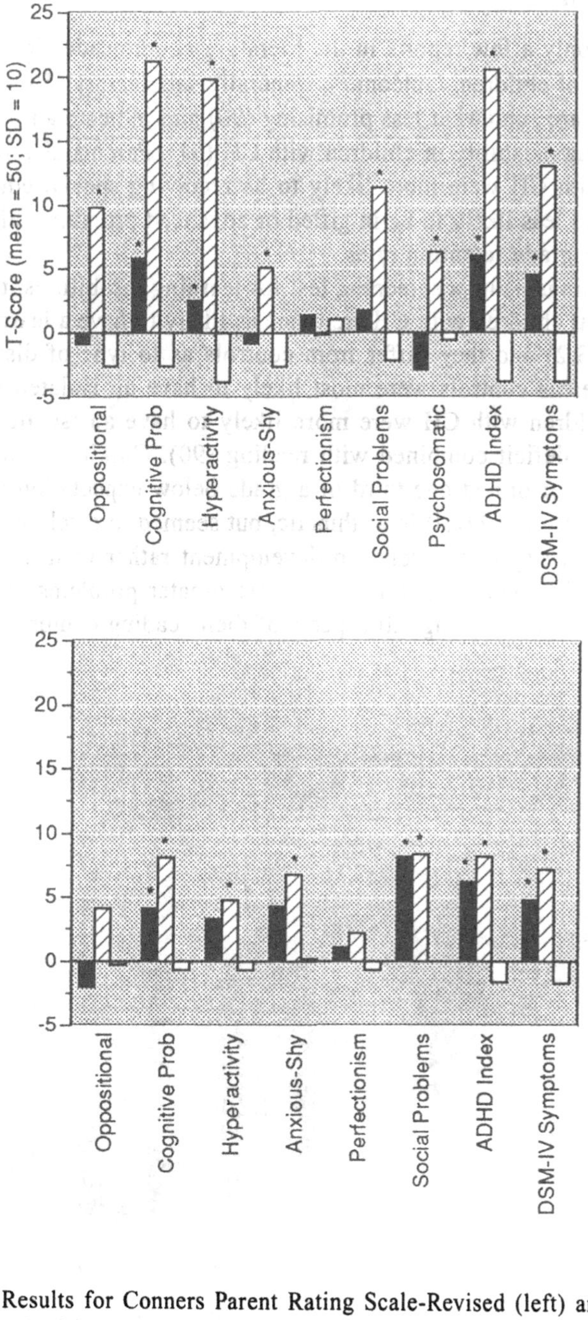

FIGURE 23.1. Results for Conners Parent Rating Scale-Revised (left) and Conners Teacher Rating Scale-Revised (right). Black bars = CH group; striped bars = ADHD group; white bars = controls. Asterisks signify a significant difference (Bonferonni correction applied) from controls. *Note*: Children with ADHD were all taking methylphenidate; hence, less severe problems were noted by teachers than parents.

Achievement

There are only a few reports in the literature about academic levels in this population of children. Outcome is generally satisfactory (58,89); however, our results are somewhat less promising (90) and indicate an increased risk of a learning disability in children with CH (91). Parents also reported that children with CH were more likely to be receiving special education than controls and less likely to be in gifted or advanced programs, although they had similar grade retention rates.

Our findings using a screening test for learning disabilities, the Einstein, indicate that children with CH are twice as likely to have a learning disability (Fig. 23.2) and they differ from controls as to type of disability (Fig. 23.3). Whereas controls were most likely to have an isolated reading disability, children with CH were more likely to have an isolated arithmetic deficit or a deficit combined with reading (90). Children with CH in the third grade performed one third of a grade below expectation and controls (who were at grade level) in arithmetic, but seemed to catch up by the sixth grade, which suggests a delay in development rather than a deficit. Even though children with CH did not indicate greater problems in mechanical reading or word decoding, all aspects of their reading comprehension were

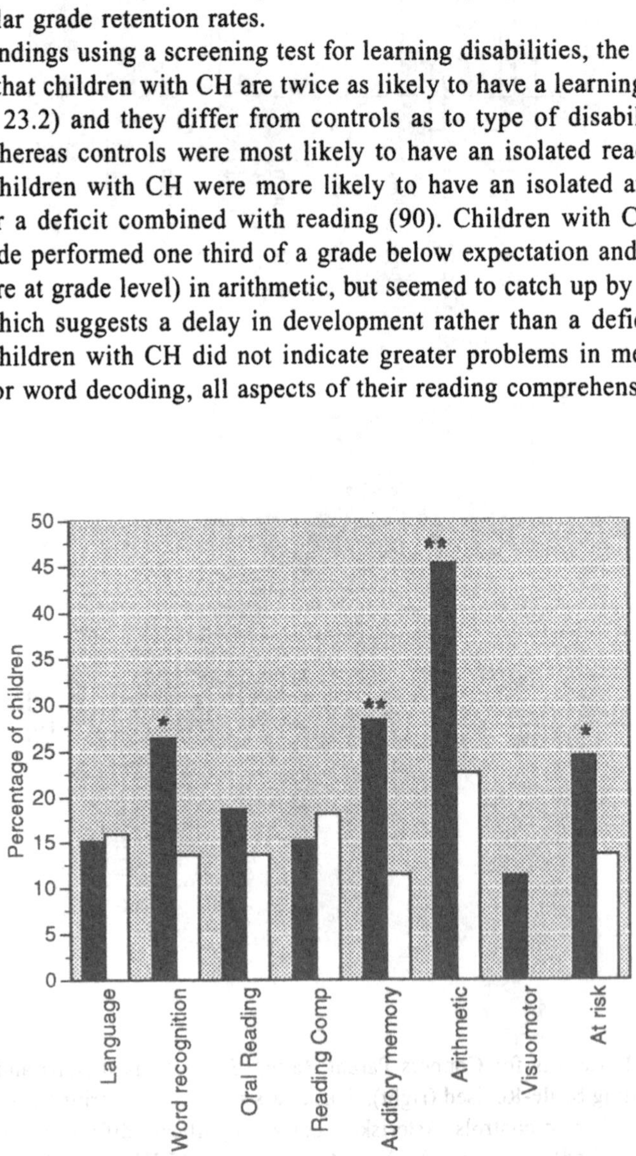

FIGURE 23.2. Proportion of children indicating problems on the Einstein Assessment of School-related Skills. Black bars = CH; white bars = controls.

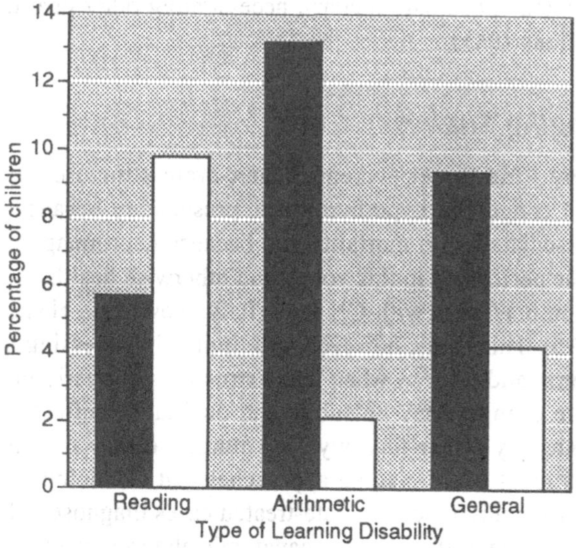

FIGURE 23.3. Proportion of third-grade children with different kinds of learning disabilities. Results are based on wide-range acheivement test-revised, cutoff scores below tenth percentile. Black bars = CH; white bars = controls.

significantly poorer than controls (91). This combination of poorer arithmetic and reading comprehension is suggestive of a nonverbal learning disability (90), which is not uncommon in other newborn disorders (92).

Behavior

Among clinically diagnosed cases treated late, increased lethargy and passivity are frequently observed. In fact, one of the classic clinical features of (untreated) CH is "the good baby syndrome." In those identified by CH screening, however, a difficult temperament is common during infancy, which reflects increased arousal levels and greater environmental sensitivity (93). We found this was associated to a greater degree with high circulating T4 levels in the months preceding the evaluation than with T4 levels at birth (93). This suggested to us that high T4 levels may have advanced the maturation of the hypothalamic-hypophyseal-adrenal axis for handling stress and stimulation.

CH is generally not associated with any major behavior problems, except increased risk of attention deficit disorder. The phenotype of their disorder, however, appears to differ from ADHD, where activity levels and impulsivity are extremely high. As many as 40% of our children with CH were reported to have poorer attention, which in several cases was benefited by psychostimulant medication. A small subset of our children demonstrated CH and ADHD as independent disorders, and several were resistant to methylphenidate therapy, necessitating other pharmacotherapeutic interventions (94).

Neuroimaging Studies

There is very little direct evidence about brain structure and function in humans with congenital hypothyroidism, presumably because this disorder is seldom associated with mortality and because neuroimaging studies cannot readily be performed in this young and otherwise healthy population. An MRI study on newborns with CH from Italy showed no changes in myelin formation (95). This study, however, was limited by assessing infants before treatment onset and prior to when many structures normally myelinate. Furthermore, the changes may be subtle and qualitative reflecting differences in myelin integrity rather than myelin volume, so they may not be detectable by traditional neuroimaging approaches and technologies.

Several case-study reports of late-treated cases diagnosed clinically have shown the presence of distinct neuroanatomic abnormalities. A study of five older late-treated hypothyroid children from India assessed with proton magnetic resonance spectroscopy showed mild cerebral atrophy in frontal and parietal lobes, which is suggestive of delayed myelination (96). This was also seen in two MRI studies of infants diagnosed with CH at 11–14 months of age (97,98). Several studies using neurophysiological procedures have reported that some parameters may be atypical in children with CH identified by newborn screening (99). Although abnormal EEGs were only seen in 7% of cases, visual evoked potential studies revealed problems suggestive of poorer visual perception in up to 64% of cases.

Summary

Early-treated congenital hypothyroidism following newborn screening is associated with significantly reduced morbidity, but there may be subtle persisting neurocognitive impairments in some of the children. Problems reflect delayed language development, poorer gross motor skills, visuospatial deficits, and selective memory and attentional problems. About 20% of children with CH may also have a hearing impairment, which contributes to poorer auditory processing and less adequate reading skill. Although some of the problems in these children with CH may be attributed to the severity, timing, and duration of their early hypothyroidism, others reflect inadequate (high) levels of circulating hormone at the time of testing. Certain attention and memory skills are particularly affected by later (high) levels of thyroid hormone. Although behavior problems are rare in these pediatric patients, there is increased risk of attention deficit disorder, which may necessitate additional pharmacological intervention.

Implications for Treatment and Management

There are a number of issues that need to be addressed in the care and management of children with CH. For those involved in their diagnosis and treatment, it is crucial that diagnosis and treatment occur promptly to prevent any delays associated with specific impairments. Although it may not yet be possible to reduce the effects of TH insufficiency during pregnancy in CH, the need to shorten the postnatal window should be paramount, regardless of distance or type of community. It is essential, therefore, that procedures are firmly in place to ensure immediate therapy in every jurisdiction. As a word of caution, because many of the follow-up studies were based on children seen in tertiary pediatric health care centres, where treatment is typically provided earlier, the findings reported in the literature may in fact be biased in favor of more positive outcome.

Children with CH should be closely and scrupulously monitored throughout infancy and childhood. The quality of their care needs to be consistently high everywhere and all health care providers should be provided strict guidelines on prudent management throughout childhood and adolescence. In Canada and the United States, many primary care physicians (who ultimately manage these children) are poorly informed as to the proper protocols for caring for these children, especially in the long term. Although some jurisdictions do provide treatment guidelines, this is often the exception. A survey has indicated that unlike other screened metabolic disorders, physicians seldom refer these patients to specialists, believing that hypothyroidism is easy to treat and they are sufficiently experienced from their adult patients, in whom the issues are actually quite different (courtesy of B. Therrell, Texas Department of Health). This practice increases the likelihood of not dealing with issues such as transient hypothyroidism, hearing problems, learning disabilities, and attention disorders.

Although guidelines are available on L-T4 therapy, there is some concern that starting dose levels may be too high and that some children may be predisposed to hyperthyroxinemia and its associated sequelae. Even though it is well recognized that euthyroidism must be achieved as soon after birth as possible to prevent mental retardation, it is important that this does not occur at the expense of other sequelae associated with extremely high thyroid hormone levels in infancy. It is also imperative that normal thyroid hormone levels be maintained continuously throughout childhood by evaluating children very frequently, especially during periods of increased growth. There is additional concern that programs of managed health in the United States may not allow for the sufficient number of visits to monitor thyroid hormone levels closely for dose changes. In Canada, cutbacks in government funding for health care may also restrict the level of care these children receive.

Another concern is the lack of public information about longer-term management of these children and support for parents. There are few pamphlets available and long-term outcome is often portrayed unrealistically. For example, under the guise of their having "normal intelligence," associated learning and attention problems may not be recognized. Unlike other pediatric disorders, there are few avenues for parent support and networking with CH, presumably because it is considered neither a serious nor a highly demanding disease. Exceptions are the highly successful programs in Michigan and Illinois, where information is shared among families and with health care specialists on dealing with children with CH. Difficulties in attention observed in this population may need additional interventions and close collaboration between endocrinologists and pediatric neuropsychiatrists.

Compliance is a critical issue, and poor compliance may account for inadequate outcome in some children (73). Although compliance does not appear to be a major issue in our experience, it has been reported that adolescents may be prone to forgetting to take their medication and so may need to be more closely monitored than realized (58). Finally, because of the association between CH and ADHD and the need for pharmaoctherapy in some cases, we recommend that pediatric endocrinologists work closely with neuropsychiatrists and psychopharmacologists to deal with these more complex and difficult cases.

As a word of caution, physicians must be cognizant that screening is not infallible, and some children may fall through the cracks or be wrongly diagnosed. Physicians must always rely on their clinical judgment and acumen and be willing to test any case that appears suspicious, which unfortunately is not always the case.

Future Research Directions

There are a number of outstanding issues on the CH population that suggest further research. The first is the need to study their *specific* cognitive deficits in greater detail, in particular their memory and attention problems and to examine the influence of exogenous (and controllable) factors such as dose levels. This information is necessary to determine the specific types of interventions they need and to prevent such problems in future children with CH. It is also important to determine whether problems in the auditory realm also exist in the visual system and in vision in particular. Are the persisting visuospatial deficits of children with CH visual or spatial in nature, which, would imply involvement (dysfunction) at different levels of the nervous system. The high incidence of learning disabilities in children with CH also warrants further study, especially as to long-term effects. Do some learning problems wane in adolescence as we observed or are they expressed in difficulties other than poor reading and arithmetic during high school? There is clearly need to document the educational levels and vocations these children achieve, especially if one is to assess the benefits of screening. The findings of potential thyroid hormone resistance in a subset of children with persistently elevated TSH levels and behavior problems also warrants additional investigation to determine who these children are, why the effects occur (e.g., is there a priming effect of an early high dose), and how best to intervene. Finally, structural and functional neuroimaging studies of children and adolescence with CH provide the opportunity to determine how thyroid hormone affects human brain development as these children provide an ideal model to study human brain maturation during a brief but critical window of development.

References

1. Burrow GN, Fisher DA, Larsen PR. Maternal and fetal thyroid function. New Engl J Med 1994;331:1072–78.
2. DeGroot LJ, Larsen PR, Henneman G. The thyroid and its diseases, sixth edition. New York: Churchill Livingstone, 1996.
3. Pop VJ, de Vries E, Anneloes L, van Baar AL, Waelkens JJ, de Rooy HA, et. al. Maternal thyroid peroxidase antibodies during pregnancy: a marker of impaired child development? J Clin Endocr Metab 1995;80:3561–66.
4. Bhatara V, Hauser P, McMillin JM. Environmental thyroid disruptors. In: Hauser P, Rovet J, eds. Thyroid diseases of infancy and childhood: effects on behavior and intellectual development. Washington DC: American Psychiatric Press, 1999.
5. Crome L, Stern J. Pathology of mental retardation. Edinburgh: Churchill Livingston, 1972.
6. Walfish PG, Ginsberg J, Rosenberg RA, Howard NJ. Results of a regional cord blood screening programme for detecting neonatal hypothyroidism. Arch Dis Child 1979;54:111–17.
7. Porterfield SP, Hendrich CE. The role of thyroid hormones in prenatal and neonatal neurological development—current perspectives. Endocrin Rev 1993;14: 94–106.
8. Porterfield SP, Stein SA. thyroid hormones and neurological development: update 1994. Endocrin Rev 1994;25:357–63.
9. Shapiro S. Metabolic and maturational effects of thyroxine in the infant rat. Endocrinol 1966;78:527–32.
10. Legrand J. Effects of thyroid hormones on central nervous system development. In: Yanat J, ed. Neurobehavioral teratolology. Amsterdam: Elsevier, 1984:331–63.
11. Potter B, Mano M, Belling G, McIntosh GH, Jua C, Cragg BC, et al. Retarded fetal brain development resulting from severe dietary iodine deficiency in sheep. Neuropath Appl Neurobiol 1982;8:303–13.
12. Nicholson JL, Altman J. Thyroid and developing cerebellum. Brain Reserch 1972;44:13–23.
13. Rosman, N, Malone, M, Helfenstein, M, Kraft, E. The effect of thyroid deficiency on myelination of the brain. Neurology 1972;22:99–106.
14. Hashimoto Y, Furukawa S, Omae F, Miyama Y, Hayashi K. Correlative regulation of nerve growth factor level and choline acetyltransferase activity by thyroxine in particular regions of infant rat brain. J Neurochem 1994;63:326–32.

15. Benda C. Mongolism and cretinism: a study of the clinical manifestations and the general pathology of pituitary and thyroid deficiency. London: Heinemann, 1941.
16. Rivkees SA, Hardin DS. Cretinism after weekly dosing with levo-thyroxine for treatment of congenital hypothyroidism. J Pediatr 1994;125:147–49.
17. Bernal J, Nunez J. Thyroid hormones and brain development. Euro J Endocrin 1995;133:390–98.
18. Brent GA. The molecular basis of thyroid hormone action. N Engl J Med 1994;331:847–53.
19. Munoz A, Rodriguez-Pena A, Perez-Castillo A, Ferreiro B, Sutcliffe JG, Bernal J. Effects of neonatal hypothyroidism on rat brain gene expression. Mol Endocrinol 1991;5:273–80.
20. Farsetti A, Desvergn B, Hallenbeck P, Robbins J, Nikodem VM. Characterization of myelin basic protein thyroid hormone response element and its function in the context of native and heterologus promotor. J Biol Chem 1992;267:15784–88.
21. Rodriguez-Pena A, Ibarrola N, Iniguez MA, Munoz A, Bernal J. Neonatal hypothyroidism affects the timely expression of myelin-associated glycoprotein in the rat brain. J Clin Invest 1993;91:812–18.
22. Nunez, J. Differential expression of microtubule components during brain development. Devel Neurosci 1986;8:125–41.
23. Fellous A, Lennon A, Francon J, Nunez J. Thyroid hormones and neurotubule assembly in vitro during brain development. Eur J Biochem 1979;101:365–76.
24. Bernal J, Rodriguez-Pena A, Iniguez MA, Ibarrola N, Munoz A. Influence of thyroid hormone on brain gene expression. Acta Med Austriaca 1992;19:32–35.
25. Bradley D, Young W, Weinberger C. Differential expression a and b thyroid hormone receptor genes in rat brain and pituitary. Neurobiology 1989;86:7250–54.
26. Madeira, MD, Sousa N, Lima-Andrade MT, Calheiros F, Cadete-Leite A, Paula-Barbosa MM. Selective vulnerability of the hippocampal pyramidal neurons to hypthyroidism in male and female rats. J Comp Neurol 1992;337:501–18.
27. Madeira M, Paula-Barbosa M. Reorganization of mossy fiber synapses in male and female hypothyroid rats: a stereological study. J Comp Neurol 1993;337:334–52.
28. Madeira M, Paula-Barbosa M, Cadete-Leite A, Tavares M. Unbiased estimate of hippocampal granule cell numbers in hypothyroid and in sex- age- matched control rats. J Hirnforsch 1988;29:643–50.
29. Madeira M, Sousa N, Lima-Andrade M, Calheiros F, Cadete-Leite A, Paula-Barbosa M. Selective vulnerability of the hippocampal pyramidal neurons to hypthyroidism in male and female rats. J Comp Neurol 1992;337:501–18.
30. Iniguez MA, De Lecea L, Guadano-Ferraz A, Morte B, Gerendasy D, Sutcliffe JG, et al. Cell-specific effects of thyroid hormone on RC3/neurogranin expression in rat brain. Endocrinology 1996;137:1032–41.
31. Bradley DJ, Towle HC, Young WS. Spatial and temporal expression of a- and b-thyroid hormone receptor mRNAs, including the b_2-subtype, in the developing mammalian nervous system. J Neurosci 1992;12:2288–302.
32. Bradley DJ, Towle HC, Young S. a and b thyroid hormone receptor (TR) gene expression during auditory neurogenesis: Evidence for TR isoform-specific transcriptional regulation *in vivo*. Proc Natl Acad Sci 1994;91:439–43.
33. Corey DP, Breakefield XO. Transcription factors in inner ear development. Proc Natl Acad Sci 1994;91:433–36.

34. Li M, Boyages SC. Detection of widespread b2 thyroid hormone receptor mRNA in rat brain using cRNA in situ hybridisation histochemistry. Thyroid 1995;5(suppl 1):S80.
35. Sjoberg M, Vennstrom B, Forrest D. Thyroid hormone receptors in chick retinal development: differential expression of mRNAs for a and N-terminal variant b receptors. Development 1992;114:39–47.
36. Strait KA, Schwartz HL, Perez-Castillo A, Oppenheimer JH. Relationship of c-erbA mRNA content to tissue triiodothyronine nuclear binding capacity and function in developing and adult rats. J Biol Chem 1990;265:10514–521.
37. Puymirat J. Effects of dysthyroidism on central catecholaminergic neurons. Neurochem Int 1985;17:969–77.
38. Savard P, Merand Y, DiPaolo T, Dupont A. Effects of thyroid state on serotonin, 5-hyroxyindolacetic acid and substance P contents in discrete brain nuclei of adult rats. Neuroscience 1983;10:1399–404.
39. Virgili M, Saverino O, Vaccari M, Barnabci O, Contestabile A. Temporal, regional and cellular selectivity of neonatal alteration of the thyroid state on neurochemical maturation in the rat. Exp Brain Res 1991;83:556–61.
40. Gould E, Butcher LL. Developing cholinergic basal forebrain neurons are sensitive to thyroid hormone. J Neurosci 1989;9:3347–58.
41. Rozanov CB, Dratman, MB. Immunohistochemical mapping of brain triiodothyronine reveals prominent localization in central noradrenergic systems. Neuroscience 1996;74:897–915.
42. Dratman MB, Pfaff DW, Kow LM. An electrophysiologic approach to the study of thyroid hormone action in brain: measurement of unit activity in pyramidal cell layer of hippocampus. Thryoid 1996;6:S59.
43. Gordon JR, Rozanov CB, Drtman MB. Triiodothyronine (T3)-localization in brainstem periventricular structures is markedly reduced in hypothyroidism resulting from sodium ipodate plus propylthiouracil treatment when compared to thyroparathyroidectomy. Thyroid 1996;6:S89.
44. Delange F, De Vijlder J, Morreale de Escobar G, Rochiccioli P, Varrone S. Significance of early diagnostic data in congenital hypothyroidism. In: Delange F, Fisher DA, Glinoer D, eds. Research in congenital hypothyroidism. Plenum: New York, 1989:225–236.
45. Levine GD, Therrell BL. Second testing for hypothyroidism. Pediatrics 1978; 86:375–76.
46. Muir A, Daneman A, Daneman D, Ehrlich RM. Thyroid screening, ultrasound and serum thyroglobulin in determining etiology of congenital hypothyroidism. Am J Dis Child 1988;142:214–16.
47. Escalante DA, Arem N, Arem R. Assessment of interchangeability of two brands of levothyroxine preparations with a third-generation TSH assay. Am J Med 1985;98:374–78.
48. Touati G, Leger J, Toublanc JE, Farriaux JP, Stuckens C, Ponte C, et al. An initial dosage of 8 mg is appropriate for the vast majority of infants with congenital hypothyroidism. In: Farriaux JP, Dhondt JL, eds. New Horizons in Neonatal Screening. Excerpta Medica, Amsterdam, 1994:145–48.
49. American Academy of Pediatrics: Newborn screening for congenital hypothyroidism: recommended guidelines. Pediatr 1993;91:1203–9.
50. Campos SP, Sandberg DE, Barrick C, Voorhess ML, MacGillivray MH. Outcome

of lower L-thyroxine dose for treatment of congenital hypothyroidism. Clin Pediatr 1995;October:514–20.
51. Dubuis JM, Glorieux J, Richer F, Deal C, Dussault J, Van Vliet G: Outcome of severe congenital hypothyroidism: closing the developmental gap with early high dose levothyroxine treatment. J Clin Endocrinol Metab 1996;81:222–27.
52. Rovet JF, Ehrlich RM. Long-term effects of L-thyroxine therapy for congenital hypothyroidism. J Pediatr 1995;126:380–86.
53. Germak J, Foley TP. Longitudinal assessment of L-thyroxine therapy for congenital hypothyroidism. J Pediatr 1990;117:211–19.
54. Ehrlich RM. Thyroxine dose for congenital hypothyroidism. Clin Pediatr 1995;34: 522–23.
55. Sack J, Frucht H, Amado O, Brish M, Lunenfeld B. Breast milk thyroxine and how cow's milk may mitigate and delay the clinical picture of neonatal hypothyroidism. Acta Paediatr Scand 1979;277(suppl):54–56.
56. Bode HH, Vanjonack WJ, Crawford JD. Mitigation of cretinism by breast-feeding. Pediatrics 1978;62:13–16.
57. Rovet JF. Does breast feeding protect the hypothyroid infant diagnosed by newborn screening? Amer J Dis Child 1990;144:319–23.
58. New England Congenital Hypothyroidism Collaborative. Correlation of cognitive test scores and adequacy of treatment in adolescents with congenital hypothyroidism. J Pediatr 1994;124:383–38.
59. Davy T, Daneman D, Walfish PG, Ehrlich R. Congenital hypothyroidism: the effect of stopping treatment at 3 years. Am J Dis Childhood 1985;139:1028–30.
60. Ehrlich RM, Rovet, JF: Screening for congenital hypothyroidism in Ontario. Contemp Pediatr 1993;Aug/Sept: 4–11.
61. Hulse J. Outcome for congenital hypothyroidism. Arch Dis Child 1984;59:23–30.
62. Bucher H, Prader A, Illig R. Head circumference, height, bone age and weight in 103 children with congenital hypothyroidism before and during thyroid hormone replacement. Helv Paediatr Acta 1985;40:305–16.
63. Heyerdahl S, Illicki A, Karlberg J, Kase BF, Larsson A. Linear growth in early treated children with congenital hypothyroidism. Acta Paediatr 1997;86:479–83.
64. Aronson R, Rovet JF, Ehrlich RM, Bailey JD. Physical development in congenital hypothyroidism detected by screening of neonates. J Pediatr 1990;116:33–37.
65. Rovet, J. Hypothyroidism. Intellectual and neuropsychological functioning. In: C. Holmes, ed. Psychoneuroendocrinology: brain, behavior, and hormonal interactions. New York: Springer Verlag, 1990:273–322.
66. Brook C. The consequences of congenital hypothyroidism. Clin Endocrinol 1995;42:431–32.
67. Grant DB. Congenital hypothyroidism. Optimal management in the light of 15 years' experience of screening. Arch Dis Child 1995;72:85–89.
68. Dattani M, Brook C. Outcomes of neonatal screening for congenital hypothyroidism. Current Opinion Pediatr 1996;8:389–95.
69. Tillotson S, Fuggle P, Smith I, Ades A, Grant D. Relation between biochemical severity and intelligence in early-treated congenital hypothyroidism: a threshold effect. Brit Med J 1994;309:440–45.
70. Simons WF, Fuggle PW, Grant DB, Smith I. Intellectual development at 10 years in early treated congenital hypothyroidism. Arch Dis Child 1994;71:232–34.
71. Rovet JF, Ehrlich RM, Sorbara DL. Neurodevelopmental outcome in infants and pre-

school children following newborn screening for congenital hypothyroidism. J Pediatr Psychol 1992;17:187–213.
72. Rovet J, Ehrlich R, Sorbara D. Intellectual outcome in children with fetal hypothyroidism. Implications for neonatal diagnosis. J Pediatr 1987;110:700–4.
73. New England Congenital Hypothyroidism Collaborative. Characteristics of infantile hypothyroidism discovered on neonatal screening. J Pediatr 1984;104:539–44.
74. Derksen-Lubsen G, Verkerk PH. Neuropsychologic development in early treated congenital hypothyroidism: analysis of literature data. Pediatr Res 1996;39: 561–66.
75. Rochiccioli R, Roge B, Alexander F, et al: Resultants du developmente psychomoteur des hypothyroidies dépistées à la naissance. Arch Fr Pediatr 1983;40:537–41.
76. Fuggle PW, Grant DB, Smith I, Murphy G. Intelligence, motor skills and behaviour at 5 years in early-treated congenital hypothyroidism. Europ J Pediatr 1991;150: 570–74.
77. Rovet J. Neuromotor deficiencies in six year old hypothyroid children identified by newborn screening. In: Pass K, ed. Proceedings 8th National Neonatal Screening Symposium and XXI Birth Defects Symposium. K. ASTPHLD, Washington D.C., November 1992:378–81.
78. Kooistra LL, Laane C, Vulsma T, Schellekens JMH, Van Der Meere JJ, Kalverboer AF: Motor and cognitive development in children with congenital hypothyroidism: a long-term evaluation of the effects of neonatal treatment. J Pediatr 1994;124:903–9.
79. Gottschalk B, Richman R, Lewandowski L. Subtle speech and motor deficits of children with congenital hypothyroidism treated early. Devel Med Child Neurol 1994;36:216–20.
80. Rovet J, Alvarez M. Thyroid hormone and attention in school-age children with congenital hypothyroidism. J Child Psychol Psychiatr 1996;37:579–85.
81. Rovet J, Alvarez M. Thyroid hormone and attention in children with congenital hypothyroidism. J Pediatr Endocrinol Metab 1996;9:63–66.
82. Kooistra L, van der Meere JJ, Vulsma T, Kalverboer AF: Sustained attention problems in children with early treated congenital hypothyroidism. Acta Paediatr 1996;85:425–29.
83. Rovet JF, Ehrlich RM, Donner E. Long-term neurodevelopmental correlates of treatment adequacy in screened hypothyroid children. Pediatr Res 1993;33:S91.
84. Rovet J, Lobaugh N, Cole S. Opposite relations of thyroid hormone and attention in children with attention deficit hypractivity disorder and congenital hypothyroidism. Thyroid 1997;7(suppl 1):S90.
85. Uziel A, Gabrion J, Ohresser M, Legrand C. Effects of hypothyroidism on the structural development of the organ of corti in the rat. Acta Otolaryngol 1981;92:469–80.
86. Deol MS. The role of thyroxine in the differentiation of the organ of corti. Acta Otolaryngol 1976;81:429–35.
87. François M, Bonfils P, Leger J, Czernichow P, Narcy P. Role of congenital hypothyroidism in hearing loss in children. J Pediatr 1994;123:444–46.
88. Rovet J, Walker W, Bliss B, Buchanan L, Ehrlich R. Long-term sequelae of hearing impairment in congenital hypothyroidism. Pediatrics 1996;128:776–83.
89. Glorieux J, Dussault, J, Van Vliet, G. Intellectual development at age 12 years of

children with congenital hypothyroidism diagnosed by neonatal screening. J Pediatr 1992;121:581–84.
90. Rovet J. Congenital hypothyroidism. In: Rourke BP, ed. Syndrome of nonverbal learning disabilities: neurodevelopmental manifestations. New York: Guilford, 1995:255–81.
91. Rovet J, Ehrlich R, Altmann D. Psychoeducational outcome in children with early-treated congenital hypothyroidism. Thyroid 1995;5(suppl 1):S84.
92. Rourke BP, ed. Syndrome of nonverbal learning disabilities: neurodevelopmental manifestations. New York: Guilford, 1995.
93. Rovet J, Ehrlich R, Sorbara D. Effect of thyroid hormone level on temperament in infants with congenital hypothyroidism detected by screening of neonates. J Pediatr 1989;114:63–68.
94. Bhatara V, Lobaugh N, Rovet J. Thyroxine therapy aggravating attention deficit hyperactivity disorder (ADHD) and other psychiatric symptoms in pediatric patients. A case series report. Thyroid 1997;7(suppl 1):S33.
95. Siragusa V, Boffelli S, Weber G, Triulzi F, Orezzi S, Scotti G, et al. Brain magnetic resonance imaging in congenital hypothyroid infants at diagnosis. Thyroid 1997; 5:761–764.
96. Gupta, Bhatia V, Poptani H, Gujral RB. Brain metabolite changes on in vivo proton magnetic resonance spectroscopy in children with congenital hypothyroidism. J Pediatr 1995;126:389–92.
97. Rivkees S, Hardin D. Cretinism after weekly dosing with levothyroxine for treatment of congenital hypothyroidism. J Pediatr 1994;125:147–49.
98. Alves C, Eidson M, Engle H, Sheldon J, Cleveland WW. Changes in brain maturation detected by magnetic resonance imaging in congenital hypothyroidism. J Pediatr 1989;115:600–3.
99. Moschini L, Costa P, Marinelli E, Maggioni G, Carta M, Fazzini C, et a. Longitudinal assessment of children with congenital hypothyroidism detected by neonatal screening. Helv Paediatr Acta 1986;41:415–24.

Author Index

Subject Index

PROCEEDINGS IN THE SERONO SYMPOSIA USA SERIES

Continued from page ii

MOLECULAR AND CELLULAR ASPECTS OF PERIIMPLANTATION PROCESSES
Edited by S.K. Dey

THE SOMATOTROPHIC AXIS AND THE REPRODUCTIVE PROCESS IN HEALTH AND DISEASE
Edited by Eli Y. Adashi and Michael O. Thorner

GHRH, GH, AND IGF-I: Basic and Clinical Advances
Edited by Marc R. Blackman, S. Mitchell Harman, Jesse Roth, and Jay R. Shapiro

IMMUNOBIOLOGY OF REPRODUCTION
Edited by Joan S. Hunt

FUNCTION OF SOMATIC CELLS IN THE TESTIS
Edited by Andrzej Bartke

GLYCOPROTEIN HORMONES: Structure, Function, and Clinical Implications
Edited by Joyce W. Lustbader, David Puett, and Raymond W. Ruddon

GROWTH HORMONE II: Basic and Clinical Aspects
Edited by Barry B. Bercu and Richard F. Walker

TROPHOBLAST CELLS: Pathways for Maternal-Embryonic Communication
Edited by Michael J. Soares, Stuart Handwerger, and Frank Talamantes

IN VITRO FERTILIZATION AND EMBRYO TRANSFER IN PRIMATES
Edited by Don P. Wolf, Richard L. Stouffer, and Robert M. Brenner

OVARIAN CELL INTERACTIONS: Genes to Physiology
Edited by Aaron J.W. Hsueh and David W. Schomberg

CELL BIOLOGY AND BIOTECHNOLOGY: Novel Approaches to Increased Cellular Productivity
Edited by Melvin S. Oka and Randall G. Rupp

PREIMPLANTATION EMBRYO DEVELOPMENT
Edited by Barry D. Bavister

MOLECULAR BASIS OF REPRODUCTIVE ENDOCRINOLOGY
Edited by Peter C.K. Leung, Aaron J.W. Hsueh, and Henry G. Friesen

MODES OF ACTION OF GnRH AND GnRH ANALOGS
Edited by William F. Crowley, Jr., and P. Michael Conn

FOLLICLE STIMULATING HORMONE: Regulation of Secretion and Molecular Mechanisms of Action
Edited by Mary Hunzicker-Dunn and Neena B. Schwartz

SIGNALING MECHANISMS AND GENE EXPRESSION IN THE OVARY
Edited by Geula Gibori

GROWTH FACTORS IN REPRODUCTION
Edited by David W. Schomberg

PROCEEDINGS IN THE SERONO SYMPOSIA USA SERIES

(Continued)

UTERINE CONTRACTILITY: Mechanisms of Control
Edited by Robert E. Garfield

NEUROENDOCRINE REGULATION OF REPRODUCTION
Edited by Samuel S.C. Yen and Wylie W. Vale

FERTILIZATION IN MAMMALS
Edited by Barry D. Bavister, Jim Cummins, and Eduardo R.S. Roldan

GAMETE PHYSIOLOGY
Edited by Ricardo H. Asch, Jose P. Balmaceda, and Ian Johnston

GLYCOPROTEIN HORMONES: Structure, Synthesis, and Biologic Function
Edited by William W. Chin and Irving Boime

THE MENOPAUSE: Biological and Clinical Consequences of Ovarian Failure: Evaluation and Management
Edited by Stanley G. Korenman

9780387989624